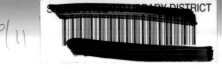
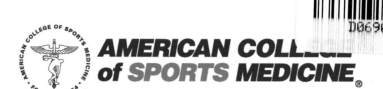

AMERICAN COLLEGE of SPORTS MEDICINE®

Complete Guide to
FITNESS
&
HEALTH

Barbara Bushman, PhD

Editor

DISCARD

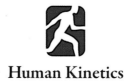

Human Kinetics

Library of Congress Cataloging-in-Publication Data

ACSM's complete guide to fitness & health / Barbara Bushman, editor.
 p. cm.
 Includes bibliographical references and index.
 ISBN-13: 978-0-7360-9337-8 (soft cover)
 ISBN-10: 0-7360-9337-0 (soft cover)
1. Exercise. 2. Physical fitness. 3. Health. I. Bushman, Barbara Ann. II. American College of Sports Medicine.
 RA781.A194 2011
 613.7'1--dc22

                          2011006563

ISBN-10: 0-7360-9337-0 (print)
ISBN-13: 978-0-7360-9337-8 (print)

The Web addresses cited in this text were current as of February 2011, unless otherwise noted.

Acquisitions Editor: Laurel Plotzke Garcia; **Developmental Editor:** Laura Floch; **Assistant Editor:** Elizabeth Evans; **Copyeditor:** Patsy Fortney; **Indexers:** Robert and Cynthia Swanson; **Permission Manager:** Martha Gullo; **Graphic Designer:** Fred Starbird; **Graphic Artist:** Kim McFarland; **Cover Designer:** Keith Blomberg; **Photographer (cover):** iStockphoto/technotr; **Photographer (interior):** Neil Bernstein, unless otherwise noted; **Photo Asset Manager:** Laura Fitch; **Visual Production Assistant:** Joyce Brumfield; **Photo Production Manager:** Jason Allen; **Art Manager:** Kelly Hendren; **Associate Art Manager:** Alan L. Wilborn; **Art Style Development:** Joanne Brummett; **Illustrations:** © Human Kinetics, unless otherwise noted; **Printer:** Versa Press

We thank the Springfield Greene County Park Board Chesterfield Family Center and the CoxHealth Fitness Center in Springfield, Missouri for assistance in providing the location for the photo shoot for this book.

Human Kinetics books are available at special discounts for bulk purchase. Special editions or book excerpts can also be created to specification. For details, contact the Special Sales Manager at Human Kinetics.

Printed in the United States of America   10   9   8   7   6   5   4   3   2   1

The paper in this book is certified under a sustainable forestry program.

Human Kinetics
Web site: www.HumanKinetics.com

United States: Human Kinetics
P.O. Box 5076
Champaign, IL 61825-5076
800-747-4457
e-mail: humank@hkusa.com

Canada: Human Kinetics
475 Devonshire Road Unit 100
Windsor, ON N8Y 2L5
800-465-7301 (in Canada only)
e-mail: info@hkcanada.com

Europe: Human Kinetics
107 Bradford Road
Stanningley
Leeds LS28 6AT, United Kingdom
+44 (0) 113 255 5665
e-mail: hk@hkeurope.com

Australia: Human Kinetics
57A Price Avenue
Lower Mitcham, South Australia 5062
08 8372 0999
e-mail: info@hkaustralia.com

New Zealand: Human Kinetics
P.O. Box 80
Torrens Park, South Australia 5062
0800 222 062
e-mail: info@hknewzealand.com

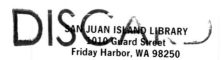

E5143

To Tobin, my wonderful husband, best friend, faithful exercise partner, and true inspiration. Without your constant and unwavering encouragement, support, love, and understanding, I could not have completed this project.

—B.B.

Contents

Preface

I f you opened this book and are reading this page, you are interested in improving your health. Congratulations on taking this step! Regardless of your current level of fitness, this book can direct you to better health by offering scientifically-based recommendations. *ACSM's Complete Guide to Fitness & Health* is different from other health and fitness books in that it relies on a solid scientific foundation and the most current research on physical activity and nutrition. Physical activity and a healthy diet are two important lifestyle factors. The *Complete Guide* provides you with steps to increase your activity as well as to make optimal nutritional decisions.

This book is divided into four parts; the first two are a framework for the last two, which provide age-specific recommendations as well as considerations for special health and medical conditions. Part I sets the stage by providing basic information on being fit, active, and healthy. Chapter 1 discusses the U.S. government's *Physical Activity Guidelines for Americans*, which are a continuing thread throughout the book. Chapter 2 explains how to safely start an exercise program and offers some simple ways to assess your current fitness level. Aerobic fitness, muscular fitness, and flexibility are the three components of a balanced exercise program. In chapter 3 you will learn about each of these along with how you can incorporate more physical activity into your daily schedule. Nutrition and a healthy diet can make a big difference in your overall health. *The Dietary Guidelines for Americans,* discussed in chapter 4, provides a framework for making positive nutritional choices. Wellness is a multidimensional concept influenced by many lifestyle factors. Chapter 5 explains how to make healthy choices in many areas in your life. Throughout the chapters in part I, you will discover your *Fitness ID* as you see how your knowledge and current fitness compare to the guidelines and assessment standards.

Part II focuses on the three components of a complete activity program—aerobic fitness (chapter 6), muscular fitness (chapter 7), and flexibility and balance (chapter 8). You will gain insight into the benefits of including particular activities into your weekly plan as well as specific exercises from which you can choose. Just being told to "be active" or "exercise more" is not helpful on a practical level. Rather, part II includes specific activity programs as well as photos and descriptions of activities that you can include in your personal plan. You will see how to develop your *Fitness ID* within your way of life and in a manner that reflects your personal interests. Whether you are just starting or looking for ways to progress, these chapters offer the information you need.

A physically active lifestyle and wise dietary choices have documented benefits. Part III provides age-specific recommendations for both physical activity and nutrition for children and adolescents (chapter 9), adults (chapter 10), and older adults (chapter 11). These chapters clearly illustrate how you can benefit from physical activity regardless of age. Nutritional issues specific to the various age groups are included to help you make the best food choices. Part III will help you evolve your *Fitness ID* as you create a balanced fitness program that fits your age as well as your current fitness level and goals.

Part IV focuses on special health and medical conditions. These chapters are for those whose *Fitness ID* may be affected by a special condition. Each chapter provides background related to a specific health or medical condition and then provides guidance in using nutrition and exercise to optimize your health. If you have heart disease, high blood pressure, or high cholesterol (addressed in chapters 12, 15, and 16), you can benefit greatly from physical activity and a healthy diet. Similarly, body weight and diabetes (addressed in chapters 13 and 14) can be controlled through exercise and diet. Other health conditions addressed in part IV are arthritis (chapter 17), pregnancy (chapter 18), and osteoporosis (chapter 19).

Many experts have contributed to this book. As editor, I am excited to provide scientifically-based guidance on how to begin, or improve, your personal exercise program. In addition, the clear, concise information on the value of good nutrition is intended to encourage you to find ways each day to make healthy food selections. Your *Fitness ID* is unique to you. This book will help you to discover, develop, evolve, and personalize that identity. Each person has the same 24 hours per day. Although schedules are busy, don't fall into the trap of neglecting your health. As you read this book, consider how an active investment in your personal fitness and health today can make your life better than you ever imagined, tomorrow and into the future.

What's your *Fitness ID?*

Acknowledgments

The time and effort put forth to make this book the best it can be have been significant. I would like to thank all of the authors of individual chapters who contributed their expertise. I am humbled by the level of knowledge these specialists have and hope the readers of this book will feel the passion they have for their topic areas. In addition, I acknowledge the contribution made by the many ACSM professionals who reviewed the chapters in this book to ensure that the material is based on the most current research. The critiques were thorough, and as a result, this book is set apart from others that may rely on opinion or individual impressions. A special thanks to Dr. Rebecca Battista, who headed up the review process so efficiently and effectively.

I would like to thank Andy Hayes, who worked closely with me to find supporting scientific articles as well as to review chapters and to assist with the photo shoot. To all the models involved with the photo shoot, I extend a huge thank-you for your patience and good humor during the rigors of multiple photos for each activity. In particular, I would like to thank Vic Pardue for his assistance with critiquing the photos and providing props in a blink of an eye. To the Springfield Greene County Park Board Chesterfield Family Center and the CoxHealth Fitness Center, I greatly appreciate your openness in allowing us to use your facilities for the photo shoot.

I also acknowledge the support and assistance given by many staff at the American College of Sports Medicine, in particular, Kerry O'Rourke and Angela Chastain. In addition, I appreciate all the work of the staff at Human Kinetics who have been involved with this book. In particular, special thanks to acquisitions editor Laurel Plotzke Garcia, developmental editor Laura Floch, and photographer Neil Bernstein. This project reflects the work of so many individuals, and, even if not named specifically, I humbly thank you for your contributions.

Barbara Bushman

Credits

Photo Andres Rodriguez/fotolia.com on page 4.

Photo iStockphoto/Alistair Scott on page 14.

Photo Tomasz Trojanowski/fotolia.com on page 44.

Photos Monkey Business/fotolia.com on pages 53, 58, 94, 116, 185, 187, 276, 304 and 315.

Photo GOL/fotolia.com on page 75.

Photo Kapu/fotolia.com on page 100.

Photo Susan Rae Tannenbaum/fotolia.com on page 106.

Photo Forgiss/fotolia.com on page 152.

Photo Felix Mizioznikov/fotolia.com on page 197.

Photo Joanna Zielinska/fotolia.com on page 198.

Photo © Elke Dennis - Fotolia.com on page 206.

Photo Wojciech Gajda/fotolia.com on page 213.

Photo iofoto/fotolia.com on page 225.

Photo falkjohann/fotolia.com on page 227.

Photo Photodisc/Getty Images on page 254.

Photo Alan Reed/fotolia.com on page 273.

Photo © Comstock/Corbis on page 282.

Photo Junial Enterprises/fotolia.com on page 289.

Photo bilderbox/fotolia.com on page 301.

Photo Xavier Lanier on page 312.

Photo Marcel Mooij/fotolia.com on page 321.

Photo Flashon Studio/fotolia.com on page 343.

Photo Bananastock on page 369.

Figure 2.1—Source: Physical Activity and Readiness Questionnaire (PAR-Q) © 2002. Used with permission from Canadian Society for Exercise Physiology www.csep.ca.

Figure 2.2—Reprinted, by permission, from American College of Sports Medicine, 2010, *ACSM's guidelines for exercise testing and prescription*, 8th ed. (Philadelphia: Lippincott Williams & Wilkins), 24.

Figure 2.3—Adapted, by permission, from American College of Sports Medicine, 2010, *ACSM's guidelines for exercise testing and prescription,* 8th ed. (Philadelphia: Lippincott Williams & Wilkins), 28.

Figure 2.6—Reprinted from U.S. Department of Health and Human Services, National Heart, Lung, and Blood Institute, 1998, *Clinical guidelines on the identification, evaluation, and treatment of overweight and obesity in adults: The evidence report.* [Online]. Available: www.nhlbi.nih.gov/guidelines/obesity/bmi_tbl.pdf [December 13, 2010].

Figure 3.2—Adapted, by permission, from B. Bushman and J.C. Young, 2005, *Action plan for menopause* (Champaign, IL: Human Kinetics), 188.

Figure 4.1—Reprinted from U.S. Department of Health and Human Services, U.S. Food and Drug Administration, 2009, How to understand and use the nutrition facts label. [Online]. Available: www.fda.gov/Food/LabelingNutrition/ConsumerInformation/ucm078889.htm [December 13, 2010].

Figure 4.2—Reprinted from U.S. Department of Health and Human Services, U.S. Food and Drug Administration, 2009, How to understand and use the nutrition facts label. [Online]. Available: www.fda.gov/Food/LabelingNutrition/ConsumerInformation/ucm078889.htm [December 13, 2010].

Figure 4.3—U.S. Department of Agriculture.

Figure 6.1—Reprinted, by permission, from B. Bushman and J.C. Young, 2005, *Action plan for menopause* (Champaign, IL: Human Kinetics), 35.

Figure 9.1(a-b)—Reprinted from Centers for Disease Control and Prevention, 2009, Individual growth charts. [Online]. Available: www.cdc.gov/growthcharts/charts.htm [December 13, 2010]. Developed by the National Center for Health Statistics in collaboration with the National Center for Chronic Disease Prevention and Health Promotion, 2000.

Figure 9.2—U.S. Department of Agriculture.

Figure 9.7—Reprinted from *Journal of Pediatrics* 146(6), W.B. Strong, R.M. Malina, C.J.R. Blimkie, et al., "Evidence based physical activity for school-age youth," 732-737, Copyright 2005, with permission from Elsevier.

Figure 10.1—Source: Centers for Disease Control and Prevention Wide-ranging Online Data for Epidemiologic Research. [Online]. Available: http://wonder.cdc.gov/data2010 [April 21, 2010].

Figure 11.3—Adapted, by permission, from R.E. Rikli and C.J. Jones, 2001, *Senior fitness test manual* (Champaign, IL: Human Kinetics), 65.

Figure 15.1—Adapted from S. Lewington, R. Clarke, N. Qizilbash, et al., 2002, "Age-specific relevance of usual blood pressure to vascular mortality: A meta-analysis of individual data for one million adults in 61 prospective studies," *The Lancet* 360: 1903-1913.

Table 2.1—Adapted from G.A. Bray, 2004, "Don't throw the baby out with the bath water," *American Journal of Clinical Nutrition* 79(3): 347-349, by permission of American Society for Nutrition.

Table 2.2—Adapted with permission from The Cooper Institute, Dallas, Texas, from *Physical Fitness Assessments and Norms for Adults and Law Enforcement*. Available online at www.cooperinstitute.org.

Table 2.3—Source: Standards for Healthy Fitness Zone, Revision 8.6 and 9.x. © 2010, The Cooper Institute, Dallas, Texas. Used with permission.

Table 2.4—Adapted with permission from The Cooper Institute, Dallas, Texas from *Physical Fitness Assessments and Norms for Adults and Law Enforcement*. Available online at www.cooperinstitute.org.

Table 2.5—Adapted from Institute for Aerobics Research, Dallas, 1994. Study population for the data set was predominantly white and college educated. A Universal DVR machine was used to measure the 1RM. Used with permission from The Cooper Institute, Dallas, Texas.

Table 2.6—Source: Canadian Physical Activity, Fitness & Lifestyle Approach: CSEP-Health & Fitness Program's Health-Related Appraisal and Counselling Strategy, 3rd edition, © 2003. Adapted with permission from the Canadian Society for Exercise Physiology.

Table 2.7—Source: Canadian Physical Activity, Fitness & Lifestyle Approach: CSEP-Health & Fitness Program's Health-Related Appraisal and Counselling Strategy, 3rd edition, © 2003. Adapted with permission from the Canadian Society for Exercise Physiology.

Table 2.8— Source: Standards for Healthy Fitness Zone, Revision 8.6 and 9.x. © 2010, The Cooper Institute, Dallas, Texas. Used with permission.

Table 2.9—Reprinted with permission from *YMCA Fitness Testing and Assessment Manual*, 4th ed. © 2000 by YMCA of the USA, Chicago. All rights reserved.

Table 4.1—Adapted, by permission, from M.H. Williams, 2007, *Nutrition for health, fitness & sport*, 8th ed. (New York: McGraw-Hill), 404. © The McGraw-Hill Companies, Inc.

Table 4.2—Adapted from U.S. Department of Agriculture, Agricultural Research Service, 2010, USDA National Nutrient Database for Standard Reference, Release 23. Nutrient Data Laboratory Home Page, www.ars.usda.gov/ba/bhnrc/ndl. [Accessed July 13, 2010].

Table 4.3—Adapted from U.S. Department of Agriculture, Agricultural Research Service, 2010, USDA National Nutrient Database for Standard Reference, Release 23. Nutrient Data Laboratory Home Page, www.ars.usda.gov/ba/bhnrc/ndl. [Accessed July 13, 2010].

Table 4.4—Adapted from U.S. Department of Health and Human Services and U.S. Department of Agriculture, 2005, *Dietary guidelines for Americans*, 6th ed. (Washington, DC: U.S. Government Printing Office), 32. Source: Agricultural Research Service (ARS) Nutrient Database for Standard Reference, Release 17.

Table 4.5—Sources: U.S. Department of Health and Human Services and National Institutes of Health, U.S. National Library of Medicine, 2010, Medline Plus. [Online]. Available: www.nlm.nih.gov/medlineplus, and Institute of Medicine, National Academy of Science, *Dietary reference intakes for calcium, phosphorous, magnesium, vitamin D, and fluoride,* 1997; *Dietary reference intakes for thiamin, riboflavin, niacin, vitamin B6, folate, vitamin B12, pantothenic acid, biotin, and choline,* 1998; *Dietary reference intakes for vitamin C, vitamin E, selenium, and carotenoids,* 2000; *Dietary reference intakes for vitamin A, vitamin K, arsenic, boron, chromium, copper, iodine, iron, manganese, molybdenum, nickel, silicon, vanadium, and zinc,* 2001; *Dietary reference intakes for water, potassium, sodium, cloride, and sulfate,* 2005; and *Dietary reference intakes for calcium and vitamin D,* 2011 (Washington, DC: National Academies Press).

Table 6.1—Adapted, by permission, from American College of Sports Medicine, 2010, *ACSM's guidelines for exercise testing and prescription,* 8th ed. (Philadelphia: Lippincott Williams & Wilkins), 166-167.

Table 6.3—Adapted, by permission, from American College of Sports Medicine, 2010, *ACSM's guidelines for exercise testing and prescription,* 8th ed. (Philadelphia: Lippincott Williams & Wilkins), 164.

Table 6.4—Source: B.E. Ainsworth, W.L. Haskell, A.S. Leon, et al., 1993, "Compendium of physical activities: Classification of energy costs of human physical activities," *Medicine & Science in Sports & Exercise* 25(1): 71-80.

Table 9.1—Reprinted with permission. *Circulation.* 2005; 112: 2061-2075. © American Heart Association, Inc.

Table 9.2—Adapted from U.S. Department of Health and Human Services, 2008, *2008 physical activity guidelines for Americans.* [Online]. Available: www.health.gov/paguidelines [December 13, 2010].

Table 9.3—Adapted from U.S. Department of Health and Human Services, 2008, *2008 physical activity guidelines for Americans.* [Online]. Available: www.health.gov/paguidelines [December 13, 2010].

Table 10.1—Adapted from U.S. Department of Health and Human Services and U.S. Department of Agriculture, 2005, *Dietary guidelines for Americans,* 6th ed. (Washington, DC: U.S. Government Printing Office), 56-65. Source: Agricultural Research Service (ARS) Nutrient Database for Standard Reference, Release 17.

Table 11.1—Adapted, by permission, from R.E. Rikli and C.J. Jones, 2001, *Senior fitness test manual* (Champaign, IL: Human Kinetics), 87.

Table 11.2—Adapted, by permission, from R.E. Rikli and C.J. Jones, 2001, *Senior fitness test manual* (Champaign, IL: Human Kinetics), 87.

Table 13.2—Reprinted from U.S. Department of Agriculture, 2005, MyPyramid food intake pattern calorie levels. [Online]. Available: www.mypyramid.gov/downloads/MyPyramid_Calorie_Levels.pdf [December 13, 2010].

Table 14.1—Adapted, by permission, from American College of Sports Medicine, 2010, *ACSM's resource manual for guidelines for exercise testing and prescription,* 6th ed. (Philadelphia: Lippincott Williams & Wilkins), 605.

Table 14.2—Adapted, by permission, from American College of Sports Medicine, 2010, *ACSM's resource manual for guidelines for exercise testing and prescription,* 6th ed. (Philadelphia: Lippincott Williams & Wilkins), 607.

Table 14.3—Adapted, by permission, from American College of Sports Medicine, 2010, *ACSM's resource manual for guidelines for exercise testing and prescription,* 6th ed. (Philadelphia: Lippincott Williams & Wilkins), 607.

Table 15.1—Adapted from U.S. Department of Health and Human Services, National Institutes of Health, National Heart, Lung, and Blood Institute, 2004, *The seventh report of the Joint National Committee on Prevention, Detection, Evaluation, and Treatment of High Blood Pressure,* 12. [Online]. Available: www.nhlbi.nih.gov/guidelines/hypertension/jnc7full.pdf [December 13, 2010].

Table 15.2—Adapted from U.S. Department of Health and Human Services, National Institutes of Health, National Heart, Lung, and Blood Institute, 2004, *The seventh report of the Joint National Committee on Prevention, Detection, Evaluation, and Treatment of High Blood Pressure,* 26. [Online]. Available: www.nhlbi.nih.gov/guidelines/hypertension/jnc7full.pdf [December 13, 2010].

Table 15.3—Adapted from U.S. Department of Health and Human Services, National Institutes of Health, National Heart, Lung, and Blood Institute, 2006, *Your guide to lowering your blood pressure with DASH,* 10. [Online]. Available: www.nhlbi.nih.gov/health/public/heart/hbp/dash/new_dash.pdf [December 13, 2010].

Table 15.4—Adapted from L.S. Pescatello, B.A. Franklin, R. Fagard, et al., 2004, "American College of Sports Medicine position stand: Exercise and hypertension," *Medicine & Science in Sports & Exercise* 36(3): 533-553.

Table 16.2—Adapted from National Institutes of Health, National Heart, Lung, and Blood Institute, 2001, *Third report of the National Cholesterol Education Program Expert Panel on Detection, Evaluation, and Treatment of High Blood Cholesterol in Adults: Adult treatment panel III: Executive summary,* 3, 16. [Online]. Available: www.nhlbi.nih.gov/guidelines/cholesterol/atp3xsum.pdf [December 13, 2010].

Table 16.3—Adapted from W.C. Willett, F. Sacks, A. Trichopoulou, et al., 1995, "Mediterranean diet pyramid: A cultural model for healthy eating," *American Journal of Clinical Nutrition* 61(6): 1402S-1406S.

Table 16.4—Adapted, by permission, from S. Roach, 2005, *Pharmacology for health professionals* (Philadelphia: Lippincott Williams & Wilkins), 244-254.

Table 16.5—Adapted from B. Fletcher, K. Berra, P. Ades, et al., 2005, "AHA scientific statement: Managing abnormal blood lipids: A collaborative approach," *Circulation* 112(20): 3184-3209.

Table 18.1—From Institute of Medicine and National Research Council of the National Academies, *Weight gain during pregnancy: Reexaminining the guidelines.* Adapted with permission from the National Academies Press, Copyright 2009, National Academy of Sciences.

Table 18.2—Adapted, by permission, from J.M. Pivarnik and L. Mudd, 2009, "Oh baby! Exercise during pregnancy and the postpartum period," *ACSM's Health & Fitness Journal* 13(3): 8-13.

Table 19.1—Adapted from Institute of Medicine, National Academy of Science, 1997, *Dietary reference intakes for calcium, phosphorous, magnesium, vitamin D, and fluoride* (Washington, DC: National Academies Press), 94, 99, 105, 111, 115.

Text, calculation to estimate aerobic capacity, page 32—Adapted, by permission, from Cureton, K.J., & Plowman, S.A. (2008). Aerobic Capacity Assessments. In G.J. Welk & M.D. Meredith (Eds.), Fitnessgram/Activitygram Reference Guide (pp. Internet Resource). Dallas, TX: The Cooper Institute.

Text, "Major Sources of SoFAS," p. 186—Adapted from U.S. Department of Agriculture and U.S. Department of Health and Human Services, 2010, *Report of the Dietary Guidelines Advisory Committee on the dietary guidelines for Americans.* [Online]. Available: www.cnpp.usda.gov/DGAs2010-DGACReport.htm [December 13, 2010].

Text, "Implementing Dietary Guidelines for Youth," p. 187—Adapted from S.S. Gidding, B.A. Dennison, L.L. Birch, et al., 2005, "Dietary recommendations for children and adolescents: A guide for practitioners: Consensus statement from the American Heart Association," *Circulation* 112(13): 2061-2075.

Text, "Ways to Decrease Sodium Intake," p. 305—Adapted from U.S. Department of Health and Human Services, National Institutes of Health, National Heart, Lung, and Blood Institute, 2006, *Your guide to lowering your blood pressure with DASH,* 17. [Online]. Available: www.nhlbi.nih.gov/health/public/heart/hbp/dash/new_dash.pdf [December 13, 2010].

Text, "Absolute Contraindications to Aerobic Exercise During Pregnancy" and "Relative Contraindications to Aerobic Exercise During Pregnancy," pp. 347-348—Exercise during pregnancy and postpartum period. ACOG Committee Opinion No. 267. American College of Obstetricians and Gynecologists. Obstet Gynecol 2002; 99: 171-173. Reprinted by permission.

part I

Fit, Active, and Healthy

Understanding what it means to be fit, active, and healthy is the first step toward discovering your personal fitness ID. Physical activity and nutrition are two lifestyle factors that can have a major impact on your fitness and health. The chapters in this section provide you with guidance in both areas so you can optimize your exercise program as well as your diet. Specific assessments are provided to help you identify your current fitness status; you can use these assessments to chart your progress in the future. In addition, you will find suggestions on setting goals, handling stress, improving your sleep, and many other aspects of life that affect your overall wellness.

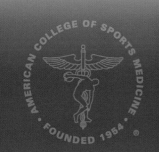
Meeting and Exceeding the Physical Activity Guidelines

Engaging in physical activity is one of the most important steps people of all ages can take to improve their health.[18] Why is exercise so important to your well-being? Children who are active are more likely to be at a healthy body weight, perform better in school, and have higher self-esteem. They are also less likely to develop risk factors for heart disease, including obesity.[2] Adults who exercise are better able to handle stress and avoid depression, perform daily tasks without physical limitation, and maintain a healthy body weight; they also lower their risk of developing a number of diseases.[18] Exercise continues to be important for older adults by ensuring quality of life and independence; regular exercise boosts immunity, combats bone loss, improves movement and balance, aids in psychological well-being, and lowers the risk of disease.[1]

Fitness has health-related and skill-related components. Although skill-related components of fitness (e.g., agility, coordination, balance, reaction time, power, and speed) *are* involved in your day-to-day activities, typically they are specifically included in training programs related to sports and athletic competition or when a situation presents itself, such as the loss of balance often observed with advancing age. The focus of this book is mainly on health-related components of physical fitness including aerobic fitness, muscular fitness, flexibility, and body composition, as follows.[1]

Physical Activity and Exercise—Same or Different?

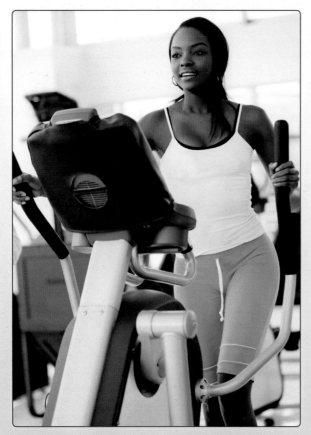

Exercise is a more specific form of physical activity.

Physical activity refers to any movement of the body that involves effort and thus requires energy above that needed at rest.[1] Day-to-day tasks such as light gardening, household chores, and taking the stairs at work are examples of baseline physical activity. Including baseline activities in your daily routine is helpful, but people who do *only* this type of activity are considered to be inactive.[18] Exercise is a more focused, or specific, form of health-enhancing physical activity. Both physical activity and exercise include movement that requires energy, but the goal of exercise is to improve or maintain physical fitness. Health-related physical fitness includes aerobic and muscular fitness as well as flexibility. Examples of health-related physical fitness exercises are brisk walking or jogging, lifting weights, and stretching. The focus of this book is exercise, but keep in mind that exercise is a type of physical activity and that the two terms are often used interchangeably.

Aerobic Fitness

Cardiorespiratory endurance refers to the functioning of your heart, blood vessels, and lungs to supply working muscles and organs with the oxygen needed during activity. Cardiorespiratory endurance is often referred to as aerobic capacity or aerobic fitness. The word *aerobic* means "with oxygen." Your body requires oxygen to perform aerobic exercises. Examples of cardiorespiratory, or aerobic, exercises are walking, jogging, running, cycling, swimming, dancing, hiking, and sports such as tennis and basketball. Chapter 6 provides details on exercises to improve your cardiorespiratory endurance and explains how these exercises benefit your health and fitness.

Muscular Fitness

Muscular fitness refers to how your muscles contract to allow you to lift, pull, push, and hold objects. Muscular fitness includes both muscular strength and muscular endurance. Consider muscular strength and muscular endurance as the two ends of the muscular fitness continuum. Strength is focused on single-effort activity such as moving a heavy box or lifting a loaded barbell. On the other end of the continuum is muscular endurance, which involves multiple contractions over time or sustained contractions. Examples of muscular endurance are lifting a small child repeatedly or holding up a child so she can see over a crowd at a parade. Repeated or sustained contractions in other activities such as yoga or rock climbing also require muscular endurance. Muscular fitness can be improved with resistance training, including lifting weights, using resistance bands or cords, and performing body-weight exercises such as push-ups and curl-ups. Chapter 7 provides details on various types and modes of activity that can help strengthen your muscles as well as specific exercises and how-to photos to help you get started or improve your current resistance training program.

Flexibility

Flexibility refers to the ability to move a joint through a full range of motion. Whether you are focusing on your golf swing or more practical aspects of daily life such as reaching for a high shelf in your closet, maintaining flexibility is important. Loss of flexibility as a result of injury, disuse, or aging can limit your ability to carry out daily activities. Flexibility can be maintained or even improved through a comprehensive stretching program. Chapter 8 outlines stretches for all the muscle groups in the body and discusses the benefits of including activities focused on stability and balance.

Body Composition

Body composition refers to the makeup of your body. The body is made up of lean tissue (including muscle) and fat tissue. Typically, the focus of body composition is the relative amounts of muscle versus fat. Although the bathroom scale can help you track your overall body weight, this measurement is general and does not reveal the amount of fat compared to muscle. Excessive amounts of body fat are related to poor health outcomes, and this is especially true for fat around the abdominal area. Chapter 13 discusses body weight management.

Of the four components of health-related fitness, the first three are part of a well-rounded exercise program, and the fourth, body composition, is influenced by both aerobic and muscular fitness exercises. This book provides activities related to aerobic and muscular fitness as well as flexibility so you can create an exercise plan that matches your goals and aspirations regardless of your age or current fitness level. Whether you are looking to begin an exercise program or optimize the time you are already investing in exercise, the upcoming chapters will show you what to include as well as how to track your progress. This book will help you balance the health-related fitness components so you can maximize the benefits from your personal exercise program.

BENEFITS OF EXERCISE

The benefits of a regular exercise program extend into many areas of life. Exercise is one intervention that is inexpensive and simple and can provide many life-enhancing advantages. Improvements in body function as a result of exercise are well documented. In addition to physiological benefits, psychological benefits can also be realized. Exercise is the best prescription! No other "product" can provide so many positive changes with so few side effects. For a comprehensive list of the health benefits related to physical activity for all age groups from children to older adults, see table 1.1.[18] The scientists working with the U.S. Department of Health and Human Services rated available evidence as strong, moderate, or weak based on the type, number, and quality of the research studies. Only the health benefits with at least moderate evidence are included in this table.

As a reader of this book, you can claim these benefits for yourself. Be encouraged! Regardless of your current level of physical activity, the information provided in the upcoming chapters will help you create a realistic, workable exercise plan that has the potential to change your life for the better. It is time to get up and get moving!

Table 1.1 **Health Benefits Associated With Regular Physical Activity**[18]

CHILDREN AND ADOLESCENTS (AGES 6 TO 17)	
Strong evidence	• Improved cardiorespiratory and muscular fitness • Improved bone health • Improved cardiovascular and metabolic health biomarkers • Favorable body composition
Moderate evidence	• Reduced symptoms of depression
ADULTS AND OLDER ADULTS (AGES 18 AND OLDER)	
Strong evidence	• Lower risk of early death • Lower risk of coronary heart disease • Lower risk of stroke • Lower risk of high blood pressure • Lower risk of adverse blood lipid profile • Lower risk of type 2 diabetes • Lower risk of metabolic syndrome • Lower risk of colon cancer • Lower risk of breast cancer • Prevention of weight gain • Weight loss, particularly when combined with reduced calorie intake • Improved cardiorespiratory and muscular fitness • Prevention of falls • Reduced depression • Better cognitive functioning (for older adults)
Moderate to strong evidence	• Better functional health (for older adults) • Reduced abdominal obesity
Moderate evidence	• Lower risk of hip fracture • Lower risk of lung cancer • Lower risk of endometrial cancer • Weight maintenance after weight loss • Increased bone density • Improved sleep quality

Physiological Benefits

Physiology deals with how the body functions. To maintain optimal function, the body must be exposed to positive stressors such as exercise. Consider a complete exercise program as including three components: aerobic fitness, muscular fitness, and flexibility. Each component contributes to ensuring that your body is operating at its optimal level. This influences your ability not only in exercise performance but also in activities of daily living.

Aerobic Fitness

When you exercise so that your heart beats faster and you breathe at a quicker rate, you are providing a positive stress on your cardiorespiratory system as well as your entire body. An inactive lifestyle does not provide this positive stress and therefore leads to inactivity-related diseases such as heart disease. A sedentary lifestyle and obesity have been described as "parallel, interrelated epidemics in the United States" related to their contribution to the risk of heart disease.[9] It is vital to find ways to fit physical activity into your daily life. Regular activity is associated with lowering risk factors related to heart disease such as high blood pressure and unhealthy cholesterol levels. If you are already somewhat active, you can further reduce your risk by engaging in additional physical activity. Heart health is discussed in more depth in chapter 12; weight management, in chapter 13; high blood pressure, in chapter 15; and high cholesterol, in chapter 16.

Physical activity also reduces the risk of type 2 diabetes.[4] Progression from prediabetes (elevated blood glucose levels that increase the risk of developing diabetes in the future) to diabetes can be delayed or even prevented by losing weight and increasing physical activity.[4] Lifestyle modifications can have a definite impact. In addition to helping people avoid type 2 diabetes, physical activity can also help control blood glucose levels in people diagnosed with either type 1 or type 2 diabetes.[18] Details on the benefits of exercise for those with diabetes are provided in chapter 14.

A dose-response relationship exists between physical activity and health. This simply means that doing some activity is better than being completely inactive and that more activity, up to a point, is better than less activity. In other words, more exercise will continue to lower the likelihood of unhealthy situations such as heart disease, overweight and obesity, and type 2 diabetes.[1] The more activity you include in your life, the lower your risk will be. Whether you are a beginner or an established exerciser, additional exercise provides added health rewards and greater fitness. Chapter 6 explains more fully the recommendations on aerobic activity as well as how you can progress over time.

Muscular Fitness

When considering muscular fitness, the first picture in your mind might be a competitive athlete with large muscles. Although increases in muscle size are possible with resistance training, for most people a more relevant reason to include resistance training is to improve muscle function in order to handle activities of daily living with less stress. For example, sufficient muscular fitness will allow you to climb stairs more easily or complete yardwork with less relative effort. Of course, improved muscular fitness will also make recreational sports and athletic endeavors more enjoyable and give you a competitive edge.

Resistance training is important for everyone throughout the lifespan. Children benefit from activities that strengthen muscles such as climbing and jumping as well as calisthenics and more organized resistance training.[10] Adults have a real need to maintain resistance training because, typically, over the course of adulthood, the amount of muscle decreases while the amount of body fat increases![2] In addition, strength training improves quality of life and limits the muscle losses typically seen with aging.

Another aspect of your health that benefits from resistance training is bone strength.[2] As muscles contract to lift, push, or pull a heavy object, a stress is placed on the bone by way of connections between muscles and bones called tendons. When a bone is exposed to this force, it responds by increasing its mass.[2] This makes bones stronger over time. Bone health is outlined in more detail in chapter 19.

Not to be ignored is the way resistance training can make you look and feel. Firm, toned muscles can inspire confidence. Stronger muscles can give you a real boost as you accomplish daily activities with greater ease and improve in competitive sports as well. For all these reasons, resistance training is an important part of your weekly activity plan. Chapter 7 outlines tools to strengthen your muscles to achieve full health and fitness benefits.

Flexibility

Many people consider flexibility to be a characteristic that you either have or you don't. Although it is true that some people naturally have a higher level of flexibility than others do, everyone has the potential to improve flexibility even if gymnast-type flexibility isn't a possibility.

Flexibility can vary greatly among people but also among the various joints in the body. The ability to have full movement at the joint, also referred to as a full range of motion, can be influenced by injury, disuse, and age. When a joint is not used throughout its normal or potential range of motion, full movement of the joint will be lost over time. The value of flexibility can be seen in daily activities such as bending to tie your shoes, looking over your shoulder to check for cars in traffic, or securing a back zipper, or in recreational activities such as swimming or golfing. For more detailed information and examples of specific stretching exercises, see chapter 8.

Conditions such as arthritis and joint pain can result in having difficulty moving the joints through their normal range of motion. Although activity is beneficial in the treatment of arthritis, 44% of people with arthritis report no leisure time activity (compared with 36% of people without arthritis).[4] Full details on flexibility as well as muscular and cardiorespiratory exercises for people with arthritis and joint pain are found in chapter 17.

Psychological Benefits

In addition to the well-established physical benefits of exercise are many psychological, or mental health, benefits. Exercise appears to provide relief from symptoms of depression and anxiety; in addition, it enhances self-esteem, provides more restful

chapter 2

Assessing Personal Fitness

I n chapter 1, you learned that physical activity and exercise can improve your health and fitness. Because physical fitness has many attributes, a wide range of tests are available to measure your personal fitness level.[1] Many of these tests require the assistance of a fitness professional, but others do not. This chapter presents a few simple tests that you can potentially do on your own. The purpose of this chapter is to show you how to assess your physical fitness and how to use fitness test results to gauge your status now and your progress in the future.

The fitness testing process includes three steps: a preparticipation screening and risk assessment; the fitness assessment, or performance of the test itself; and an interpretation of test results.[1] Each step provides you with information about yourself that can be used to develop a safe and effective exercise program.

PREPARTICIPATION SCREENING AND RISK ASSESSMENT

Preparticipation screening is an important part of the fitness assessment process. This is the first step in learning about your personal health and gaining a sense of the exercises you can do to improve your physical fitness. Preparticipation screening consists of both self-guided and professionally-guided questionnaires and may also include consultations with your health care provider to be sure that you are ready for both fitness testing and physical activity.

Most physical fitness tests are very safe. Before starting, though, you should reflect on your current health status by using a preparticipation health screening, such as the one in this section. If you have questions or concerns regarding your ability to complete a given test, consulting with your health care provider is recommended.

Preparticipation Screening

Figure 2.1 shows the Physical Activity Readiness Questionnaire, more commonly known by its abbreviation, PAR-Q. The PAR-Q is a very simple questionnaire that can help you assess your physical readiness for exercise. Be sure to read both pages carefully. If you answer yes to any of the seven questions on the first page of the PAR-Q, you should check with your health care provider before you begin to exercise or participate in any of the exercise tests described in this chapter.

Other screening questionnaires have been published over the years that are more suited for administration by your health care provider. These questionnaires are often more detailed or focused on a certain condition or population, such as athletes or pregnant women. All of them do the same thing, though—assess readiness for regular exercise, exercise testing, or both. If you have any questions, check with your health care provider.

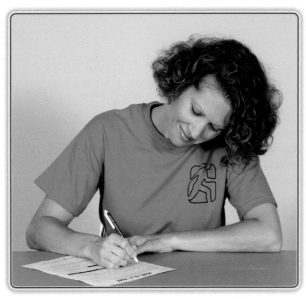

Preparticipation screening is an important first step in assessing your fitness.

Risk Assessment

Whether you are using a self-guided questionnaire or consulting with your health care provider, the goal of preparticipation screening is to verify your physical readiness for exercise testing or future physical activity. In addition to determining physical activity readiness, preparticipation screening also provides a risk stratification. Although it may sound like an intimidating term, risk stratification is really nothing more than a classification of your risk for diseases that could affect your ability to exercise.[1]

Physical Activity Readiness
Questionnaire - PAR-Q
(revised 2002)

PAR-Q & YOU

(A Questionnaire for People Aged 15 to 69)

Regular physical activity is fun and healthy, and increasingly more people are starting to become more active every day. Being more active is very safe for most people. However, some people should check with their doctor before they start becoming much more physically active.

If you are planning to become much more physically active than you are now, start by answering the seven questions in the box below. If you are between the ages of 15 and 69, the PAR-Q will tell you if you should check with your doctor before you start. If you are over 69 years of age, and you are not used to being very active, check with your doctor.

Common sense is your best guide when you answer these questions. Please read the questions carefully and answer each one honestly: check YES or NO.

YES	NO		
☐	☐	1.	**Has your doctor ever said that you have a heart condition <u>and</u> that you should only do physical activity recommended by a doctor?**
☐	☐	2.	**Do you feel pain in your chest when you do physical activity?**
☐	☐	3.	**In the past month, have you had chest pain when you were not doing physical activity?**
☐	☐	4.	**Do you lose your balance because of dizziness or do you ever lose consciousness?**
☐	☐	5.	**Do you have a bone or joint problem (for example, back, knee or hip) that could be made worse by a change in your physical activity?**
☐	☐	6.	**Is your doctor currently prescribing drugs (for example, water pills) for your blood pressure or heart condition?**
☐	☐	7.	**Do you know of <u>any other reason</u> why you should not do physical activity?**

If you answered

YES to one or more questions

Talk with your doctor by phone or in person BEFORE you start becoming much more physically active or BEFORE you have a fitness appraisal. Tell your doctor about the PAR-Q and which questions you answered YES.

- You may be able to do any activity you want — as long as you start slowly and build up gradually. Or, you may need to restrict your activities to those which are safe for you. Talk with your doctor about the kinds of activities you wish to participate in and follow his/her advice.
- Find out which community programs are safe and helpful for you.

NO to all questions

If you answered NO honestly to <u>all</u> PAR-Q questions, you can be reasonably sure that you can:
- start becoming much more physically active – begin slowly and build up gradually. This is the safest and easiest way to go.
- take part in a fitness appraisal – this is an excellent way to determine your basic fitness so that you can plan the best way for you to live actively. It is also highly recommended that you have your blood pressure evaluated. If your reading is over 144/94, talk with your doctor before you start becoming much more physically active.

DELAY BECOMING MUCH MORE ACTIVE:
- if you are not feeling well because of a temporary illness such as a cold or a fever – wait until you feel better; or
- if you are or may be pregnant – talk to your doctor before you start becoming more active.

PLEASE NOTE: If your health changes so that you then answer YES to any of the above questions, tell your fitness or health professional. Ask whether you should change your physical activity plan.

<u>Informed Use of the PAR-Q</u>: The Canadian Society for Exercise Physiology, Health Canada, and their agents assume no liability for persons who undertake physical activity, and if in doubt after completing this questionnaire, consult your doctor prior to physical activity.

No changes permitted. You are encouraged to photocopy the PAR-Q but only if you use the entire form.

NOTE: If the PAR-Q is being given to a person before he or she participates in a physical activity program or a fitness appraisal, this section may be used for legal or administrative purposes.

"I have read, understood and completed this questionnaire. Any questions I had were answered to my full satisfaction."

NAME _____

SIGNATURE _____   DATE_____

SIGNATURE OF PARENT _____   WITNESS _____
or GUARDIAN (for participants under the age of majority)

Note: This physical activity clearance is valid for a maximum of 12 months from the date it is completed and becomes invalid if your condition changes so that you would answer YES to any of the seven questions.

© Canadian Society for Exercise Physiology   Supported by: 🍁 Health Canada Santé Canada

continued on other side...

Figure 2.1   Physical Activity and Readiness Questionnaire (part 1)

Source: Physical Activity and Readiness Questionnaire (PAR-Q) © 2002. Used with permission from the Canadian Society for Exercise Physiology www.csep.ca.

PAR-Q & YOU

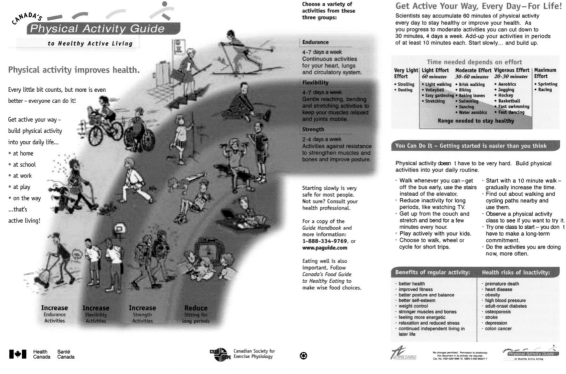

Choose a variety of activities from these three groups:

Endurance
4-7 days a week
Continuous activities for your heart, lungs and circulatory system.

Flexibility
4-7 days a week
Gentle reaching, bending and stretching activities to keep your muscles relaxed and joints mobile.

Strength
2-4 days a week
Activities against resistance to strengthen muscles and bones and improve posture.

Starting slowly is very safe for most people. Not sure? Consult your health professional.

For a copy of the *Guide Handbook* and more information:
1-888-334-9769, or **www.paguide.com**

Eating well is also important. Follow *Canada's Food Guide to Healthy Eating* to make wise food choices.

Get Active Your Way, Every Day – For Life!

Scientists say accumulate 60 minutes of physical activity every day to stay healthy or improve your health. As you progress to moderate activities you can cut down to 30 minutes, 4 days a week. Add-up your activities in periods of at least 10 minutes each. Start slowly... and build up.

	Time needed depends on effort			
Very Light Effort	**Light Effort** *60 minutes*	**Moderate Effort** *30-60 minutes*	**Vigorous Effort** *20-30 minutes*	**Maximum Effort**
• Strolling • Dusting	• Light walking • Volleyball • Easy gardening • Stretching	• Brisk walking • Biking • Raking leaves • Swimming • Dancing • Water aerobics	• Aerobics • Jogging • Hockey • Basketball • Fast swimming • Fast dancing	• Sprinting • Racing
	Range needed to stay healthy			

You Can Do It – Getting started is easier than you think

Physical activity doesn't have to be very hard. Build physical activities into your daily routine.

- Walk whenever you can – get off the bus early, use the stairs instead of the elevator.
- Reduce inactivity for long periods, like watching TV.
- Get up from the couch and stretch and bend for a few minutes every hour.
- Play actively with your kids.
- Choose to walk, wheel or cycle for short trips.
- Start with a 10 minute walk – gradually increase the time.
- Find out about walking and cycling paths nearby and use them.
- Observe a physical activity class to see if you want to try it.
- Try one class to start – you don't have to make a long-term commitment.
- Do the activities you are doing now, more often.

Benefits of regular activity:	Health risks of inactivity:
• better health • improved fitness • better posture and balance • better self-esteem • weight control • stronger muscles and bones • feeling more energetic • relaxation and reduced stress • continued independent living in later life	• premature death • heart disease • obesity • high blood pressure • adult-onset diabetes • osteoporosis • stroke • depression • colon cancer

Source: Canada's Physical Activity Guide to Healthy Active Living, Health Canada, 1998 http://www.hc-sc.gc.ca/hppb/paguide/pdf/guideEng.pdf
© Reproduced with permission from the Minister of Public Works and Government Services Canada, 2002.

FITNESS AND HEALTH PROFESSIONALS MAY BE INTERESTED IN THE INFORMATION BELOW:

The following companion forms are available for doctors' use by contacting the Canadian Society for Exercise Physiology (address below):

The **Physical Activity Readiness Medical Examination (PARmed-X)** – to be used by doctors with people who answer YES to one or more questions on the PAR-Q.

The **Physical Activity Readiness Medical Examination for Pregnancy (PARmed-X for Pregnancy)** – to be used by doctors with pregnant patients who wish to become more active.

References:
Arraix, G.A., Wigle, D.T., Mao, Y. (1992). Risk Assessment of Physical Activity and Physical Fitness in the Canada Health Survey Follow-Up Study. **J. Clin. Epidemiol.** 45:4 419-428.
Mottola, M., Wolfe, L.A. (1994). Active Living and Pregnancy, In: A. Quinney, L. Gauvin, T. Wall (eds.), **Toward Active Living: Proceedings of the International Conference on Physical Activity, Fitness and Health**. Champaign, IL: Human Kinetics.
PAR-Q Validation Report, British Columbia Ministry of Health, 1978.
Thomas, S., Reading, J., Shephard, R.J. (1992). Revision of the Physical Activity Readiness Questionnaire (PAR-Q). **Can. J. Spt. Sci.** 17:4 338-345.

For more information, please contact the:

Canadian Society for Exercise Physiology
202-185 Somerset Street West
Ottawa, ON K2P 0J2
Tel. 1-877-651-3755 • FAX (613) 234-3565
Online: www.csep.ca

The original PAR-Q was developed by the British Columbia Ministry of Health. It has been revised by an Expert Advisory Committee of the Canadian Society for Exercise Physiology chaired by Dr. N. Gledhill (2002).

Disponible en français sous le titre «Questionnaire sur l'aptitude à l'activité physique - Q-AAP (revisé 2002)».

 © Canadian Society for Exercise Physiology   Supported by: Health Canada Santé Canada

---

Figure 2.1 Physical Activity and Readiness Questionnaire (part 2)
Source: Physical Activity and Readiness Questionnaire (PAR-Q) © 2002. Used with permission from the Canadian Society for Exercise Physiology www.csep.ca.

Commonly, three disease types are considered during risk stratification: cardiovascular, pulmonary, and metabolic.[1] As you will learn in other chapters, diseases in these categories can affect your physical fitness but do not necessarily preclude you from exercising. In fact, a great many people would be at a lower risk for disease if they exercised regularly.

Having completed preparticipation screening, the next step is to determine how much of an impact the presence of these diseases or your risk for developing them has on your plans to become more physically active.[1] To ensure safety, high-risk people should undergo exercise testing under the supervision of a physician before beginning an exercise program. Moderate-risk people should be supervised by a physician if the tests involve maximal levels of exertion. In contrast, low-risk, apparently healthy people do not require the presence of a physician during testing.

To determine your risk level, follow the three steps outlined in figure 2.2 as follows:

1. Check for known disease.
2. Check for signs or symptoms of disease.
3. Count the number of cardiovascular risk factors.

You addressed the first two steps, in part, when you completed the preparticipation screening. For a more complete assessment, check your status compared to the lists of known diseases as well as signs and symptoms in figure 2.2. If you have one of these diseases or have any of the major signs or symptoms of these diseases, you are considered to be high risk.

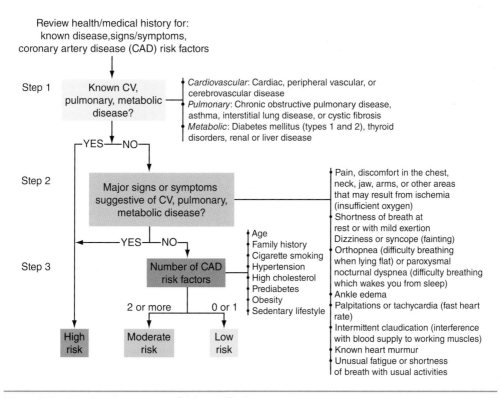

Figure 2.2 Step-by-step process of risk stratification.

Reprinted by permission from American College of Sports Medicine, 2010, p. 24.

Because the cardiovascular system is so important to the physiology of exercise and physical activity, cardiovascular disease risk is carefully evaluated in the third step. Note that the list of eight risk factors in figure 2.2 includes factors over which you have no control (e.g., age, family history) as well as those you can control (e.g., smoking, sedentary behavior). The number of risk factors determines whether you are considered to be at a low or moderate risk of developing heart disease.[1] To assess your status, read through the eight risk factors in figure 2.3 and check "Yes" or "No" in the "Are you at risk?" column.

In summary, if you answered no to all questions on the PAR-Q and have no known disease or signs or symptoms, then you are either at low or moderate risk depending on the number of cardiovascular risk factors you identified in figure 2.3. Low-risk people can complete any of the fitness tests in this chapter. Moderate-risk people should avoid maximal levels of exertion (unless under a physician's supervision). For example, a low-risk person could complete the 1.5-mile (2.4 km) run test, whereas a moderate-risk person might instead select the 1-mile (1.6 km) walk test, which would be a lower level of exertion. When completing the fitness assessments or beginning your exercise program, always use common sense and do not push beyond what your current fitness level allows.

If you answered yes to any of the questions on the PAR-Q or already know you have a cardiovascular, metabolic, or pulmonary disease or have identified that you have specific signs or symptoms as shown in figure 2.2, you should meet with your health care provider before undergoing any of the fitness assessments in this chapter or before beginning an exercise program. The recommendation to meet with your health care provider does not necessarily mean that you cannot exercise; actually, exercise may very well be part of your treatment plan.

The risk stratification process sometimes works in reverse—that is, if you are at high risk, rather than preventing you from exercise testing or being physically active, your health care provider may refer you to a fitness professional for exercise testing and prescription as part of your treatment. You should approach the prescription of exercise as an enjoyable, low-cost opportunity to improve your health. You just might be surprised by the results you obtain in a short period of time!

A CLOSER LOOK
George

To determine his readiness to exercise, George answered the questions in the PAR-Q. Although he answered no to all of them, his responses to questions posed in figure 2.3 affirm that he is indeed sedentary but not obese. Of course, being 65 years old, George meets another risk factor—age. Thus, he has two risk factors for cardiovascular disease (sedentary lifestyle and age). Looking at the risk stratification chart in figure 2.2, George is best classified as being at moderate risk. George decides to meet with his physician about his new exercise plans. George's physician encourages George to perform several of the tests described in this chapter, but suggests that he not perform the more vigorous 1.5-mile run at this point. Rather, he suggests that George estimate his aerobic capacity using the moderate-intensity walking test instead.

FIGURE 2.3

Risk Factor Scoring Checklist

Risk Factors	Definition	Are You At Risk?
Age	45 years of age or older for men; 55 years of age or older for women	___ Yes ___ No
Family history	Heart attack, bypass surgery, or sudden cardiac death before the age of 55 years in father, brother, or son, or before the age of 65 in mother, sister, or daughter	___ Yes ___ No
Cigarette smoking	Current smoker or quit within the last six months	___ Yes ___ No
High blood pressure[a]	Systolic blood pressure over 140 mmHg *or* diastolic blood pressure over 90 mmHg, confirmed on two separate occasions *or* on blood pressure lowering medication	___ Yes ___ No
Unhealthy cholesterol[b]	LDL 130 mg/dl or above *or* HDL less than 40 mg/dl *or* total cholesterol 200 mg/dl or above *or* on cholesterol-lowering medication. (*Note:* You will subtract 1 from your total score below, if your HDL cholesterol is 60 mg/dl or higher.)	___ Yes ___ No
Prediabetes[c]	Fasting glucose (sugar) between 100 to 126 mg/dL *or* impaired glucose tolerance, confirmed on two separate occasions	___ Yes ___ No
Obesity	Body mass index [d] of over 30 kg/m^2 or waist girth of over 102 cm (40 in.) for men or 88 cm (35 in.) for women	___ Yes ___ No
Sedentary lifestyle	Anyone not participating in at least 30 minute of moderate-intensity physical activity on at least three days of the week for the past three months	___ Yes ___ No
Add the number of "Yes" answers you checked and then subtract 1 from your score if your HDL cholesterol is 60 mg/dL or higher. Following is your risk based on your score: • *Low risk*—risk score of no more than 1 • *Moderate risk*—risk score of 2 or greater • *High risk*—known disease or signs or symptoms (see figure 2.2)		_____ Risk score

[a]Blood pressure includes two numbers. The top number is the systolic blood pressure and the bottom number is the diastolic blood pressure.

[b]Cholesterol is recorded with varying degrees of specificity. You may only know your total cholesterol level, and that can be helpful in determining risk. LDL cholesterol is the "bad" cholesterol with regard to coronary heart disease, so high values are a concern. The HDL cholesterol is the good cholesterol and thus is a concern if it is low, but is a good situation if it is high.

[c]The blood glucose measures will require a visit to your health care provider because these are more advanced tests. High levels of glucose are a concern.

[d]A description of body mass index is provided on page 26 of this chapter. Body mass index incorporates both height and weight into a single value expressed in units kilograms per squared meters (kg/m^2).

Adapted by permission from American College of Sports Medicine, 2010, p. 28.

FITNESS ASSESSMENT

Chapter 1 identified both health-related and skill-related components of fitness. Skill-related physical fitness is indeed important, but is generally related to sports. For example, a coach may want to assess the agility and speed of his soccer players. This chapter provides health-related physical fitness assessments, including those for heart rate, body composition, cardiorespiratory fitness, muscular fitness, and flexibility. The equipment needed for these tests is minimal, and you do not have to perform them all in one day.

If you want to perform more than one of these tests on a certain day, you should follow the order of testing presented in this section to optimize accuracy.[1] When you check your progress after a couple of months, test yourself just as you did during your initial assessment. Keeping the order of testing the same ensures that any changes in your results are attributable to your new activity program.

Assessing Heart Rate

Perhaps the simplest fitness assessment is that of heart rate, which is reported in beats per minute. Heart rate naturally increases during exercise. The higher the intensity, the faster your heart must beat to bring oxygen and nutrients to your working muscles. As you gain fitness, however, your heart rate will be lower at rest as well as in response to a given level of exercise. Your heart can now do the same job while beating slower because it is able to push out more blood with each heartbeat. This is evidence of your body adapting to the exercise and improvement in your cardiorespiratory fitness. Heart rate can be measured from just about any artery of the body (see *Where to Find Your Heart Beat* for an explanation of the two most common sites).

Resting heart rate is best assessed first thing the morning before you get out of bed. Be sure you have a stopwatch or clock nearby that displays time in seconds. Locate one of the arteries described previously, and simply count the number of

---

Where to Find Your Heart Beat

You can determine your heart rate by finding a location on your body where an artery (a blood vessel carrying blood from the heart to the rest of the body) is close to the surface of the skin so you can feel your pulse, which is the slight surge in blood flow that occurs when the heart contracts. Common locations are the radial artery in the wrist (see figure 2.4a) and the carotid artery in the neck (see figure 2.4b). Use the tips of your middle and index fingers to feel your pulse. If you use the carotid, be sure to keep the pressure light. Too much pressure at this location can alter your heart rate artificially.

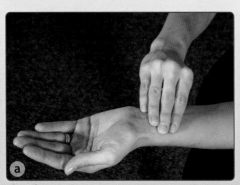

Figure 2.4 *(a)* Radial and *(b)* carotid pulse locations.

beats (pulses) you feel for one minute. For most adults, the resulting number is between 60 and 100, but if your heart rate is lower than 60 or higher than 100 after multiple resting measurements, you should mention this to your health care provider.

Exercise heart rate is just as easy to measure as resting heart rate, but you must work quickly to get an accurate measurement. Because heart rate steadily returns to a resting rate once you break from physical activity, finding your pulse and beginning your count immediately upon stopping is important. Take your pulse for 15 seconds and multiply the resulting number by 4. The answer is your exercise heart rate in beats per minute.

If manually taking your pulse is too difficult, consider making an investment in a heart rate monitor (an example is shown in figure 2.5). A heart rate monitor allows for a constant real-time readout of your heart rate. It includes a transmitter (worn

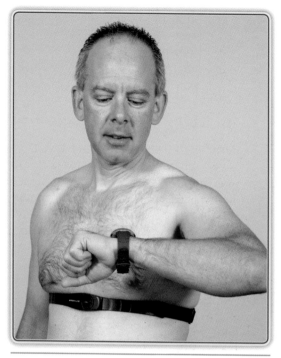

Figure 2.5 Heart rate monitor.

around the chest) that electronically communicates with a receiver that looks like a wristwatch, where the heart rate is displayed in beats per minute. The cost of heart rate monitors varies widely depending on their features (e.g., programmable heart rate zones, memory features to download to a computer after a workout, time-keeping functions). The simplest models that display only heart rate typically cost around $25. They are very durable and allow for easy checks of your heart rate during exercise.

Assessing Body Composition

Many of the body composition assessment techniques available require special equipment and training. Although more technical assessments do provide more complete insight, for a general gauge of your personal health, two simple measurements can provide valuable information—body mass index and waist circumference.

Body Mass Index

Body mass index (BMI) is a simple test you can complete on your own. The results are helpful as you monitor your progress toward improved physical fitness. BMI reflects your body weight in relationship to your height and is expressed in the measurement units of kilograms per squared meters (kg/m^2).

To determine your BMI, see figure 2.6. After finding your height in inches along the far left column, follow that line across until you find the column corresponding to your weight in pounds. Look at the top of that column for your BMI in kg/m^2 as well as a rough interpretation of that number. Note that, ideally, BMI should be less than 25 kg/m^2. For more information on BMI as it pertains to weight management,

FIGURE 2.6

Body Mass Index (BMI) Calculator

	Normal						Overweight					Obese										Extreme Obesity														
BMI	19	20	21	22	23	24	25	26	27	28	29	30	31	32	33	34	35	36	37	38	39	40	41	42	43	44	45	46	47	48	49	50	51	52	53	54
Height (inches)												**Body weight (pounds)**																								
58	91	96	100	105	110	115	119	124	129	134	138	143	148	153	158	162	167	172	177	181	186	191	196	201	205	210	215	220	224	229	234	239	244	248	253	258
59	94	99	104	109	114	119	124	128	133	138	143	148	153	158	163	168	173	178	183	188	193	198	203	208	212	217	222	227	232	237	242	247	252	257	262	267
60	97	102	107	112	118	123	128	133	138	143	148	153	158	163	168	174	179	184	189	194	199	204	209	215	220	225	230	235	240	245	250	255	261	266	271	276
61	100	106	111	116	122	127	132	137	143	148	153	158	164	169	174	180	185	190	195	201	206	211	217	222	227	232	238	243	248	254	259	264	269	275	280	285
62	104	109	115	120	126	131	136	142	147	153	158	164	169	175	180	186	191	196	202	207	213	218	224	229	235	240	246	251	256	262	267	273	278	284	289	295
63	107	113	118	124	130	135	141	146	152	158	163	169	175	180	186	191	197	203	208	214	220	225	231	237	242	248	254	259	265	270	278	282	287	293	299	304
64	110	116	122	128	134	140	145	151	157	163	169	174	180	186	192	197	204	209	215	221	227	232	238	244	250	256	262	267	273	279	285	291	296	302	308	314
65	114	120	126	132	138	144	150	156	162	168	174	180	186	192	198	204	210	216	222	228	234	240	246	252	258	264	270	276	282	288	294	300	306	312	318	324
66	118	124	130	136	142	148	155	161	167	173	179	186	192	198	204	210	216	223	229	235	241	247	253	260	266	272	278	284	291	297	303	309	315	322	328	334
67	121	127	134	140	146	153	159	166	172	178	185	191	198	204	211	217	223	230	236	242	249	255	261	268	274	280	287	293	299	306	312	319	325	331	338	344
68	125	131	138	144	151	158	164	171	177	184	190	197	203	210	216	223	230	236	243	249	256	262	269	276	282	289	295	302	308	315	322	328	335	341	348	354
69	128	135	142	149	155	162	169	176	182	189	196	203	209	216	223	230	236	243	250	257	263	270	277	284	291	297	304	311	318	324	331	338	345	351	358	365
70	132	139	146	153	160	167	174	181	188	195	202	209	216	222	229	236	243	250	257	264	271	278	285	292	299	306	313	320	327	334	341	348	355	362	369	376
71	136	143	150	157	165	172	179	186	193	200	208	215	222	229	236	243	250	257	265	272	279	286	293	301	308	315	322	329	338	343	351	358	365	372	379	386
72	140	147	154	162	169	177	184	191	199	206	213	221	228	235	242	250	258	265	272	279	287	294	302	309	316	324	331	338	346	353	361	368	375	383	390	397
73	144	151	159	166	174	182	189	197	204	212	219	227	235	242	250	257	265	272	280	288	295	302	310	318	325	333	340	348	355	363	371	378	386	393	401	408
74	148	155	163	171	179	186	194	202	210	218	225	233	241	249	256	264	272	280	287	295	303	311	319	326	334	342	350	358	365	373	381	389	396	404	412	420
75	152	160	168	176	184	192	200	208	216	224	232	240	248	256	264	272	279	287	295	303	311	319	327	335	343	351	359	367	375	383	391	399	407	415	423	431
76	156	164	172	180	189	197	205	213	221	230	238	246	254	263	271	279	287	295	304	312	320	328	336	344	353	361	369	377	385	394	402	410	418	426	435	443

Reprinted from U.S. Department of Health and Human Services, National Heart, Lung, and Blood Institute, 1998.

see chapter 13. To account for differences in growth patterns, youth between the ages of 2 and 20 typically do not use BMI but rather BMI-for-age charts (see chapter 9 for information on how to interpret the results).

Concerns related to health are linked to a BMI of 25 kg/m^2 or above; a BMI of 30 kg/m^2 or above is associated with high blood pressure, concerns with cholesterol levels, and coronary heart disease.[1] Because BMI does not take into account the amount of body fat compared to muscle, it is not a perfect predictor of risk. For example, a lean, muscular athlete would not be at a higher health risk even though the athlete's BMI would likely be higher than that of a normal person of the same height.

Waist Circumference

People have different patterns of body fat distribution, and these patterns correspond to different risk levels for disease. The location of body fat accumulation influences your health risk.[1] The risk is lower for those who have fat distributed more around the hips and thighs (called gynoid obesity and commonly referred to as a pear-shaped physique) than for those who carry fat on the trunk or abdominal area (called android obesity, commonly called an apple-shaped physique). Because of the concern with abdominal obesity, waist circumference alone can help identify whether you are at risk of health concerns.

Waist circumference is measured using a measuring tape. You could also use a string or long belt to take your measurement and then lay it along a ruler or yardstick. See figure 2.7 to guide your placement of the tape. You may need a partner to help you keep the tape level, but taking the measurement is easy. Just stand relaxed and breathe normally.

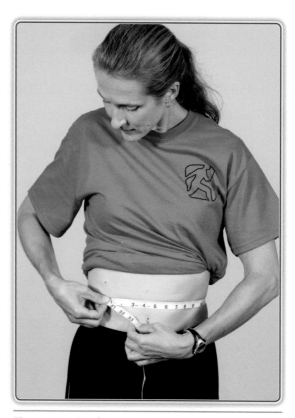

Figure 2.7 Site for measuring waist circumference.

Table 2.1 Interpretation of Waist Circumference for Adults

Risk category	WAIST CIRCUMFERENCE (IN INCHES AND CENTIMETERS)	
	Men	Women
Very low	Less than 31.5 in. (80 cm)	Less than 27.5 in. (70 cm)
Low	31.5–39.0 in. (80–99 cm)	27.5–35 in. (70–89 cm)
High	39.5 to 47.0 in. (100–120 cm)	35.5–43.0 in. (90–109 cm)
Very high	Greater than 47.0 in. (120 cm)	Greater than 43.0 in. (110 cm)

Adapted by permission from Bray, 2004, p. 348.

Take a horizontal measure at the narrowest part of your torso above your navel but below your rib cage. Use the ranges in table 2.1 to interpret your measurements in centimeters or inches. Lower risk for heart disease is noted for women with a waist circumference of 35 inches (89 cm) or less and for men with a waist circumference of 39 inches (99 cm) or less.[1]

Using BMI and waist circumference provides indirect, but quick insight into body composition. Other more advanced measurements are also available but require consultation with a fitness professional. One method, for example, is skinfold measurements, which involve measuring "pinches" of fat just under the skin at various locations to estimate the overall amount of fat in the body. Another method is bioelectrical impedance, which estimates the amount of fat in the body by measuring the resistance to electrical flow through body tissues. Both of these methods provide more precise information on the composition of the body, but unfortunately, also require special equipment and can be influenced by hydration status.

Assessing Aerobic Fitness

Aerobic fitness is typically assessed by looking at maximal oxygen consumption, also called $\dot{V}O_2$max. $\dot{V}O_2$max is a marker of your body's ability to take in and use oxygen. The higher this value is, the better your aerobic fitness is. Complex laboratory tests can most precisely determine your $\dot{V}O_2$max, but you can get a reasonable estimate from simple tests, such as the Rockport One-Mile Fitness Walking Test or the 1.5-mile run test, both of which are described in this section.

Select one of these tests based on your current activity and perceived fitness level. The walking test is more appropriate if you are planning to begin an exercise program after a period of inactivity or currently engage in more moderate levels of exercise. If you are healthy and more active, the run test is a better option. Each test and the associated calculations produce an estimation of your aerobic capacity. Use that result and the numbers provided in table 2.2 to determine your fitness level by age and sex.

Rockport One-Mile Walking Test

The Rockport One-Mile Walking Test is a way to estimate $\dot{V}O_2$max. To complete this test, you should have the ability to walk one mile continuously. Choose a day without windy weather for testing. Ideally, you should perform the One-Mile Walking Test using an outdoor or indoor running track so that you can be certain that the distance you walk is no more or less than one mile. A standard quarter-mile track would be ideal (four laps on the inside lane), but many tracks are metric. If you are on a 400-meter track, then you will need to complete four laps on the inside lane plus an additional 9.3 meters (equal to approximately 31 feet). If a track is not available, any measured course will work as long as the surface is smooth and the course is flat. Grab a comfortable pair of shoes and a stopwatch. Walk the course as rapidly as you can without jogging or running, and record the time it takes for you to complete the mile. You also need to take your pulse as previously described immediately after you complete the mile walk.

Computing your results from the Rockport One-Mile Walking Test takes a bit of work, but the math is very simple when you plug results into one of the formulas shown here (numbers in bold are constant in the equations and thus are predetermined):

Males

139.150	
MINUS (**0.1692** × ___	weight in kilograms)
MINUS (**0.3877** × ___	age in years)
MINUS (**3.2649** × ___	time in minutes)
MINUS (**0.1565** × ___	heart rate in beats per minute)
= ___	AEROBIC CAPACITY

Females

132.835	
MINUS (**0.1692** × ___	weight in kilograms)
MINUS (**0.3877** × ___	age in years)
MINUS (**3.2649** × ___	time in minutes)
MINUS (**0.1565** × ___	heart rate in beats per minute)
= ___	AEROBIC CAPACITY

To obtain your weight in kilograms, multiply your weight in pounds by 0.454. For the time factor, you might wonder how to account for the number of seconds. For example, suppose you completed the one-mile walk in 14 minutes and 25 seconds. The 25 seconds needs to be expressed as a fraction (decimal number) of a minute. To do that, simply divide the number by 60 (because there are 60 seconds in a minute). In this case, 25 seconds would be about 0.42 of a minute, so you would use the number 14.42 in your calculation of aerobic capacity.

The answer you calculate is your aerobic capacity and refers to the amount of oxygen your body can use each minute—more specifically, the number of milliliters of oxygen your body uses per unit of body weight every minute (mL/kg/min). The more oxygen your body can use, the better your aerobic fitness level is. Once you have determined your aerobic capacity, find your fitness classification level in table 2.2.

1.5-Mile Run Test

Just as the Rockport One-Mile Walking Test is a way to estimate aerobic capacity, so too is the 1.5-mile (2.4 km) run. Because of the higher intensity and longer distance of this test, it is not appropriate for beginners, anyone with symptoms of or known heart disease, or anyone with risk factors or other health concerns as determined by a health screening or a health care provider.

To perform this test, choose a day without windy weather and use an outdoor or indoor running track. If you are on a quarter-mile track, this will involve six laps in the inside lane. If you are using a 400-meter track, this will involve six laps plus an additional 14 m (46 feet) to complete the full distance of 1.5 miles. Grab a comfortable pair of running shoes and a stopwatch. Because this test requires you to run as fast as you can for 1.5 miles, you should walk a lap or two to warm up. At the track, run as rapidly as you can for 1.5 miles, timing yourself to the nearest second. For this test, there is no need to record your heart rate. This test is challenging, so be sure to walk a lap or two to cool down after completion, and rehydrate as needed soon after.

The math used to interpret your results is much simpler than that for the Rockport One-Mile Walking Test. Use the following formula to estimate your aerobic capacity:

Aerobic capacity = (**483** ÷ _time in minutes_) + **3.5**

As with the One-Mile Walking Test, this calculated value is an estimate of your aerobic capacity, or $\dot{V}O_2$max. Because the number itself may not have much meaning, be sure to consult table 2.2 to check on your status compared to others of your age and sex.[1] The higher the value, the better!

Other assessments are available for younger as well as older people. For youth, a shorter-distance run test is often used (see _One-Mile Run Test for Youth_). Although some older adults may be comfortable completing the one-mile walk or 1.5-mile run tests, another option is a 6-minute walk test.[4] Details on this test are outlined in chapter 11 on page 234. Focusing on a time rather than a particular distance covered allows older adults of all abilities to assess their fitness.

Table 2.2 **Fitness Levels for Aerobic Capacity* in Males and Females**

	AGE					
Males	**20-29**	**30-39**	**40-49**	**50-59**	**60-69**	**70-79**
Superior	55.5 or higher	54.1 or higher	52.5 or higher	49.0 or higher	45.7 or higher	43.9 or higher
Excellent	51.1 to 55.4	48.3 to 54.0	46.4 to 52.4	43.3 to 48.9	39.6 to 45.6	36.7 to 43.8
Good	45.6 to 51.0	44.1 to 48.2	42.4 to 46.3	39.0 to 43.2	35.6 to 39.5	32.4 to 36.6
Fair	41.7 to 45.5	40.7 to 44.0	38.4 to 42.3	35.5 to 38.9	32.3 to 35.5	29.4 to 32.3
Poor	38.0 to 41.6	36.7 to 40.6	34.8 to 38.3	32.0 to 35.4	28.7 to 32.2	25.7 to 29.3
Very poor	37.9 or lower	36.6 or lower	34.7 or lower	31.9 or lower	28.6 or lower	25.6 or lower
	AGE					
Females	**20-29**	**30-39**	**40-49**	**50-59**	**60-69**	**70-79**
Superior	49.6 or higher	47.4 or higher	45.3 or higher	41.0 or higher	37.8 or higher	37.2 or higher
Excellent	43.9 to 49.5	42.4 to 47.3	39.6 to 45.2	36.7 to 40.9	32.7 to 37.7	30.6 to 37.1
Good	39.5 to 43.8	37.7 to 42.3	35.9 to 39.5	32.6 to 36.6	29.7 to 32.6	28.1 to 30.5
Fair	36.1 to 39.4	34.2 to 37.6	32.8 to 35.8	29.9 to 32.5	27.3 to 29.6	25.9 to 28.0
Poor	32.3 to 36.0	30.9 to 34.1	29.4 to 32.7	26.8 to 29.8	24.6 to 27.2	23.5 to 25.8
Very poor	32.2 or lower	30.8 or lower	29.3 or lower	26.7 or lower	24.5 or lower	23.4 or lower

*Aerobic capacity or $\dot{V}O_2$max expressed in mL/kg/min.

Adapted with permission from The Cooper Institute, Dallas, Texas, from _Physical Fitness Assessments and Norms for Adults and Law Enforcement_. Available online at www.cooperinstitute.org.

Assessing Muscular Fitness

Muscular fitness includes both muscular strength and muscular endurance, which are the two ends of the muscular fitness continuum. Having information on both will give you a complete picture of your muscular fitness.

Muscular Strength

Muscular strength is the maximum amount of force that a muscle or muscle group can produce. For example, the ability to move a heavy piece of furniture when rearranging a room demonstrates muscular strength, as does lifting a loaded barbell. Two common assessments of muscular strength are the bench press test and the leg press test, both of which give snapshots of upper-body and lower-body strength. These tests require special equipment and the supervision of a certified fitness professional to ensure appropriate test implementation. For both tests, the goal is to lift as much weight as you possibly can with good form one time only. The resulting number is your 1-repetition maximum, or rep max (typically abbreviated as 1RM). This can be rather technical and time consuming to determine. An easier method is to estimate your rep max by lifting a weight multiple times

One-Mile Run Test for Youth

The FITNESSGRAM is an assessment for children that emphasizes personal fitness for health rather than comparisons among children.[3] With this philosophy in mind, healthy ranges are given rather than fitness rankings. Youth are considered in the "healthy fitness zone" or "needs improvement" zone. For boys and girls between the ages of 10 and 17, a one-mile run test is used (if a child cannot run this entire distance, encourage walking at a fast pace). For the one-mile run test, the calculation to estimate aerobic capacity ($\dot{V}O_2$max) takes into account BMI as well as the time to complete the one-mile run or see www.cooperinstitute.org/youth/fitnessgram/hfz-tables.cfm.

Boys

108.94
PLUS (**0.21** ×   age in years)
MINUS (**0.84** ×   BMI)
MINUS (**8.41** ×   mile time in minutes)
PLUS (**0.34** ×   mile time in minutes ×   mile time in minutes)
=   ESTIMATED $\dot{V}O_2$MAX

Girls

108.94
MINUS (**0.84** ×   BMI)
MINUS (**8.41** ×   mile time in minutes)
PLUS (**0.34** ×   mile time in minutes ×   mile time in minutes)
=   ESTIMATED $\dot{V}O_2$MAX

Calculation adapted by permission from Cureton and Plowman, 2008.

Note that this estimation can only be used for run times of 13 minutes or less. If the child requires more than 13 minutes to complete the one-mile run, then simply enter "13" into the formula for the mile time. See table 2.3 for the healthy fitness zone for boys and girls between the ages of 10 and 17.[3]

Table 2.3 **FITNESSGRAM Standards for Aerobic Capacity Based on the One-Mile Run***

Age	Boys	Girls
10	40.2 or higher	40.2 or higher
11	40.2 or higher	40.2 or higher
12	40.3 or higher	40.1 or higher
13	41.1 or higher	39.7 or higher
14	42.5 or higher	39.4 or higher
15	43.6 or higher	39.1 or higher
16	44.1 or higher	38.9 or higher
17	44.2 or higher	38.8 or higher

*The values listed represent the healthy fitness zone and indicate the child has a sufficient fitness level to provide important health benefits. Being below the value listed indicates a need for improvement.
Source: Standards for Healthy Fitness Zone, Revision 8.6 and 9.x. © 2010, The Cooper Institute, Dallas, Texas. Used with permission.

(following a general warm-up) and doing some mathematical calculations[2] as follows:

- Multiply the number of repetitions you can perform for a given exercise by 2.5. (*Note:* If you can lift a particular weight more than 20 times, it would be more accurate to repeat the assessment with a higher weight after taking a 10-minute rest.)
- Subtract that number from 100. The resulting number reflects the percentage of your theoretical 1-repetition maximum.
- Take that number and divide it by 100 to produce a decimal value.
- Divide the weight you lifted by that decimal value. The resulting weight is your estimated 1-repetition maximum weight.

To compare yourself with others of your age and sex, take your estimated rep max weight and divide it by your body weight. You can use the resulting number to interpret your muscular fitness in conjunction with tables 2.4 and 2.5. Notice that the ratio of weight lifted to body weight is the same whether you use pounds or kilograms.

For a more general approach to assessing muscular strength, you can also simply track your progress over time within your resistance training program. As you gain strength, a weight you could lift only 10 times initially you can now lift more often before fatiguing, or you may be lifting a heavier weight for those same 10 repetitions. Either way, you are showing improvements in strength.

Table 2.4 Interpretations of Upper-Body Strength for Males and Females*

Males	AGE					
	20 or younger	20–29	30–39	40–49	50–59	60+
Superior	1.76 or higher	1.63 or higher	1.35 or higher	1.20 or higher	1.05 or higher	.94 or higher
Excellent	1.34–1.75	1.32–1.62	1.12–1.34	1.00–1.19	.90–1.04	.82–.93
Good	1.19–1.33	1.14–1.31	.98–1.11	.88–.99	.79–.89	.72–.81
Fair	1.06–1.18	.99–1.13	.88–.97	.80–.87	.71–.78	.66–.71
Poor	.89–1.05	.88–.98	.78–.87	.72–.79	.63–.70	.57–.65
Very poor	.88 or lower	.87 or lower	.77 or lower	.71 or lower	.62 or lower	.56 or lower

Females	AGE					
	20 or younger	20–29	30–39	40–49	50–59	60+
Superior	.88 or higher	1.01 or higher	.82 or higher	.77 or higher	.68 or higher	.72or higher
Excellent	.77–.87	.80–1.00	.70–.81	.62–.76	.55–.67	.54–.71
Good	.65–.76	.70–.79	.60–.69	.54–.61	.48–.54	.47–.53
Fair	.58–.64	.59–.69	.53–.59	.50–.53	.44–.47	.43–.46
Poor	.53–.57	.51–.58	.47–.52	.43–.49	.39–.43	.38–.42
Very poor	.52 or lower	.50 or lower	.46 or lower	.42 or lower	.38 or lower	.37 or lower

*Bench press weight ratio = weight lifted divided by body weight.

Adapted with permission from The Cooper Institute, Dallas, Texas, from *Physical Fitness Assessments and Norms for Adults and Law Enforcement.* Available online at www.cooperinstitute.org.

Table 2.5 Interpretations of Lower-Body Strength for Males and Females*

| Males | AGE | | | | |
	20–29	30–39	40–49	50–59	60+
Well above average	2.27 or higher	2.07 or higher	1.92 or higher	1.80 or higher	1.73 or higher
Above average	2.05–2.26	1.85–2.06	1.74–1.91	1.64–1.79	1.56–1.72
Average	1.91–2.04	1.71–1.84	1.62–1.73	1.52–1.63	1.43–1.55
Below average	1.74–1.90	1.59–1.70	1.51–1.61	1.39–1.51	1.30–1.42
Well below average	1.73 or lower	1.58 or lower	1.50 or lower	1.38 or lower	1.29 or lower

| Females | AGE | | | | |
	20–29	30–39	40–49	50–59	60+
Well above average	1.82 or higher	1.61 or higher	1.48 or higher	1.37 or higher	1.32 or higher
Above average	1.58–1.81	1.39–1.60	1.29–1.47	1.17–1.36	1.13–1.31
Average	1.44–1.57	1.27–1.38	1.18–1.28	1.05–1.16	.99–1.12
Below average	1.27–1.43	1.15–1.26	1.08–1.17	.95–1.04	.88–.98
Well below average	1.26 or lower	1.14 or lower	1.07 or lower	.94 or lower	.87 or lower

*Leg press weight ratio = weight lifted divided by body weight.

Adapted from Institute for Aerobics Research, Dallas, 1994. Study population for the data set was predominantly white and college educated. A Universal DVR machine was used to measure the 1RM. Used with permission from The Cooper Institute, Dallas, Texas.

A CLOSER LOOK
George

George wanted to know whether he was in shape enough to bike to work on weekdays. Although George found that he was in reasonably good aerobic shape, he still wanted to know if he had the muscular fitness to make the rides. It turns out that the road he will take to work is relatively flat, and the distance is only about 2 miles (3.2 km), but George remains curious about his strength and ability to use his muscles over the course of those 2 miles. These attributes make up muscular fitness.

To find his actual rep max, George would require some assistance from a fitness professional. In addition, this test would very fatiguing because it requires maximal exertion and could result in soreness afterward. Alternatively, George decided to estimate his rep max from the steps outlined on page 33. He found that he could bench press 120 pounds (54.5 kg) six times (but not seven). To estimate his rep max from this value, he goes through the following steps:

1. Multiply the number of repetitions by 2.5: *6 × 2.5 = 15.*
2. Subtract this value from 100 to determine the percentage of his theoretical rep max: *100 − 15 = 85.*
3. Take that outcome and divide by 100 to produce a decimal value: *85 ÷ 100 = 0.85.*
4. Divide the weight lifted by that decimal value to determine the estimated rep max: *120 ÷ 0.85 = 141.*

George's estimated rep max is 141 pounds (64 kg). To compare himself to others of his age and sex, he divides this value by his body weight (141 ÷ 179 = 0.79). This value can be checked in table 2.4—as you can see his upper-body strength is in the "Good" category. For the leg press, the procedure is the same as that of the bench press. To see where George would rank if his estimated rep max were 270 pounds (123 kg), check table 2.5. If the weight lifted (270 lb) is divided by George's weight (179 lb), the result is 1.5. For a 60+-year-old male, this is in the "Average" category.

Muscular Endurance

Muscular endurance is the ability of a muscle or muscle group to exert a force repeatedly over time or to maintain a contraction for a period of time. Consider an assembly line worker who must move objects from one location to another; the person's movements do not require maximal effort, but the muscles must respond again and again over time. Another example of muscular endurance is holding a full bag of groceries; the muscle contraction must be maintained to prevent the produce from rolling down the street. Repeated or sustained muscle contractions are found in many sports and recreational activities, such as mountain biking, yoga, and martial arts. Like muscular strength, muscular endurance can be different in different muscle groups, but there are a couple of commonly used muscular endurance tests that will help you gauge how much force your muscles can generate over time. These involve curl-ups and push-ups.

The curl-up test is used to assess the endurance of your abdominal muscles. You will need a stopwatch, a ruler, and masking tape to conduct this test. Place two pieces of masking tape on the floor, parallel to each other. Use the ruler to be sure that the tape strips are 4 inches (10 cm) apart. To perform the test, assume the starting position depicted in figure 2.8a, and move to the full range of motion shown in figure 2.8b. Note that your knees should be bent at a 90-degree angle with your feet flat on the floor. There is no need to perform a full sit-up with this test. See how many curl-ups you can perform with controlled movements (your rate should be 25 per minute, which is about one curl-up every 2.5 seconds). You can verify correct form by sliding your fingers in conjunction with your upper-body movements between the two pieces of tape as shown. Continue without pausing for up to a minute or to a maximum of 25 curl-ups.[1] Check your score in table 2.6. This reflects the ability of your abdominal muscles to contract repeatedly over time and thus serves as a marker of muscular endurance.

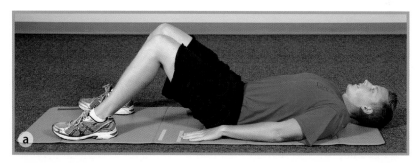

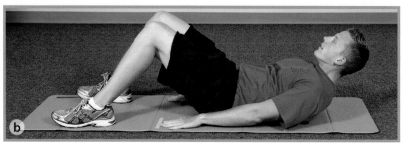

Figure 2.8 Curl-up.

Table 2.6 Curl-Up Test Norms for Males and Females

Males	AGE				
	20–29	30–39	40–49	50–59	60–69
Excellent	25 or more	25 or more	25 or more	25 or more	25 or more
Very good	21–24	18–24	18–24	17–24	16–24
Good	16–20	15–17	13–17	11–16	11–15
Fair	11–15	11–14	6–12	8–10	6–10
Needs improvement	10 or fewer	10 or fewer	5 or fewer	7 or fewer	5 or fewer
Females	AGE				
	20–29	30–39	40–49	50–59	60–69
Excellent	25 or more	25 or more	25 or more	25 or more	25 or more
Very good	18–24	19–24	19–24	19–24	17–24
Good	14–17	10–18	11–18	10–18	8–16
Fair	5–13	6–9	4–10	6–9	3–7
Needs improvement	4 or fewer	5 or fewer	3 or fewer	5 or fewer	2 or fewer

Adapted by permission from Canadian Society for Exercise Physiology, 2003.

The push-up test may be something you remember from elementary school, and it is still in use today. The goal is to perform as many push-ups as possible until you can no longer perform another with proper form. It is important to perform these exercises as shown so you can determine an accurate categorization using table 2.7. Notice in figures 2.9 and 2.10 that there are two ways to perform the push-up used for the test, one for males and another for females. Proper form includes keeping your back straight and pushing up to a straight-arm position and then returning down until the chin touches the floor. For males the toes are the rear pivot point, but for females, the knees are in contact with the ground.

Table 2.7 Push-Up Test Norms for Males and Females

Males	AGE				
	20–29	30–39	40–49	50–59	60–69
Excellent	36 or more	30 or more	25 or more	21 or more	18 or more
Very good	29–35	22–29	17–24	13–20	11–17
Good	22–28	17–21	13–16	10–12	8–10
Fair	17–21	12–16	10–12	7–9	5–7
Needs improvement	16 or fewer	11 or fewer	9 or fewer	6 or fewer	4 or fewer
Females	AGE				
	20–29	30–39	40–49	50–59	60–69
Excellent	30 or more	27 or more	24 or more	21 or more	17 or more
Very good	21–29	20–26	15–23	11–20	12–16
Good	15–20	13–19	11–14	7–10	5–11
Fair	10–14	8–12	5–10	2–6	2–4
Needs improvement	9 or fewer	7 or fewer	4 or fewer	1 or none	1 or none

Adapted by permission from Canadian Society for Exercise Physiology, 2003.

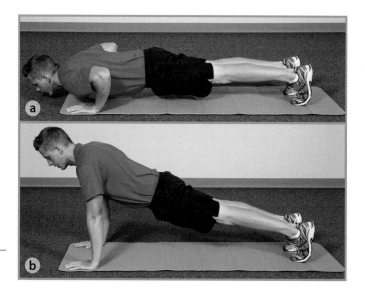

Figure 2.9
Push-up for males.

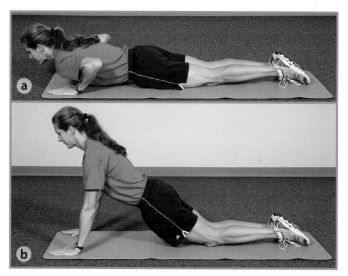

Figure 2.10
Push-up for females.

A CLOSER LOOK

George

George performed the curl-up test and was pleased to see that he was able to complete 18 curl-ups in one minute. Note from table 2.6 that this places George in the "Very good" category for a man of his age. George also completed the push-up test. He was able to complete 15 push-ups with good form. After checking table 2.7, George was pleased to note that he is in the middle of the "Very good" category for this test as well.

Having completed tests for muscular strength and muscular endurance, George has a better sense of his physical fitness on those attributes. Although exercises such as the bench press and curl-up seem to have nothing to do with biking to work, they do correlate well with the movements needed for biking. George should feel confident that with his high scores on these tests, he may very well be ready to make these rides.

As with aerobic fitness, alternative assessments of muscular fitness are available for youth and older adults. See *Muscular Fitness Assessments for Youth* for details on curl-up and push-up tests for kids. Two additional tests have been specifically developed to assess muscular fitness in older adults. The chair stand test is used to assess lower-body strength, which is important in daily activities such as climbing stairs; walking; and getting out of a chair, bathtub, or car.[4] An arm curl test is used to assess upper-body strength, which is important for daily activities such as carrying groceries or grandchildren. These two tests are described in detail in chapter 11 on pages 233 and 234.

Muscular Fitness Assessments for Youth

The FITNESSGRAM includes healthy fitness zone ranges for curl-ups and push-ups.[3] A few modifications of the adult versions of these tests are needed. For the curl-up test, the two pieces of tape used to help guide the extent of the curl-up are placed 3 inches (7.6 cm) apart for 5- to 9-year-olds and 4.5 inches (11.4 cm) apart for 10- to 19-year-olds. Heels must stay in contact with the mat, and no pauses or rest periods are allowed (see figure 2.11 for an example of a youth performing a curl up). Movement should be controlled (about one curl every three seconds or a total of 20 per minute). If the heels come up, the fingers do not touch the far tape, or the child is unable to maintain a continuous cadence, the test is over and the final count should be recorded (a total of 75 curl-ups is considered maximal). Healthy ranges are found in table 2.8.

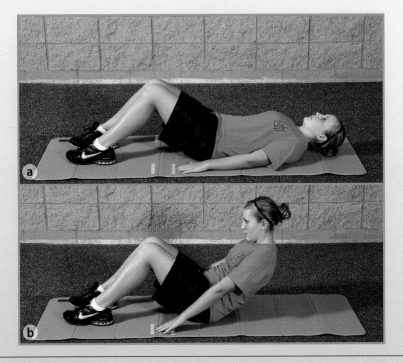

Figure 2.11 Curl-up for youth.

For the push-up test, the hands are placed slightly wider than the shoulders and the legs are out straight (see figure 2.12). The back should remain in a straight line from head to toes throughout the test. The body is lowered until the elbows are at a 90-degree angle and the upper arms are parallel with the floor. Then, arms should be straightened fully to return to the starting position. The test is continued as long as these form requirements are met and the movement is continuous (no rest stops are allowed). Record the maximal number completed. Boys and girls follow the same protocol. Healthy ranges are found in table 2.8.

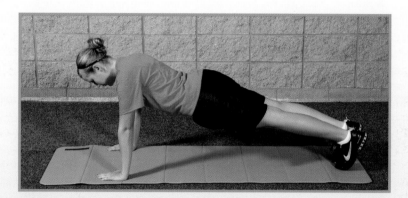

Figure 2.12 Push-up for youth.

Table 2.8 FITNESSGRAM Standards for Healthy Fitness Zone* for Curl-Ups and Push-Ups for Boys and Girls

Age	CURL-UP		PUSH-UP	
	Boys	Girls	Boys	Girls
5	2 or more	2 or more	3 or more	3 or more
6	2 or more	2 or more	3 or more	3 or more
7	4 or more	4 or more	4 or more	4 or more
8	6 or more	6 or more	5 or more	5 or more
9	9 or more	9 or more	6 or more	6 or more
10	12 or more	12 or more	7 or more	7 or more
11	15 or more	15 or more	8 or more	7 or more
12	18 or more	18 or more	10 or more	7 or more
13	21 or more	18 or more	12 or more	7 or more
14	24 or more	18 or more	14 or more	7 or more
15	24 or more	18 or more	16 or more	7 or more
16	24 or more	18 or more	18 or more	7 or more
17	24 or more	18 or more	18 or more	7 or more
17+	24 or more	18 or more	18 or more	7 or more

*The values listed represent the healthy fitness zone and indicate the child has a sufficient fitness level to provide important health benefits. Being below the value listed indicates a need for improvement.

Source: Standards for Healthy Fitness Zone, Revision 8.6 and 9.x. © 2010, The Cooper Institute, Dallas, Texas. Used with permission.

Assessing Flexibility

Flexibility refers to the range of motion possible in joints. Numerous joints exist in the body with major joints involving the knees, hips, and shoulders. Many factors affect joint range of motion, but good flexibility is an important dimension of physical fitness throughout the lifespan.

To assess flexibility completely, you would have to measure the range of motion of all major joints of the body. Over the years, one fitness test, called the sit-and-reach test, has been developed to index flexibility. Using a yardstick and some tape, the test is simple enough to perform, but the results provide only a general overall score and do not take into account differences in limb length or differences in flexibility at the various joints involved. Nonetheless, because the sit-and-reach test involves many joints of the body, it is considered to be reasonably good for assessing general flexibility.

Set up a spot on the floor for your sit-and-reach test. Place a yardstick on the floor and a 12-inch (30.5 cm) piece of tape across the yardstick at the 15-inch (38 cm) mark. Sit upright on the floor placing the heels of your feet (with shoes removed) against the inner edge of the taped mark so your heels are about 10 to 12 inches (25.4 to 30.5 cm) apart as shown in figure 2.13a. Exhale as you reach forward between your feet to touch as far down the yardstick as you can, as shown in figure 2.13b. Make several attempts and record your longest measure. Do not bounce into the stretch, but rather, bend forward slowly and hold the final position for a couple of seconds. It is best to perform some aerobic exercise as a warm-up before this test. Use table 2.9 to interpret the results of your sit-and-reach test. How flexible are you?

The sit-and-reach test for children and adolescents is implemented in a slightly different format (see *Sit-and-Reach Test for Youth*). In addition, many older adults

Table 2.9 **Interpretations of Sit-and-Reach Test Results for Males and Females***

Males	AGE					
	18–25	26–35	36–45	46–55	56–65	66 and older
Well above average	22 in. or higher	21 in. or higher	21 in. or higher	19 in. or higher	17 in. or higher	17 in. or higher
Above average	19–21 in.	17–20 in.	17–20 in.	15–18 in.	13–16 in.	13–16 in.
Average	17–18 in.	15–17 in.	15–16 in.	13–14 in.	11–13 in.	10–12 in.
Below average	14–16 in.	13–14 in.	13–14 in.	10–12 in.	9–10 in.	8–9 in.
Well below average	13 in. or lower	12 in. or lower	12 in. or lower	9 in. or lower	8 in. or lower	7 in. or lower

Females	AGE					
	18–25	26–35	36–45	46–55	56–65	66 and older
Well above average	24 in. or higher	23 in. or higher	22 in. or higher	21 in. or higher	20 in. or higher	20 in. or higher
Above average	21–23 in.	20–22 in.	19–21 in.	18–20 in.	17–19 in.	17–19 in.
Average	19–20 in.	19–20 in.	17–18 in.	16–17 in.	15–16 in.	15–17 in.
Below average	17–18 in	16–18 in.	15–16 in.	14–15 in.	13–14 in.	13–14 in.
Well below average	16 in. or lower	15 in. or lower	14 in. or lower	13 in. or lower	12 in. or lower	12 in. or lower

* If you have recorded your result in cm, divide that value by 2.54 to determine the number of inches; compare the number of inches you could reach to those within the table.

Reprinted with permission from *YMCA Fitness Testing and Assessment Manual,* 4th ed. © 2000 by YMCA of the USA, Chicago. All rights reserved.

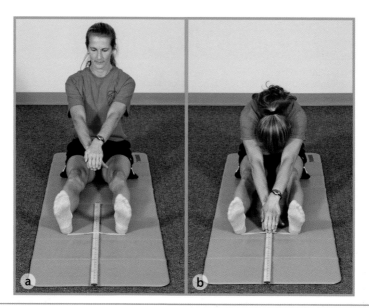

Figure 2.13 Sit-and-reach.

have functional limitations that make it difficult to get down and then up again from the standard sit-and-reach test position of sitting on the floor with legs extended. The chair sit-and-reach test allows for the assessment of lower-body flexibility while seating in a chair.[4] Details on this test and what the score means are included in chapter 11 on pages 236 and 237.

You may have been surprised by the number of steps required to assess your personal fitness. Just as fitness includes many aspects, so do the tests for determining how fit you really are. In this chapter, George's example was used throughout to help you understand preparticipation screening, risk stratification, and fitness testing. Some of his results were better than others. Each person has areas of strengths and areas that need improvement. When you know your strengths and weaknesses, you can adjust your current exercise program to address areas in need of improvement while maintaining in areas that you already have a good level of fitness. Additional information on tracking progress for youth, adults, and older adults is found in chapters 9, 10, and 11, respectively.

A CLOSER LOOK
George

In recent years, George has noticed that his range of motion has been decreasing, particularly in his shoulders. Aerobic exercise, such as biking to work, may help him increase his flexibility, but where does he stand now?

When George performed the sit-and-reach test, he found that he was indeed inflexible. He was only able to reach to the 9-inch (22.9 cm) mark, even after a warm-up and several tries. Using table 2.9, he learned that this score placed him in the "Below average" category for men his age. Perhaps George can have his bike shop make adjustments to his bike to account for his relative inflexibility, but regular exercise and renewed attention to his stretching program is bound to help him improve his range of motion.

Sit-and-Reach Test for Youth

The sit-and-reach test used in the FITNESSGRAM uses a 12-inch-high (30.5 cm) box and a yardstick.[3] The yardstick is place on the box with the zero end of the yardstick facing the child and the 9-inch (22.9 cm) mark at the nearest edge of the box. One foot is placed against the box and the other is flat on the floor next to the knee of the straight leg (see figure 2.14a). The child reaches forward with back straight and head up (see figure 2.14b). After measuring one side, have the child reverse the position of the legs and repeat.

Record the number of inches for both the right and left sides to the nearest half inch (1.3 cm). Rather than determining a range, the test establishes a standard score to be met (or not). For boys ages 5 to 17, this is 8 inches (20.3 cm). For girls the standard increases with age: for 5- to 10-year-olds the standard is 9 inches (22.9 cm), for 11- to 14-year-olds it is 10 inches (25.4 cm), and for 15- to 17-year-olds it is 12 inches (30.5 cm). This test focuses more on hamstring flexibility; the adult test also assesses low back flexibility.

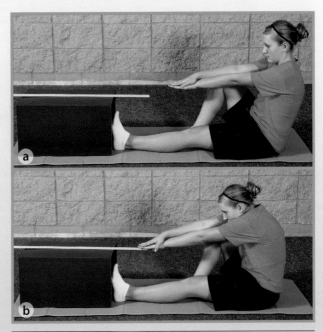

Figure 2.14   Sit-and-reach for youth.

Although this chapter outlines some simple assessments you can perform on your own with minimal equipment and assistance from others, you should never hesitate to consult with your health care provider or seek help from a certified fitness professional if you have questions or desire more advanced testing. In no time at all, you will find that the exercise you do will pay off as your physical fitness improves. The simple assessments included in this chapter can be used to track your progress over time.

chapter 3

ACSM's Program for Balanced Fitness

Getting started with an exercise program or finding ways to improve what you are already doing can seem like a daunting task. To simplify the process of developing a lifelong exercise habit, this *Complete Guide* proposes that you take two steps. The first is to examine your goals and consider how an exercise program can fit into your life. The second is to determine the specifics of what to include in your personal exercise program.

Rather than being an exact formula, an exercise prescription is more like my mother-in-law's recipes. She gives some general guidelines along with a list of ingredients, but then it gets interesting. She suggests adding a bit more of one ingredient if you prefer a spicier dish, or using a substitution if you are short on a particular ingredient. She hesitates to give exact measurements, as if she believes that doing so would ruin the cooking experience. The dish resulting from her type of recipe is individualized.

Your exercise program will be based on solid guidelines and a list of ingredients, but then you will be presented with options to allow you to make the exercise program your own. You are unique in terms of your health status, your current level of activity, and your fitness goals. This chapter discusses the basic guidelines and components of an exercise program (aerobic fitness, muscular fitness, and flexibility) and then provides some insights into how to individualize that program.

FITNESS CATEGORIES

A balanced exercise program is like a sturdy three-legged stool. If one leg is weak or too short, the stool isn't stable. In the same way, ignoring one of the exercise components will put your fitness program out of balance. Each health-related component of physical fitness—aerobic fitness, muscular fitness, and flexibility and balance—is important and must be considered. Although you may have a slightly different focus than someone else, to meet your own personal health or fitness goals, you need to address each of these fitness components.

Aerobic Fitness

Aerobic fitness is also known as cardiorespiratory endurance. Aerobic activities are those that require oxygen to provide energy and are typically described as involving large-muscle groups used in a repeated or rhythmic fashion. Probably the most popular aerobic exercise is walking. Other examples are jogging, running, bicycling, swimming, using aerobic equipment (e.g., elliptical machines, stair climbers), tennis, and team sports (e.g., basketball, soccer). When you are engaged in these activities, you can feel your breathing rate go up as your body strives to bring needed oxygen to your working muscles.

In chapter 2, two basic tests were described to help you estimate your level of aerobic fitness (the one-mile walking test on page 28 and the 1.5-mile run test on page 29). Either of these tests can provide a simple estimate of your body's ability to take in and use oxygen, referred to as $\dot{V}O_2$max. By determining your current $\dot{V}O_2$max, you can better determine the focus you need to place on aerobic fitness. The lower your $\dot{V}O_2$max is, the more attention you should give to improving your aerobic fitness.

You should engage in aerobic exercise three to five days per week. The intensity (i.e., how hard you are working) will depend on your fitness level. Refer back to your fitness assessment from chapter 2 and consider your current level of activity as outlined in table 3.1 for guidance on aerobic activity targets (for now, focus

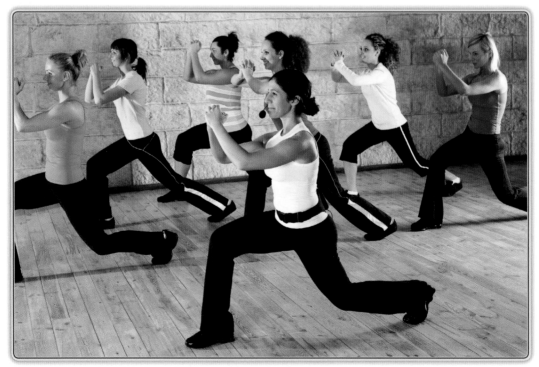

Group exercise classes are one way to build aerobic fitness.

Table 3.1 Aerobic and Resistance Training Targets Based on Activity Status

Activity status	Aerobic training focus	Resistance training focus
Beginner (inactive with no or minimal physical activity and thus deconditioned)	*No prior activity*: Focus is on light to moderate-level activity for 20–30 minutes over the course of the day. Accumulating time in 10-minute bouts is an option. Overall, your target is 60–150 minutes per week. *Minimal prior activity* (i.e., once you have met the target level of 60-150 minutes): Focus is on light- to moderate-level activity for 30–60 minutes per day. Accumulating time in 10-minute bouts is an option. Overall, your target is 150–200 minutes per week.	Select six exercises (one targeting each of the following muscle groups: hips and legs, chest, back, shoulders, low back, and abdominals). Begin with one set of 8–12 repetitions twice per week. Your target is one or two sets of 8–12 repetitions done two or three days per week. (*Note:* For older adults, 10–15 repetitions per set is recommended.)
Intermediate (sporadically active but without an optimal exercise plan and thus moderately deconditioned)	*Fair to average fitness:* Focus is on moderate activity for 30–90 minutes per day. Overall, your target is 200–300 minutes per week.	Select 10 exercises (one targeting each of the following muscle groups: hips and legs, quadriceps, hamstrings, chest, back, shoulders, biceps, triceps, low back, and abdominals). Your target is two sets of 8–12 repetitions on two or three days per week. (*Note:* For older adults, 10–15 repetitions per set is recommended.)
Established (regularly engaging in moderate to vigorous exercise)	*Regular exerciser* (moderate to vigorous): Focus is on moderate- to vigorous-intensity activity for 30–90 minutes per day. Overall, your target is 200–300 minutes per week.	You can continue with the intermediate plan (but simply add more weight as you adapt), or you may want to consider splitting your workout and focusing more on specific muscle groups on a given day (more information on this option is given in chapter 7).

on the aerobic training column; resistance training will be discussed in the next section).[1]

Details on how to determine your intensity level are provided in chapter 6. The point of examining these recommendations is to highlight the ranges with regard to frequency, intensity, and time. The options are almost unlimited.

Muscular Fitness

Muscular fitness training is typically referred to as resistance training and addresses both muscular strength and muscular endurance. Muscular strength is the maximum amount of force a muscle or muscle group can produce. Muscular endurance is the ability of a muscle or muscle group to exert a force repeatedly over time or to maintain a contraction for a period of time. Most activities involve aspects of both; thus, in this book the term *muscular fitness* is generally used.

Muscular fitness can be improved with resistance training, and examples of specific exercises are provided in chapter 7. In general, your program should include exercises for the major muscle groups—chest, shoulders, arms, upper and lower back, abdomen, hips, and legs.[1] You should also train opposing muscle groups to maintain muscle balance, which will help you avoid injury (e.g., include both low back exercises and abdominal exercises).

Your resistance training program consists of repetitions and sets. A repetition refers to the act of lifting a weight one time; lifting the weight multiple times in succession is called a set. Each muscle group should be trained in sets. You can repeat a given exercise, or you can select different exercises that target the same muscle group. The number of repetitions and sets will depend on your goals.

A CLOSER LOOK
Suzie and John

Suzie and John are at different stages in life and meet their exercise goals by participating in very different types of activity. Neither program is better than the other, but rather, each is appropriate to the goals and purpose of the person.

Suzie

Suzie is a 55-year-old elementary school teacher. She is in apparently good health but has not maintained a regular exercise program for the last 10 years. She has a goal of completing a 5K (3.1 miles) fund-raising walk at her school to benefit a family in need. She has three months to prepare. To determine her baseline, she completed the Rockport one-mile walking test (see page 28 in chapter 2) on a marked course at her school. She was disappointed to see that her time of 15:45 along with her heart rate of 120 beats per minute and body weight of 140 pounds (63.6 kg) placed her in the "Fair" category for aerobic fitness.

Suzie decided it was time to take charge of her aerobic fitness. She started out walking in her neighborhood for 10 minutes before school, 10 minutes at lunchtime with her students, and 10 minutes in her neighborhood after work. Initially, her pace was leisurely, but over the course of the first month, she first increased the time and then gradually increased the pace of her walking. Now, two months later, she is completing 15 minutes of brisk walking before work and 20 minutes after work, along with 15 minutes of more leisurely walking with her students during lunch. On the weekends, she and her husband enjoy walking a 3-mile (4.8 km) trail at the local nature center. In total, Suzie is now engaging in aerobic activity of moderate intensity for about 200 minutes per week and was able to easily complete her 5K walk for the fund-raiser.

John

John is a 32-year-old accountant. He was a competitive runner in high school and has continued to be active over the years, enjoying competing in local 10K races (6.2 miles). He now participates in many activities in addition to running. He joined a local fitness center and enjoys swimming as well as using the various pieces of aerobic-training equipment (elliptical machine, rowing machine, and stair climber).

Because his workdays are very hectic, John has developed the habit of exercising early in the morning. Over the years, he has found this to be the best way to adhere to his exercise program. By completing his workout before heading to his office, he feels energized and does not have to worry about how to fit in his exercise routine at the end of a long, busy day with clients. He exercises for at least 50 minutes before work each day; he does aerobic activity on Mondays, Wednesdays, and Fridays and resistance training on Tuesdays and Thursdays. He also joins friends for a longer hike at a nearby state park or rides his bike at least an hour on either Saturday or Sunday. This provides him with over 200 minutes per week of moderate- to high-intensity activity.

Getting Started With a Resistance Training Program[4]

1. Make a commitment.
   - Exercise will take time and effort. Expect to resistance train 20 to 45 minutes, two or three times per week.
   - You may be a little sore initially or when adding a new activity, but it will pass.
2. Find a good resource.
   - Learn 8 to 10 different exercises to strengthen all the major muscle groups.
   - Seek the help of a professional or a good book (e.g., chapter 7 in the book you are currently reading!) to learn the appropriate body position and lifting technique for each exercise.
3. Develop a routine.
   - Perform 8 to 15 repetitions for each set, and complete two to four sets of each exercise. If you cannot do at least eight repetitions, the weight is too heavy.
   - Breathe once for each repetition; inhale when relaxing and exhale when lifting.
   - Always move the weight slowly.
   - Rest approximately two minutes between sets, or do an exercise focused on a different muscle group.
4. Progress as you improve.
   - If you can exceed 15 repetitions, the weight is too light; gradually increase the resistance. Initially, you will make more frequent adjustments.
5. Rest and grow.
   - Do not do resistance training of the same muscle group on two consecutive days.
   - Rest to give your body time to recuperate.
   - You will become stronger—typically 25% to 100% stronger in each muscle group.
   - Research shows that the biggest improvements are in the first few months.

In addition, the relative intensity of the resistance training session is another factor. To improve muscular fitness, you have to apply an overload, or stress beyond typical use, to the muscle or muscle group. For additional information on how to get started with a resistance training program, see *Getting Started With a Resistance Training Program.*

Table 3.1 offers guidance regarding resistance training for beginning, intermediate, and established exercisers. Note that you may be doing aerobic exercise regularly (and thus be in the "Established" category) but may be a beginner when it comes to resistance training. For this reason, you should consider each component separately.

Flexibility and Balance

Flexibility is the ability to move a joint through its full range of motion, or in other words, the amount of movement possible given the structure of the joint. To improve flexibility, you need to include stretching exercises in your exercise program.

Stretching refers to exercises that move joints, along with the related muscles, tendons, and ligaments, through their range of motion. Include stretching in your exercise program at least two to three days per week. Typically, about 10 minutes will allow you to stretch the major muscle groups (neck, shoulders, back, pelvis, hips, and legs).[1] Chapter 8 includes more information about stretching, along with specific examples of stretches.

In addition to flexibility, adult exercise programs should also address balance. Your nervous system interacts with your muscles to move your body as well as to optimize agility and balance. Aging can result in a loss of balance and agility, thus leading to an increased risk of falling. Balance-enhancing activities, often referred to as neuromuscular exercises (because of the brain/nerve and muscle connection), are recommended for adults in the form of activities such as tai chi, Pilates, and yoga, and for older adults who are at risk of falling or who have impairments in mobility.[1] Chapter 8 includes a number of activities that can be included in balance training.

CREATING A BALANCED PROGRAM

Creating an exercise program is not difficult, but it requires some thought and planning. The first step is often the hardest. If you have been reading from the beginning of this book, you have seen compelling evidence regarding the health-related benefits of physical activity. Knowledge is good, but now it is time to develop an action plan by assessing where you are in your life and how you can find the motivation to move forward (see *Self-Assessment Questions* for a list of questions to ask yourself).

Reviewing Your Fitness Assessments

The fitness assessments in chapter 2 provide some very helpful baseline information. Knowing where you stand with regard to aerobic and muscular fitness as well as your level of flexibility is a good starting point. If you were pleasantly surprised with the outcome of your assessments, be encouraged to continue and to find additional ways to maintain or improve your fitness. If you were unhappy with some of your fitness assessment results, do not be discouraged. No matter what your current level of fitness is, you can always improve. This is true whether you are currently inactive or already active.

Fitness assessments also provide evidence of improvement over time. Repeating the assessments periodically can provide objective evidence of your improvement, or can show you areas that may need some extra attention. If you are a beginner, you may want to include assessments more frequently (every two to four months) because the feedback will help you adjust your program. If you are a more established exerciser, you will not experience substantial changes and thus may only want to conduct assessments two or three times a year. Progress charts for children, adults, and older adults appear in chapter 9 (page 204), chapter 10 (page 218), and chapter 11 (page 242), respectively. Enter your score along with the ranking for each item in the appropriate chart. Ideally, you will see your scores, or rankings, slowly improve over time. If you aren't seeing progress in a particular area, you may need to increase your focus on that fitness component. If you are already at a good level of fitness, then seek to maintain it.

Although the scores and rankings from fitness assessments are useful in establishing a baseline as well as in marking your progress, your reasons for becoming active are not likely linked to a number on a chart. More likely, your wake-up call was realizing that lack of fitness prevents you from engaging fully in life activities. Consider the following examples:

Aerobic Fitness

- Do you find yourself breathless going up a short flight of stairs?
- Do you avoid social or recreational situations that may involve physical activity?
- Are you unable to keep up with peers in sport competitions or recreational activities?

Muscular Fitness

- Are you unable to lift a full bag of groceries from your vehicle?
- Do you struggle to hold your child or grandchild?
- Are you limited in your recreational pursuits by a lack of strength?

Flexibility

- Are you unable to reach over your shoulder to fasten a zipper?
- Do you find it difficult to look behind you to check for traffic when driving?
- Do you have to modify your movements (e.g., a golf swing) to compensate for limited joint mobility?

Body Composition

- Are your clothes tighter than they were last year?
- Do you feel unhappy with your appearance because of weight gain?
- Does added body fat limit your enjoyment of recreational activities such as jogging or cycling?

Although assessing each of the components of fitness is encouraged, acknowledge that you are more than a score! Your quest for improved health and fitness relates to how you function on a daily basis. Make the changes you need to fulfill your potential. The scores or rankings provided by the fitness assessments are simply intended to help you monitor your progress.

Setting Goals

Goal setting is one of the most important aspects of successful behavior change. Without goals, you cannot develop a plan because you don't know where you want to go! It would be like going on a trip but never identifying the geographic location of your final destination. To succeed, you need to develop both long-term and short-term goals. Long-term goals are like your final destination; short-term goals are the individual routes that will get you there.

Short-terms goals are those that can be realistically accomplished within a brief period of time—this week, this month. For example, if you have been totally inactive, a short-term goal might be to walk around the neighborhood for 10 minutes each night after work for the upcoming week. This short-term goal has some valuable characteristics that you can remember with the acronym SMART, as follows:[4]

- *Specific*: The activity has been clearly defined both in terms of length and location. The goal is unambiguous in what is desired.
- *Measurable*: At the end of the week, you can reflect back on whether you walked each day after work. This is better than a goal such as, "I want to get in better shape," which would be hard to measure.
- *Action-based*: The goal includes an activity rather than generalities or an outcome, such as improving fitness or losing weight. It is focused on what you will actually be doing.
- *Realistic*: The location for the activity is convenient, and the length of the walk is not excessive. Too often, goals are so far out of reach that they become a source of discouragement rather than encouragement. Your goals should be relevant to you and firmly based in the reality of what you can accomplish.
- *Time-anchored*: This goal is linked with a specific time frame. Rather than being too open-ended, the goal specifies the upcoming week. Without a time-

centered approach, you might be tempted to procrastinate starting or moving forward with an exercise program.

SMART short-term goals can provide wonderful encouragement and focus. In addition, they can instill a sense of self-confidence that you *can* perform the activity. By creating a series of short-term goals, you can build toward your long-term goals.

Long-term goals are those that that you can achieve in the future—three months to a year from now. With careful planning, meeting your short-term goals should lead to accomplishing your long-term goals. Consider the consumer profile on page 46: Suzie had a long-term goal of completing a 5K fund-raising walk. She had three months to prepare for this event. Meeting short-term goals of increasing the time she spent walking and then increasing her pace (intensity) ultimately prepared her to complete her long-term goal of the 5K event. She gradually increased her activity over that time period, which allowed her to fulfill her long-term goal. Once she completed her 5K walk, she needed to develop another goal to keep her moving forward. Without goals, it is easy to fall into a rut or even to lose focus entirely. Setting new goals helps you focus on continual improvement.

Setting both short-term and long-term goals in each of the fitness areas will allow you to individualize your exercise program. You may already be walking on a regular basis but now see that you have neglected your muscular fitness or flexibility (like Suzie from page 48). By including goals in all areas, you can maintain your balance. As you identify your own strengths and weaknesses, you can focus additional attention on the areas in which you struggle and maintain your fitness in the areas in which you already have a solid foundation.

On a final note, writing down your goals is helpful. There is a saying: It's a dream until you write it down, and then it's a goal. Putting the words on paper can provide an opportunity to reflect on what you really want to accomplish with your exercise program. This also gives you a reference point. Keep your short-term goals prominently visible. Some people write their goals in their schedule books or post them on a note board, mirror, or even the refrigerator. Find a method that works for you, one that allows you to see the goals as a reminder of the actions you want to take. You can check off completed short-term goals and add new ones as you progress toward your long-term goals.

Sticking With Your Plan

With your goals for aerobic and muscular fitness along with flexibility and body composition written down, you now need to plan for success. To reap health and fitness benefits, your exercise plan needs to become a regular part *of* your life . . . *for* your life. A number of skills and strategies that experts have identified as helpful for promoting physical activity[2] are outlined in this section.

Creating a Decisional Balance Sheet

Changing your life by adding exercise to an already busy day is a major decision. As with any big decision, creating a list of the pros and cons can be very productive. Consider the things that support your decision to increase your activity level while also acknowledging the factors that may inhibit that change. This is called a decisional balance sheet (see figure 3.1 for an example).

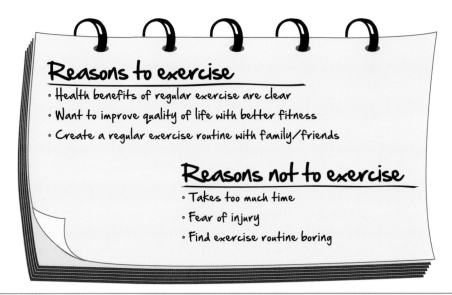

Reasons to exercise
- Health benefits of regular exercise are clear
- Want to improve quality of life with better fitness
- Create a regular exercise routine with family/friends

Reasons not to exercise
- Takes too much time
- Fear of injury
- Find exercise routine boring

Figure 3.1   Sample decisional balance sheet.

As you examine your own list of factors impeding your commitment to regular exercise, consider how you might modify them to move them to the pro side of the list, or at least how you might address them. For example, the extra time that a regular exercise program takes cannot be denied. However, you can modify your perspective on the time spent. You can think of your exercise time as a time to clear your mind and unwind from the stresses of school, work, or home responsibilities. You may select aerobic activities such as treadmill walking or stationary biking that allow you to read or watch television—activities you find rewarding but typically don't take time to enjoy.

If you have a jam-packed schedule, consider breaking your exercise routine into multiple shorter bouts. In the consumer profile on page 46, Suzie split her exercise into three shorter time periods throughout the day. She took advantage of her lunch break to add extra activity into her day and in doing so also served as an excellent role model for her students who enjoyed walking with her at school. Others, like John, find that an early morning routine works best. Although you may need to adjust your bedtime, morning workouts ensure you exercise before the hectic schedule of the day takes over.

Another common concern is the fear of injury or even death with increased physical activity. As discussed in chapter 2, certain health-related situations may require you to meet with your health care provider to ensure the safety of your exercise program. This is the reason for completing the preparticipation screenings outlined in chapter 2. For most apparently healthy people, starting with light to moderate intensity and progressing slowly will minimize the likelihood of injury as well as heart attack or death. The health benefits of a regular physical activity program are greater than the risk of adverse events for almost everyone.[5]

Finally, if you find your current exercise routine boring—find other options! Your exercise program should include activities you enjoy. Consider adding more variety or joining a group exercise class. Listening to music or stopping by your local library for a downloadable book can provide mental variety even if you keep your activity the same. Of course, when using a headset, be sure to be indoors or in a controlled environment so you do not become distracted from observing traffic or others around you.

Gaining Social Support

Social support is a very strong motivator. Consider the encouragement provided by a spouse who supervises a young child so the other spouse can head outside for a run or attend a group exercise session at a local health club. Research shows that active and ongoing support from significant others helps people stick with their exercise programs.[3] Parents who model an active lifestyle are providing a wonderful example for their children. Even better is to be active together as a family. A family outing to a local park can be a great stress reliever as well as an opportunity for everyone to be active. Physical activity is important throughout the lifespan. Developing active habits early in life will have lifelong benefits.

Participating in group activities—with family members, friends, or local groups—can also be a strong motivator to stay active. Most communities have clubs or associations of people with similar interests (e.g. cycling, running, mall walking, ballroom dancing). These are wonderful opportunities to meet new people and find real enjoyment in your exercise program.

If your family or close friends do not support your desire to be active, seek out other support systems. Some people, when facing their own health problems, may feel threatened by your resolution to move forward to better health. Don't let others sabotage your plans. Find an exercise partner or another fitness class member who values activity as much as you do. By encouraging each other, you can generate the motivation to continue. Hopefully, over time, your example will persuade your family members and friends to join you in a physically active lifestyle.

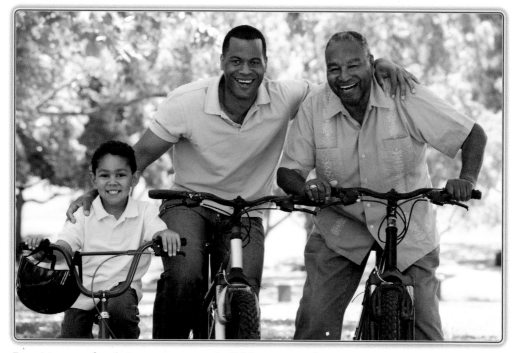

Exercising as a family is a great way to build fitness together.

Dealing With Setbacks

Will you experience setbacks in your exercise program? Very likely. Life situations arise that may disrupt your physical activity plan. Don't let this be discouraging. Instead, plan for it! Your exercise program is not an all-or-none endeavor. For example, when traveling for business, you may become stuck in the airport with a delayed flight. Rather than sit and fret about the delay (over which you have no control), take a brisk walk around the terminal. When traveling, consider staying in hotels that have fitness rooms. Although often not ideal, typically you can find activities that will complement your program. If there is no fitness room, walk the halls or consider doing some calisthenics and stretching in your room. Ask the hotel staff about safe places to walk or jog in the neighborhood.

When sickness, travel, family responsibilities, work obligations, and other unavoidable situations arise, realize they are just short-term holdups to your exercise program, not permanent derailments. Have a return plan of action in place. When faced with a setback, you might have to reverse your timeline a bit. For example, after an illness, you should start back slowly rather than jumping right back to where you left off. Although you may feel frustrated at losing fitness, be encouraged that you are able to start again and build back up.

Maintaining Motivation

Motivation can be described as a mental process that links a thought or feeling to an action. *You* are the one to make the decision to engage in physical activity each day. What motivates you? Some people are motivated by external factors such as pleasing a family member, a friend, or even an employer. Although it is helpful to have support from those around you, if the external focus is your only reason to exercise, it often leads to feelings of guilt or frustration if you don't feel as though you measure up to someone else's standards. In contrast, internal motivation focuses on what *you* want—to look better, feel better, get healthier, or learn a new activity.

Ultimately, motivation cannot be generated from someone else. Rather, motivation is about mobilizing that drive for action that already exists within you. Motivation is a mental process that can lead to positive lifestyle or behavior change. Motivation involves linking your intellectual understanding or feeling with action-oriented steps. This book provides the steps to start or to improve your exercise program, but in the end, the drive to action rests within you (for more information on motivation, see chapter 5).

Checking Progress

Keeping tabs on your exercise program will help keep you on track. Just as regular car maintenance gives you worry-free driving, taking a few moments to check your body's progress will ensure that you are still on course to meet your goals. One way to do this is to write down what you have accomplished each week. The weekly log in figure 3.2 provides space to record your activity in each of the three areas (aerobic fitness, muscular fitness, and flexibility). In addition, at the bottom of the form is a space to record a summary of the week's workouts and to write down some goals for the upcoming week, including things you may want to change.

FIGURE 3.2

Sample Activity Log

Day	A–M–F*	Time or distance	Comments (heart rate, rating of perceived exertion, health status, environmental conditions, etc.)
Sunday			
Monday			
Tuesday			
Wednesday			
Thursday			
Friday			
Saturday			
Weekly summary	A → # workouts = _____ ; # minutes = _____ M → # workouts = _____ ; # minutes = _____ F → # workouts = _____ ; # minutes = _____		
Next week's goal:			

*A = aerobic; M = muscular; F = flexibility.

Adapted by permission from Bushman and Young, 2005, p. 188.

From ACSM, 2011, *ACSM's complete guide to fitness & health* (Champaign, IL: Human Kinetics).

If logbooks aren't your style, consider simply jotting your exercise accomplishments in your schedule book or calendar. On the first day of each month, take a moment to look back over the previous month. This isn't elaborate but does give you the opportunity to reflect on what you have accomplished.

━━━━ ▪▪▪▪ ━━━━

Deciding to take charge of your health and to improve your fitness is a powerful resolution. Understanding the basic components of fitness—aerobic fitness, muscular fitness, and flexibility—gives you the tools you need. With tools in hand, you must reflect on what is important to you. Putting your goals down on paper and examining your reasons for exercising will give you a perspective that will allow you to create an exercise program that is right for you. Your exercise program will not be static but will likely change over time as you continue to develop new and more challenging goals.

chapter 4

Nutrition for Better Health and Fitness

Eating well, in combination with participating in a regular exercise program, is a positive step you can take to prevent and even reverse some diseases. Though nutrition is a broad science, this chapter focuses on some of the basics, along with how to make healthy choices in your daily food intake and how those choices can influence your ability to be active.

Too often, people associate nutrition and diet with restriction and unappealing options (note that the word *diet* simply refers to what you eat, not a particular weight loss plan). This chapter presents a positive view of nutrition and offers suggestions for taking control of your diet to improve how you feel. By providing your body with needed calories and nutrients, you will fully fuel your body for physical activity and exercise, as well as for competition, if you are so inclined. Just as a car needs quality fuel to run smoothly, your body needs a balance of nutrients to function optimally.

The *Dietary Guidelines for Americans*, published jointly by the U.S. Department of Health and Human Services and the U.S. Department of Agriculture, provides general guidance regarding nutrition for people 2 years of age and older. The Dietary Guidelines provide advice about how good dietary practices can promote health and prevent chronic disease.

The *Dietary Guidelines for Americans* includes the following key recommendations:[26, 28]

- Balance calories to manage weight:
    - With a focus on preventing or reducing overweight and obesity, improve eating and physical activity behaviors.
    - Control total calorie intake to manage body weight.
    - Increase physical activity and reduce time spent in sedentary behaviors.

- Maintain appropriate calorie balance throughout life (childhood, adolescence, adulthood, pregnancy and breastfeeding, and older age).
- Reduce some foods and food components:
  - Reduce sodium intake to less than 2300 mg (or even lower, to 1500 mg, adults 51 or older, and for those of any age who are African American or have hypertension, diabetes, or chronic kidney disease).

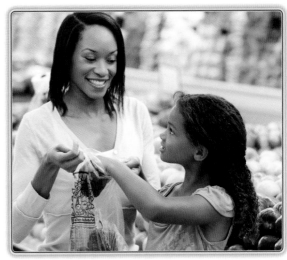

People of all ages can benefit from healthy foods.

  - Consume less than 10% of calories from saturated fatty acids; replace with monounsaturated and polyunsaturated fatty acids. Keep trans fatty acid consumption as low as possible (limit synthetic sources such as solid fats and partially hydrogenated oils).
  - Reduce intake of calories from solid fats and added sugars.
  - Limit consumption of refined grains, especially those that contain solid fats, added sugars, and sodium.
  - Consume alcohol in moderation if at all (moderation is considered up to one drink per day for women and two drinks per day for men).
- Foods and nutrients to increase (while staying within calorie needs):
  - Increase intake of fruits and vegetables.
  - Select a variety of vegetables, especially dark-green and red and orange vegetables and beans and peas.
  - Consume whole grains for at least half of all grains consumed.
  - Increase intake of fat-free or low-fat milk and milk products.
  - Choose a variety of lower-fat protein foods (e.g., seafood, lean meat and poultry, eggs, beans and peas, soy products, unsalted nuts and seeds).
  - Increase seafood consumption by substituting for some meat and poultry.
  - Use oils to replace solid fats where possible.
  - Choose foods that provide more potassium, dietary fiber, calcium, and vitamin D (e.g., vegetables, fruits, whole grains, milk, and milk products).
- Build healthy eating patterns
  - Develop an eating pattern that meets your nutrient needs over time while remaining at an appropriate calorie level.
  - Account for all foods and beverages consumed and assess how they fit within a total healthy eating pattern.
  - Follow food safety recommendations when preparing and eating foods to reduce the risk of foodborne illnesses.

Nutrition and Overall Health

Researchers of nearly all chronic diseases have studied the role of nutrition (the term *chronic* is used to refer to diseases that often begin at a younger age and develop over time). Six of the top 13 causes of death are related to poor nutrition and inactivity. By rank, these are heart disease (number 1), cancer (2), stroke (3), type 2 diabetes (6), chronic liver disease or cirrhosis (12), and high blood pressure (13).[20] Obesity is related to many of these causes of death, and although some have a genetic component, most are related to poor nutrition and lack of exercise, both of which are lifestyle habits.

Chronic diseases resulting from poor nutrition also lead to other disabilities, resulting in further loss of independence. For example, type 2 diabetes is one of the leading causes of blindness and amputation. Hip fractures are typically a result of osteoporosis, and people who suffer from a hip fracture are more likely to die within one year of their fracture or require long-term care.[21] Approximately 69% of people who have a first heart attack, 77% of those who have a first stroke, and 74% of those with congestive heart failure have blood pressure higher than 140/90 mm Hg (i.e., hypertension).[3] Obesity is an epidemic, with about a third of adults in the United States considered obese.[8] Furthermore, about 17% of American children and teenagers (2 to 19 years of age) are considered obese.[22]

Researchers have reported that unhealthy eating and sedentary behavior cause from 310,000 to 580,000 deaths per year in the United States. Because most Americans consume diets too high in total fat, trans fat, saturated fat, sodium, and sugar, and too low in whole grains, fruits, vegetables, and fiber, poor health and death are often related to poor nutrition. The combination of unhealthy diets and inactivity are the leading causes of death in the United States, above tobacco and alcohol use, and far above drug use and motor vehicle accidents.[18] In addition, the health care costs of poor nutrition and inactivity are astronomical. Healthier diets could save billions of dollars in medical costs per year, and also prevent lost productivity and, most important, loss of life.

Good nutrition and physical activity are the two most beneficial "medicines" you can use to prevent disease and live a good-quality life. Take control! You owe it to yourself to treat your body well.

These guidelines are an excellent place to start on the path to a healthier diet. The next step is to look at the nutrients and distribution you need to meet your energy needs.

DETERMINING CALORIE NEEDS

Because total calorie requirements are addressed throughout this chapter, this section explains the factors that influence your daily caloric needs and shows you how to estimate the number of calories you need. Total energy expenditure (TEE) is the total number of calories your body needs on a daily basis and is determined by the following:

- Your basal metabolic rate (BMR)
- The thermic effect of food (also known as dietary-induced thermogenesis)
- The thermic effect of your physical activity

What is a Calorie?

A calorie is defined as the heat required to raise the temperature of 1 gram of water 1 degree Celsius. Because this is a relatively small amount, scientists use the larger unit Calories (uppercase C), also called a kilocalorie (abbreviated as kcal). The Calorie, or kilocalorie, is equal to 1,000 calories. Food labels in the United States display Calories, or kilocalories. This is all pretty technical and does not reflect typical usage in everyday language. In this book, the word *calories* refers to Calories, or kilocalories (i.e., 1,000 calories), which is common usage.

Basal metabolic rate is defined as the energy required to maintain your body at rest (e.g., breathing, circulation). To precisely determine your BMR, you would need to fast from 8 to 12 hours and then undergo a laboratory test in which you sit quietly for about 30 minutes while the air you exhale is analyzed. This determines how many calories you are burning at rest. Basal metabolic rate is 60% to 75% of total energy expenditure. Typically, the larger and more muscular a person is, the higher the BMR is.

The thermic effect of food is the energy required to digest and absorb food. The thermic effect of food is measured in a similar way as BMR, although the measurement time is usually about four hours after you consumed a meal. The thermic effect of food is 10% to 15% of your total energy expenditure.

The thermic effect of activity is the amount of energy required for physical activity. It can be measured in a laboratory when you are exercising on a stationary bike or treadmill. The thermic effect of activity is the most variable of the three major components of total energy expenditure because it can be as low as 15% for sedentary people and as high as 80% for athletes who train six to eight hours per day.

One other component of total energy expenditure that plays a role is non-exercise activity thermogenesis (NEAT), which is energy expended in unplanned physical activity. This can include taking the stairs instead of the elevator, sitting on a balance ball at your desk, parking farther from your destination in a parking lot, fidgeting, and other calorie-burning activities.

Although determining your energy needs in a laboratory is precise, you do not need to go to that expense to estimate the number of calories you use. Some methods of estimation require first calculating your BMR based on your age, sex, height, and weight[13, 19] and then adding in the thermic effects of food and of activity, but this can be rather time-consuming. For general purposes, some simple math will allow you to quickly estimate your energy needs. See table 4.1 for the estimated daily caloric intake needed to maintain your current weight. In the first column, find the activity level that best represents your current status. If you know your body weight in pounds, multiply that number by the estimated number of calories per pound in the second column; if you know your weight in kilograms, look at the third column in the table.

Table 4.1 Approximate Daily Caloric Intake per Unit of Body Weight Needed for Maintaining Desirable Body Weight

Activity level	Calories per pound of body weight	Calories per kilogram of body weight
Very sedentary (restricted movement such as a patient confined to home)	13	29
Sedentary (most Americans, office job, light work)	14	31
Moderate activity (weekend recreation)	15	33
Very active (meet ACSM standards for vigorous exercise three times per week)	16	35
Competitive athlete (daily vigorous activity in high-energy sport)	17 or more	38 or more

Adapted, by permission, from M.H. Williams, 2007, *Nutrition for health, fitness & sport*, 8th ed. (New York: McGraw-Hill), 404. © The McGraw-Hill Companies, Inc.

DETERMINING NUTRIENT NEEDS

Nutrients include carbohydrates, proteins, fats, vitamins, minerals, and water. The first three—carbohydrates, proteins, and fats—are found in larger ("macro") quantities in the body and thus are referred to as macronutrients. Vitamins and minerals are found in smaller (micro) amounts and are referred to as micronutrients.

Macronutrients

Macronutrients (carbohydrates, proteins, and fats) provide energy for daily activities and during exercise, recreational activity, and sport training. They provide slightly different numbers of calories per gram, as follows:

- Carbohydrates provide about 4 calories per gram.
- Proteins provide about 4 calories per gram.
- Fats provide about 9 calories per gram.

A CLOSER LOOK
Brenda

Brenda is a 41-year-old, 145-pound (66 kg) woman who wants to maintain her current body weight. She exercises regularly and meets the guidelines for vigorous activity described in this book. Therefore, she is in the "Very active" category. After consulting table 4.1, she verifies that 16 calories per pound are about what a "very active" person needs. She then multiplies her body weight by 16 to estimate how many calories she needs each day. She calculates this to be 2,320 calories (145 pounds × 16 calories per pound).

Take a moment to do this calculation based on your body weight and activity level. Keep in mind that your final estimate is just that—an estimate. Your actual daily calorie needs may vary somewhat, but this provides an approximate starting point. To maintain your body weight, this is about how many calories you should consume. To lose or gain weight, you will need to adjust your food intake accordingly.

These values show clearly that on a gram-per-gram basis, fat is much denser with regard to calories than carbohydrate or protein. This is the reason a food high in fat provides more calories than a food lower in fat. Chapter 13 provides additional information on the macronutrients as they pertain to weight management. Although alcohol is not a required nutrient, it has its own unique calorie content of 7 calories per gram.

Carbohydrates

Although some diets (e.g., the Atkins diet) seem to suggest that carbohydrates are the villain when it comes to weight management, carbohydrates are actually vital for the optimal functioning of your body. For example, your brain and central nervous system rely on blood glucose (sugar) for energy. Carbohydrates are also an important source of energy during physical activity. Without sufficient carbohydrate in your diet, you will not be able to fully enjoy a vigorous workout or competition because your body will not have the fuel it needs to perform.

Carbohydrates exist in the form of sugars, starches, and fiber. Sugars are naturally found in items such as fruit and milk products. Sugar is also added to various products to add flavor and taste. Cutting down on products with added sugar is recommended (e.g., candy, nondiet soda, and fruit drinks). These are rather obvious, but checking food labels can reveal added sugars that aren't as obvious, which are called many different names, including brown sugar, corn sweetener, corn syrup, dextrose, high-fructose corn syrup, glucose, honey, lactose, maltose, malt syrup, molasses, and sucrose. Be especially careful when these items are listed as one of the first few ingredients on the food label because components are listed in the order of predominance by weight.[3]

Focusing on fruits, vegetables, and whole grain products maximizes the health benefits of carbohydrates. Starches are a more complex form of carbohydrate that the body can use for energy and are found in products such as vegetables, dried beans, and grains. Consumption of whole grains can help prevent cardiovascular disease, type 2 diabetes, and other chronic diseases mainly because they are high in vitamins and minerals, as well as antioxidants.[15, 23]

The third category of carbohydrate—fiber—includes parts of food that the body cannot break down and absorb. Sources of fiber include vegetables, fruits, and whole grains. Consuming higher-fiber foods promotes greater feelings of fullness as well as bowel health. Higher-fiber diets have been found to reduce the risk of diabetes, colon cancer, and obesity.[28] Table 4.2 provides examples of good sources of carbohydrates, including the contribution made by fiber.

Approximately 45% to 65% of your calorie intake should be from carbohydrates.[10] This is a relatively wide range to account for the variety of nutritional approaches while avoiding deficiencies or adverse health consequences. The Daily Value listed on food labels (see the full discussion later in this chapter beginning on page 64) is based on 60% of the calorie intake. If you are active, or if you are a competitive athlete, keeping your carbohydrate intake near the upper end of this range will provide sufficient fuel for your working muscles. Now that you know about how many calories you need per day, as figured from table 4.1 on page 61, you can determine how much carbohydrate is recommended. For example, for someone who needs 2,500 calories per day, approximately 1,125 to 1,625 calories should be from carbohydrate. This would be calculated as follows:

2,500 calories per day × 0.45 (45%) = 1,125 calories from carbohydrate

2,500 calories per day × 0.65 (65%) = 1,625 calories from carbohydrate

To determine the number of grams of carbohydrate you need, recall that each gram of carbohydrate supplies 4 calories. Simply take the number of calories from carbohydrates and divide by 4 to determine how many grams you need:

1,125 calories ÷ 4 calories per gram = 281 grams from carbohydrate

1,625 calories ÷ 4 calories per gram = 406 grams from carbohydrate

Table 4.2 **Sources of Carbohydrates and Fiber**

Food	Serving size	Carbohydrate per serving (g)	Fiber per serving (g)
Grains			
Raisin bagel	1 whole	36	2
Whole grain bread	1 slice	13	2
Raisin bran cereal	1 oz (28 g)	47	7
Brown rice	1 cup	45	4
Spaghetti	1 cup	43	3
Fruits			
Banana, sliced	1 cup	34	4
Blueberries	1 cup	21	4
Figs, dried	2 figs	24	4
Grapefruit juice	6 fl oz (177 ml)	72	<1
Vegetables			
Beans (dry), cooked	1 cup	45–55	13–19
Baked beans, canned	1 cup	47	18
Carrots, cooked	1 cup	13	5
Sweet potato	1 cup	54	5
Dairy			
Milk, low or nonfat	1 cup	12	0
Yogurt, plain, skim milk	8 oz (227 g)	17	0
Cottage cheese, nonfat	1 cup	10	0

Adapted from U.S. Department of Agriculture, Agricultural Research Service, 2010.

Reading Food Labels

Food labels are important windows of information for products that have them (fruits and vegetables do not). Because there is not enough room to place all the nutrient information on a food label, the label provides only a quick look at the nutrient content. Reading labels, however, can be confusing; the following clarifies the information labels provide. See figure 4.1 for an example of a food label.

Serving Size

Serving size is usually the first item listed on a food label. Serving sizes are standardized for similar foods. Pay close attention to the serving size, because, in some cases, food companies package items in a set of two (i.e., the serving size is half of the total amount in the package). Consider a regular-size bag of microwave popcorn. If you eat the whole bag, you have consumed two or three servings of popcorn! Because the calories listed reflect a single serving, you need to do some multiplication to determine how many calories you actually consumed. Paying attention to the serving size will help you track your calorie intake and avoid overeating and gaining weight over time.

Calories and Calories From Fat

You should always check the total number of calories provided in a food item, as well as the total number of calories from fat. Paying attention to serving size is key to determining your overall calorie intake of each food item. As a quick guide to calorie intake, consider the following:[27]

- a food item providing 40 calories per serving is considered "low calorie."
- a food item providing 100 calories per serving is considered "moderate calorie."
- a food item providing 400 calories or more per serving is considered "high calorie."

Throughout the course of a typical day, you will likely consume food items in various categories. As long as you keep your eye on the total calories you consume over the course of the day, you will be able to remain in energy balance (i.e., your consumed calories will match the number of calories you expend).

Percent Daily Value

Another item to pay attention to on a food label is the "% Daily Value" (%DV) listed for certain nutrients on all food labels. These values are based on a 2,000-calorie diet. Daily values are recommended levels of intake. For some nutrients (e.g., total fat, saturated fat, cholesterol, and sodium), it is better to aim to consume less than the recommended amount; however, for others, such as total carbohydrate and dietary fiber, it is important to try to consume at least the recommended amount. In general, a %DV of less than 5% is considered low, and 20% or greater is considered high.[27]

When looking at the section of the label focused on fat, note that both saturated and trans fats are listed. You should restrict trans fats as much as possible from your diet and consume no more than 10% of total calorie intake in the form of saturated fat. Similarly, keeping cholesterol and sodium levels in check is important. For carbohydrate, the subcategories of dietary fiber and sugars are listed. You should try to increase, rather than limit, your intake of dietary fiber.

The bottom of the label contains a footnote with the Daily Values for diets of 2,000 and 2,500 calories per day. Although this might not be a direct match to the calories you need on a daily basis, it does provide general guidance and covers a wide range of people. The footnote presents the recommended dietary information for important nutrients (e.g., fat, sodium, fiber). This footnote is only on larger food packages and does not change from food product to food product.

Sample Food Label for
Macaroni and Cheese

Nutrition Facts

1. Start here →

Serving Size 1 cup (228g)
Servings Per Container 2

Amount Per Serving

2. Check calories

Calories 250   Calories from Fat 110

6. Quick Guide
to % DV

	% Daily Value*
Total Fat 12g	18%
Saturated Fat 3g	15%
Trans Fat 3g	
Cholesterol 30mg	10%
Sodium 470mg	20%
Potassium 170mg	5%
Total Carbohydrate 31g	10%
Dietary Fiber 0g	0%
Sugars 5g	
Protein 5g	

• 5% or less
is low

• 20% or more
is high

3. Limit these
nutrients

4. Get enough
of these
nutrients

Vitamin A	4%	• Vitamin C	2%
Calcium	20%	• Iron	4%

* Percent Daily Values are based on a 2,000 calorie diet. Your daily values may be higher or lower depending on your calorie needs:

5. Footnote

	Calories:	2,000	2,500
Total Fat	Less than	65g	80g
Sat Fat	Less than	20g	25g
Cholesterol	Less than	300mg	300mg
Sodium	Less than	2,400mg	2,400mg
Potassium		3,500mg	3,500mg
Total Carbohydrate		300g	375g
Dietary Fiber		25g	30g

Figure 4.1   Sample food label.
Reprinted from U.S. Department of Health and Human Services, U.S. Food and Drug Administration, 2009.

Proteins

Proteins are made of small units called amino acids, which are considered the building blocks of the body. Proteins promote muscle growth and are required for many body functions including assistance with chemical reactions and hormones. Even though proteins can provide 4 calories per gram, you typically do not use protein for energy unless you are deficient in your intake of carbohydrate or fat. This is so the proteins you consume can be used to promote growth and for normal body functions. See table 4.3 for the protein content of various foods.

Proteins should account for about 10% to 15% of total calories (AMDR is 10% to 35% for adults; see *What Do All the Abbreviations Mean?* on page 70 for a definition of AMDR).[10] As with carbohydrate, a range is provided to account for differences in diet and to suggest a safe upper limit. Depending on your total calorie intake, you may be near the low or high end of this range. Your personal protein requirement is based on your body weight; you should consume approximately 0.36 grams of protein for each pound of body weight. Simply multiply your body weight in pounds by 0.36 to determine approximately how many grams of protein you need to consume each day. If you know your body weight in kilograms, multiple that value by 0.8.[2] For example, for a 150-pound person, this would be figured as shown:

150 × 0.36 = 54 grams protein × 4 calories per gram= 216 calories from protein

Note that protein requirements are increased for athletes and are different depending on the sport, the intensity and frequency out of the workout, and how experienced the athlete is. Typical recommendations for strength-trained athletes (e.g., American football players, bodybuilders) and endurance athletes (e.g., marathon runners) are between 0.55 and 0.77 grams of protein per pound of body weight (or 1.2 to 1.7 grams of protein per kilogram of body weight).[2] Because many Americans already consume more than the recommended daily allowance for protein, athletes or other highly active people may already be consuming adequate protein.

Table 4.3 Protein Content of Various Foods

Food	Serving size	Protein per serving (g)
Meat (including turkey, pork)	3 oz (85 g)	24
Fish (including trout, perch, haddock, flounder, tuna)	3 oz (85 g)	20–22
Beans (including pinto, kidney, black, navy)	1 cup	13–15
Yogurt, plain, skim milk	8 oz (227 g)	13
Cinnamon-raisin bagel	4 in. (10 cm) bagel	9
Peanuts	1 oz (28 g)	8
Hard-boiled egg	1 large	6
Raisin bran cereal	1 cup	5
Whole wheat bread	1 slice	4
Sweet potato	1 potato	3
Squash	1 cup	2
Orange	1 cup	2
Banana	1 banana	1

Adapted from U.S. Department of Agriculture, Agricultural Research Service, 2010.

Alex

Alex is a 34-year-old computer programmer who enjoys running at a local park during his lunch hour as well as more extended run training on the weekends as he prepares for a half marathon. He also does some resistance training a couple of nights each week with friends at a local gym. Although he is happy with his current exercise regimen, he knows his diet is very high in fat and far from optimal. As a first step, he determines how many calories he needs and then what targets he should have for various nutrients.

To provide an estimate of his calorie needs, he checks table 4.1 for the number of calories he needs per unit of his body weight. He is in the "Very active" category given his running and resistance training activities. Thus he will take his body weight (188 lb, or 85 kg) and multiply it by 16.

188 × 16 = 3,008 calories

To keep things simple for calculating, he rounds this off to 3,000 calories needed per day. Next he determines the amount of calories he needs to consume from carbohydrate, fat, and protein. He starts with protein because this is best based on his body weight. Because of his higher level of endurance training, he selects 0.55 grams per pound of body weight for his target. He takes his body weight and multiplies it by 0.55:

188 × 0.55 = 103 grams of protein

To check the percentage of calories from protein, he multiplies the grams by 4 (because there are 4 calories per gram of protein):

103 × 4 = 412 calories from protein

Alex determines that about 14% of his calories should be from protein (412 calories from protein divided by 3,000 total calories = 0.14, which is the decimal representation of 14%).

For carbohydrate, Alex selects 60% of calories, and so the remaining 26% should come from fat. He calculates these as follows:

3,000 calories × 0.60 = 1,800 calories from carbohydrate

3,000 calories × 0.26 = 780 calories from fat

These calculations provide Alex with some general targets to help create balance in his diet. Not every meal has to fall precisely within these percentages; rather, this is more appropriate to consider over the course of the entire day. Some meals may be higher in protein, whereas others may have more fat or carbohydrate. Alex needs to reflect on the foods and beverages consumed over the course of the day rather than becoming too focused on each food item or meal.

Fats

Fats, also called lipids, are provided in the diet from such sources as animal protein, butter, oils, nuts, and many refined products. Fats are often thought of as bad, a myth perpetuated by the many fat-free products flooding store shelves. However, fats are needed in appropriate amounts for normal functioning in the body.[2] For example, lipids are the main component of each cell in your body. In addition, fat is a major source of energy, especially when you are at rest or performing low- to moderate-intensity physical activity. Excessive consumption of fat is unhealthy, but concerns also arise when fat intake is too low. A balanced approach to fat intake will provide the necessary amount of fat for optimal health.

Fats are present in a number of forms, including saturated fats, monounsaturated fats, and polyunsaturated fats. These designations have to do with the chemical structure of the fat. Trans fats are found naturally in some animal products (mainly meat and dairy products), but also are a result of a manufacturing process called hydrogenation. Hydrogenation changes the structure of a fat to make it more stable, and as a result more like saturated fats (which are solid at room temperature). Food companies hydrogenate fat to increase the shelf life of the product, to make it taste more like butter, and to save money because it is less expensive to hydrogenate oil than it is to use butter.

In general, health concerns result from consuming too much saturated and trans fats. Trans fats have been shown to increase the bad cholesterol in blood (low-density lipoprotein cholesterol, or LDL-C), even more so than saturated fats. Sources of trans fats include animal products, margarine, and snack foods. The good news is that, as a result of health concerns, the food industry is reformulating many products to remove or at least reduce the amount of trans fats. Many restaurants have also now gone "trans fat free." Companies that make processed food products are required to list the amount of trans fat in their products. Although some products have labels that state they are "trans fat free," this actually means that they contain no more than 0.5% trans fat.

Monounsaturated fats, such as olive oil, canola oil, avocados, walnuts, and flax-seeds, have been shown to be protective against heart disease and type 2 diabetes. That is not to say that you can consume as much monounsaturated fat as you want; however, selecting monounsaturated fats instead of saturated fats may lead to better health (e.g., healthier blood cholesterol levels).

Polyunsaturated fats, such as safflower oil, corn oil, and fish oils, have also been shown to be protective against many diseases. Fish oils (eicosapentaenoic [EPA] and docosahexaenoic [DHA]) have been shown to decrease inflammation within the body, and may protect against heart disease, type 2 diabetes, and arthritis. This does not mean that EPA and DHA are protective against everything, but they are important to overall health. Therefore, you should try to consume 2 to 3 ounces (57 to 85 g) of fatty fish (e.g., tuna, salmon, and sardines) at least two days per week.[26] Fish oil supplements may also be warranted (consult with your health care provider to see if this is appropriate for you).

Saturated fats are found in products such as butter, cheese, meat, palm oil, and whole milk. Because of the increased risk of disease associated with saturated fats, less than 10% of your calories should come from saturated fat,[26] with an even better target of less than 7%.[28] Trans fats also should be limited to as little as possible.[26] Because of the focus on saturated and trans fats, the nutrition labels on food products include total fat as well as the amount of saturated and trans fats (see figure 4.1 on page 65).

Although not technically a fat, cholesterol is in the lipid family and is found in animal products. Your body needs a certain amount of cholesterol, and thus, even if your diet contained none, the liver would produce what your body needs. The problem arises when cholesterol levels in the blood become too high. Total blood cholesterol levels, as well as LDL-C levels, are definite predictors of heart disease (for more information, see chapter 16). Although you consume cholesterol in your diet, a major factor influencing your blood cholesterol is the amount of saturated and trans fats you consume. Thus, limiting saturated fat intake to no more than 10% of your calories is recommended (no more than 7% is even better) as well as keeping your consumption of cholesterol to less than 300 milligrams per day.[26, 28]

Total fat intake should be between 20% and 35% of calories.[26] Most of these calories should come from monounsaturated and polyunsaturated fats (e.g., fish, nuts, vegetable oils), and your consumption of saturated fat should be limited. For example, for someone with a target of 2,500 calories per day, total fat intake should be between 20% and 35% of total calories. In this example, a target of 28% is selected (middle of the range). This would be approximately 700 calories from fat. This would be calculated as follows:

$$2,500 \times 0.28 = 700 \text{ calories}$$

To keep saturated fat at no more than 10% of total calories, the calories from saturated fat would total only 250, determined as follows:

$$2,500 \times 0.10 = 250 \text{ calories from saturated fat}$$

To determine how many grams this represents, the calories from fat can be divided by 9 (recall that each gram of fat provides 9 calories). Thus, in this example, total fat would be around 78 grams ($700 \div 9 = 78$), and saturated fat would no more than around 28 grams ($250 \div 9 = 28$).

Some of the food groups contributing to saturated fat intake are cheese, beef, milk products, frozen desserts, snack foods (e.g., cookies, cakes, doughnuts, potato chips), butter, salad dressings, and eggs.[26] Making small changes in the foods you select could result in meaningful decreases in the saturated fat and calories you consume (see table 4.4 for some comparisons).

Table 4.4 Food Selection Alternatives for Lower Saturated Fat Consumption

Food	Higher-fat option	Lower-fat option
Cheddar cheese (1 oz or 28 g)	Regular cheddar cheese (6 g saturated fat; 114 calories)	Low-fat cheddar cheese (1.2 g saturated fat; 49 calories)
Milk (1 cup)	Whole milk, 3.24% (4.6 g saturated fat; 146 calories)	Low-fat milk, 1%* (1.5 g saturated fat; 102 calories)
Frozen desserts (1/2 cup)	Regular ice cream (4.9 g saturated fat; 145 calories)	Low-fat frozen yogurt (2.0 g saturated fat; 110 calories)
Ground beef (3 oz, or 85 g, cooked)	Regular ground beef, 25% fat (6.1 g saturated fat; 236 calories)	Extra-lean ground beef, 5% fat (2.6 g saturated fat; 148 calories)
Chicken (3 oz, or 85 g, cooked)	Fried chicken, leg with skin (3.3 g saturated fat; 212 calories)	Roasted chicken, breast no skin (0.9 g saturated fat; 140 calories)
Fish (3 oz, or 85 g)	Fried fish (2.8 g saturated fat; 195 calories)	Baked fish (1.5 g saturated fat; 129 calories)

*Skim milk would decrease the saturated fat to 0 grams and only 80 calories.

Adapted from U.S. Department of Health and Human Services and U.S. Department of Agriculture, 2005, p. 32.

What Do All The Abbreviations Mean?

Understanding what you need in your diet can be difficult. Clarity can be provided by examining the dietary reference intakes (DRIs) and acceptable macronutrient distribution range (AMDR), which are reference values and ranges for the amounts of nutrients your body needs. This looks like alphabet soup; however, each set of standards is helpful.[9, 10]

DRI

DRI is an umbrella term. It includes the estimated average requirement (EAR), the recommended dietary allowance (RDA), the adequate intake (AI), and the tolerable upper intake level (UL). The DRIs are focused on the nutrition requirements of healthy people (i.e., they focus on 97% of the population). The DRIs are set by a committee established by the Food and Nutrition Board of the National Academy of Sciences.

- EAR—The nutrient values established when there is enough scientific information. Once an EAR is established, an RDA can be established for that particular nutrient.
- RDA—Target values established by scientists with a focus on preventing nutrition-related diseases.
- AI—Values set for nutrients when there is not enough scientific evidence to support establishing the RDA.
- UL—The upper limits established for nutrients to prevent toxic consumption levels.[11] These were set because so many people take vitamin and mineral supplements.

AMDR

AMDR is not under the main umbrella of DRIs, but rather provides ranges for the amount of carbohydrates, fats, and proteins (i.e., macronutrients) you should consume. The macronutrients are given in a range because the requirements vary among people more than those of the micronutrients (i.e., vitamins and minerals, which are covered by the DRI).

It is not necessary to obtain 100% of the established DRI for every nutrient every day; however, it is good to strive for at least 70% of the established DRI per day for each nutrient.[9, 10] As you will see later in this chapter, the AMDR also provides guidance for dietary choices. All of the nutritional choices you make on a daily basis can make a difference for your health.

Micronutrients

Micronutrients include vitamins and minerals. Minerals and vitamins, although part of energy-yielding reactions in your body, cannot provide energy directly. Many have antioxidant, or cell-protecting, functions (e.g., vitamins A, C, and E; copper; iron; selenium; and zinc). It is important to consume the DRI amounts for vitamins and minerals (or at least obtain 70% of the DRI) to maintain overall health.[9, 10] It is beyond the scope of this chapter to discuss all the vitamins and minerals in detail; however, table 4.5 provides a listing of the major vitamins and minerals, including common sources as well as concerns with consuming too much or too little.

Table 4.5 **Vitamins and Minerals**

VITAMINS				
Requirement (adult)*	**Function**	**Deficiency**	**Toxicity**	**Examples of food sources**
Thiamin (vitamin B1): 1.2 mg/day for males; 1.1 mg/day for females	Needed for carbohydrate and protein metabolism and functioning of the heart, muscles, and nervous system	Weakness, fatigue, psychosis, nerve damage	Not identified	Fortified breads and cereals, whole grains, lean meats (e.g., pork), fish, soybeans
Riboflavin (vitamin B2): 1.3 mg/day for males; 1.1 mg/day for females	Needed for energy production and red blood cell production	Fatigue, sore throat, and swollen tongue (all rare)	Not identified	Lean meats, eggs, nuts, green leafy vegetables, milk and milk-based products, fortified cereals
Niacin (vitamin B3): 16 mg/day for males; 14 mg/day for females	Needed for energy production and health of digestive system, skin, and nerves	Pellagra (symptoms include diarrhea, dementia, and dermatitis)	Liver damage, peptic ulcers, skin rashes, skin flushing	Poultry, dairy products, fish, lean meats, nuts, eggs
Pantothenic Acid (Vitamin B5): 5 mg/day	Needed for energy production	Typically no toxicity	Diarrhea (rare)	Eggs, fish, milk and milk products, lean beef, legumes, broccoli
Biotin: 30 µg/day	Needed for energy production	Typically no toxicity	Diarrhea (rare)	Eggs, fish, milk and milk products, lean beef, legumes, broccoli
Vitamin B6: 1.3 mg/day for ages 19-50; 1.7 mg/day for males and 1.5 mg/day for females age 51 and above	Needed for protein metabolism, immune and nervous system functions	Dermatitis, sore tongue, depression, confusion	Neurological disorders and numbness	Beans, nuts, legumes, eggs, meats, fish, whole grains, fortified breads and cereals
Folate: 400 µg/day	Need for cellular growth, replication, regulation, and maintenance	Diarrhea, fatigue, headache, sore tongue, poor growth	Not identified	Beans and legumes, citrus fruits, whole grains, dark green leafy vegetables, poultry, shellfish
Vitamin B12: 2.4 µg/day	Needed in red blood cell formation, neurological function, role with metabolism	Anemia, numbness, weakness, loss of balance	Not identified	Eggs, meat, poultry, shellfish, milk and milk products
Vitamin C: 90 mg/day for males; 75 mg/day for females	Needed for its antioxidant properties, iron absorption, and role with connective tissues (skin, bones, and cartilage)	Dry/splitting hair, gingivitis, dry skin, depressed immune function, slow wound healing	Gastrointestinal disturbances (cramps and diarrhea)	Citrus fruits, red and green peppers, tomatoes, broccoli, greens
Vitamin A: 900 µg/day for males; 700 µg/day for females	Important role in vision as well as healthy teeth, bones, and skin	Night blindness, decreased immune function	Toxic at higher doses, birth defects	Eggs, milk, cheese, liver, kidney (also, beta carotene, which can be turned into a form of Vitamin A, is found in orange and dark green vegetables)
Vitamin D: 5 µg/day for ages 19-50; 10 µg/day for ages 51-70; 15 µg/day for ages 71 and above	Needed for calcium absorption and for bone growth and remodeling	Osteoporosis	Kidney stones, and calcium deposits in heart and lungs	Skin exposure to sunlight, fish, fortified milk
Vitamin E: 15 mg/day	Needed for its antioxidant properties and important role in immune function	Deficiency is rare	Increase risk of death at higher doses (400 IU or higher)	Wheat germ, nuts, seeds, vegetable oils
Vitamin K: 120 µg/day for males; 90 µg/day for females	Major role in blood clotting	Excessive bleeding due to clotting impairment, more likely to bruise	Not identified	Green vegetables, dark colored berries

(continued)

Table 4.5 (continued)

MINERALS				
Requirement (adult)*	Function	Deficiency	Toxicity	Examples of food sources
Calcium: 1000 mg/day for ages 19-50; 1200 mg/day for ages 51 and above	Needed for bone growth and maintenance, muscular contractions, cardiovascular and nervous system functions, hormone and enzyme secretion	Numbness, muscle cramps, convulsions, lethargy, abnormal heart rhythms, low bone mineral density	High amounts for a long time can increase risk of kidney stones	Milk, cheese, yogurt, leafy green vegetables
Iron: 8 mg/day for males; 18 mg/day for females ages 19-50; 8 mg/day for females age 51 and above	Major role in oxygen transport in the blood	Iron deficiency anemia, lack of energy, headache, dizziness, weight loss	Fatigue, dizziness, nausea, vomiting, weight loss, shortness of breath	Dried beans, eggs, liver, lean red meat, oysters, salmon, whole grains
Zinc: 11 mg/day for males; 8 mg/day for females	Major role in energy production, immune function, and wound healing	Slow growth, impaired immune function, hair loss, delayed healing of wounds, problems with sense of taste and smell	Vomiting, abdominal cramps, diarrhea, and headaches can occur with large amount of supplements	Beef, pork, lamb, peanuts, peanut butter, legumes
Chromium: 30-35 µg/day for males; 20-25 µg/day for females (lower amount for age 51 and above)	Enhances the function of insulin and involved with the metabolism of fat and carbohydrates	Impaired glucose tolerance	Not identified from dietary sources	Beef, liver, eggs, chicken, bananas, spinach, apples, green peppers
Magnesium: 400-410 mg/day for males; 310-320 mg/day for females (lower amount for ages 19-30)	Major role in proper muscle and nerve function	Muscle weakness, sleepiness (all rare)	No set upper limit for dietary intake	Dark green leafy vegetables, nuts, whole grains, soy products
Selenium: 55 µg/day	Helps with antioxidant function to prevent cellular damage	Joint/bone disease, mental retardation (all rare)	Selenosis (gastrointestinal upsets, hair loss, fatigue, irritability, some nerve damage) (rare)	Vegetables, fish, shellfish, grains, eggs, chicken, liver
Copper: 900 µg/day	Role in the formulation of red blood cells as well as healthy blood vessels, nerves, immune system, and bones	Anemia and osteoporosis	Poisonous in large amounts	Organ meats (kidneys, liver), oysters and other shellfish, whole grains, beans, nuts, potatoes, dark leafy greens
Iodine: 150 µg/day	Major role in the metabolism of cells and in normal thyroid function	Goiter or hypothyroidism	Reduced functioning of the thyroid gland (rare)	Iodized salt, seafood (e.g., cod, sea bass), kelp
Phosphorus: 700 mg/day	Major role in the formulation of bones and teeth, also involved in the utilization of fats, carbohydrates and protein for growth and maintenance of cells, and for energy production	Rare (available widely in the food supply)	Deposits in muscle (rare)	Milk and milk products, meat

* Requirements vary for different ages and status (e.g. pregnancy, lactation). For more information on specific requirements, see http://fnic.nal.usda.gov and then find the DRI under "Topics A-Z" on the top navigation bar.

Sources: U.S. Department of Health and Human Services and National Institutes of Health, U.S. National Library of Medicine, 2010, and Institute of Medicine, National Academy of Science, 1997, 1998, 2000, 2001, 2005, and 2011.

Tiffany

Tiffany, age 48, is looking to decrease her overall calorie intake but also wants to ensure that she is consuming adequate calcium. She knows dairy products are excellent sources of calcium but wonders which of two milk options would fit best in her nutrition plan: 2% milk or nonfat (skim) milk. Which one would be preferred to optimize calcium intake while minimizing caloric intake? A 1-cup serving of each provides the same amount of calcium, vitamins, carbohydrate, and protein, but the 2% milk has a third more calories than the nonfat milk, all coming from added fat (see figure 4.2, for a comparison of the food labels for the two). Tiffany selects the nonfat milk because it provides her with the same amount of calcium at a lower number of calories.

Reduced-Fat Milk
(2% Milkfat)

Nutrition Facts

Serving Size 1 cup (236ml)
Servings Per Container 1

Amount Per Serving

Calories 120	Calories from Fat 45

% Daily Value*

Total Fat 5g	8%
Saturated Fat 3g	15%
Trans Fat 0g	
Cholesterol 20mg	7%
Sodium 120mg	5%
Total Carbohydrate 31g	10%
Dietary Fiber 0g	0%
Sugars 11g	
Protein 9g	

Vitamin A 10%	•	Vitamin C 4%

Calcium 30% • Iron 0% • Vitamin D 25%

* Percent Daily Values are based on a 2,000 calorie diet. Your daily values may be higher or lower depending on your calorie needs.

Nonfat Milk

Nutrition Facts

Serving Size 1 cup (236ml)
Servings Per Container 1

Amount Per Serving

Calories 80	Calories from Fat 0

% Daily Value*

Total Fat 0g	0%
Saturated Fat 0g	0%
Trans Fat 0g	
Cholesterol 5mg	7%
Sodium 120mg	5%
Total Carbohydrate 11g	4%
Dietary Fiber 0g	0%
Sugars 11g	
Protein 9g	

Vitamin A 10%	•	Vitamin C 4%

Calcium 30% • Iron 0% • Vitamin D 25%

* Percent Daily Values are based on a 2,000 calorie diet. Your daily values may be higher or lower depending on your calorie needs.

Figure 4.2 Comparison of two milk products.
Reprinted from U.S. Department of Health and Human Services, U.S. Food and Drug Administration, 2009.

You may be feeling overwhelmed thinking about consuming each of the macronutrients *and* the micronutrients (all the vitamins and minerals) each day. However, if you consume a diet that is varied, includes five to eight servings of fruits and vegetables per day, and is composed mostly of whole foods and less of processed foods, you will be doing your body well. You may also feel daunted by the idea of consuming five to eight servings of fruits and vegetables per day, but remember that these servings include fruits *and* vegetables (not five to eight servings of each!), and that a serving can be a medium banana, 4 ounces (113 ml) of 100% fruit juice, 1/2 cup of broccoli, and the like. The website MyPyramid.gov can help you better understand serving sizes, as well as your particular requirements (see figure 4.3 for a quick peek at the premise behind the pyramid). When making food choices, consider the following simple guidelines:

- Whole grain is better than processed or white grain.
- More color is better than less color (e.g., dark green leafy vegetables, deep red vegetables and fruits, and dark blue or purple fruits have more vitamins and minerals than those with less color).
- Less-processed foods are best.

Often, contemplating how to improve your diet is difficult because it is hard to know where to start. As with any change, focus on short-term and long-term goals, as discussed in chapter 3. Consider a person, like Alex, who has a long-term goal of cutting down on fat intake as well as improving the nutrient content of his diet (e.g., increasing his consumption of whole grains, fruits, and vegetables). A short-term goal might be: *I will pack my lunch (including vegetable sticks, lean meat sandwich on whole wheat bread, piece of fruit, and a yogurt cup) rather than stopping at fast-food restaurants each day for the upcoming week.* This is a SMART goal. It is *specific* in terms of the activity as well as the time frame. At the end of the week, Alex can reflect on whether he packed a lunch (*measurable*). It provides for specific action to be taken (i.e., it is *action-based*) and is an activity that can be accomplished without excessive difficulty (i.e., it is *realistic*). A specific time frame is provided so that the action starts now rather than being too open-ended (i.e., it is *time-anchored*). Following are other examples of short-term goals:

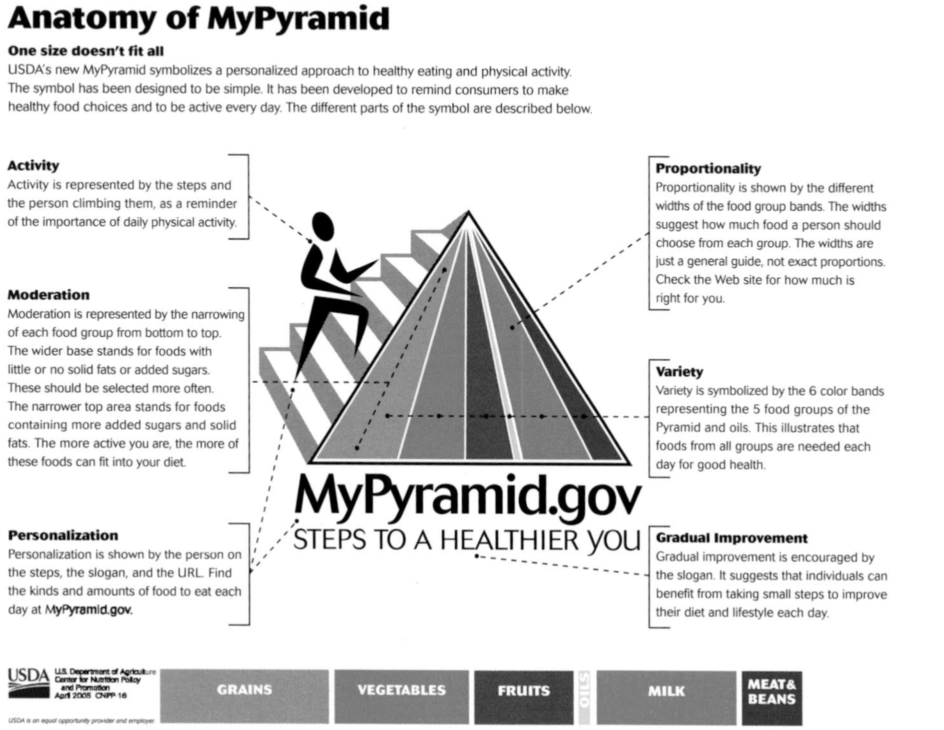

Figure 4.3 Anatomy of MyPyramid.
U.S. Department of Agriculture

- To stop at a local farmer's market each weekend for the next month to select enough fruit to provide at least two selections each day
- To include a salad with Romaine lettuce, tomatoes, onions, peppers, and carrots, topped with low-fat vinaigrette dressing, for dinner on at least two days during the upcoming week
- To replace an afternoon candy bar from the vending machine with a piece of fruit and some almonds

Building on short-term goals, and maintaining those healthy behaviors, will ultimately result in success at reaching the long-term goal.

Water

Water is a required nutrient for all living beings. Water is important for hydration; however, it may be valuable for disease prevention as well. For example, researchers have found a relationship between water intake and reduction of gallstones and kidney stones as well as between water intake and colon cancer.[5, 6, 16, 25] Similarly, maintaining a sufficient intake of water while flying may help reduce the risk of blood clots.[12]

With respect to physical activity, water is important for hydration. When you are active, you need to remain in a euhydrated (balanced) state.[24] The DRI for water is 2.7 liters (90 oz) per day for women and 3.7 liters (125 oz) per day for men.[9] Water

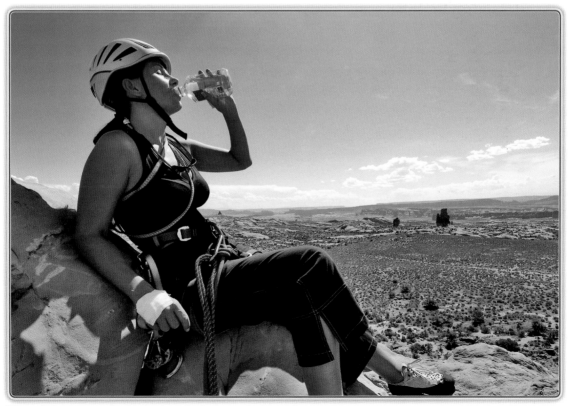

Water is important for hydration during physical activity.

balance means that you are replacing the fluid you lose through sweating and urine production. Hydration does not just occur from drinking water. Water can be gained from food, which makes up about 20% of total water intake, and as well as from other beverages. Thus, although water is an excellent source of fluid, other beverages, such as tea, milk, coffee and 100% juice, can also fulfill your fluid needs.[9]

Sweating during exercise is one way the body tries to cool you.[1] Sweat is composed of water as well as other substances such as electrolytes (sodium, potassium, and chloride).[17] The amount of electrolytes in sweat varies among people depending on sweat rate, fitness level, electrolyte intake, as well as the temperature of the environment. Sodium (salt) is one electrolyte you may have noticed dried on your skin after prolonged sweating. Replacement of sodium lost in the sweat is not an issue for most people, considering that, in general, Americans consume far more salt than their bodies need (see chapter 15 for insight into how sodium intake can influence blood pressure).

Nutrition and Weight

When you consume basically the same number of calories as you expend, your body weight remains relatively stable. If you want to gain or lose weight, you must manipulate this balance between calories consumed and calories expended.

Gaining Weight

Some people have a difficult time gaining weight. This can be a result of a higher-than-normal basal metabolic rate or a high physical activity level. When weight gain is a goal, the focus is on gaining muscle and not fat weight. To do this in a healthy way, you should consume more frequent meals with healthy snacks. For example, in addition to three main meals, consume three snacks per day. Consuming about 300 to 500 calories per day more would result in about a 1-pound (0.45 kg) per week weight gain. Healthy snacks include yogurt, peanut butter and jelly sandwiches, cereal with milk, fruit smoothies, and turkey sandwiches. It is also important to continue to exercise to ensure that the weight gain is mostly muscle. In particular, resistance training will be an important factor for building muscle (see chapter 7 for more information on resistance training). Although it will take some time, the slower the weight gain, the more likely it will be to be muscle gain and not fat or water gain.

Losing Weight

Weight loss is a more common goal than gaining weight. Losing weight involves a negative energy balance. This can be achieved by increasing exercise and decreasing caloric intake. See chapter 13 for more details on weight loss.

You should start focusing on water balance before you are active by consuming fluids in advance of your exercise bout.[24] While you are exercising, your goal should be to avoid excessive dehydration. For shorter workouts (less than an hour), consuming water will be fine.[24] For longer workouts, consider using a sport performance beverage that provides fluids as well as some carbohydrate and sodium.[14] Ideally, by consuming adequate fluids, you can avoid dehydration. One simple way to check your hydration status is to look at the color of your urine; it should be a clear, pale yellow color.[4] Another way to track fluid lost during exercise is to check your body weight before and after your workout. For each pound (0.45 kg) lost during exercise, you should consume about 16 to 20 ounces (475 to 600 ml) of water or sport performance beverage.[24]

Understanding the importance of macronutrients, micronutrients, water, and the *Dietary Guidelines for Americans* provides a framework for improving your diet. Knowing how to read labels and how to calculate your energy needs will help you make healthy choices regarding your diet. A healthy diet should include a wide variety of foods that you enjoy. Following the *Dietary Guidelines for Americans* is a good start to working toward consuming a healthy, varied, and nutrient-dense diet that will help prevent disease and give you more energy each day.

chapter 5

Adopting and Maintaining Healthy Habits

Living a healthy lifestyle is a significant challenge. This challenge has two equally important components: adopting healthy habits and maintaining them. Whether your focus is on physical activity, diet, sleep, or stress management, starting and continuing with healthy lifestyle habits are key to your overall wellness. The good news is that better health is within your reach.

DEFINING WELLNESS

How do you define wellness? If this question was asked of 10 people, 10 different definitions would likely result. Each person defines wellness based on personal experiences and perspectives. In the past, conceptions of wellness focused on being free of illness, disease, and debilitating conditions. Instead of focusing on avoiding negative conditions, contemporary views of wellness suggest an approach to health that focuses on balancing many aspects, or dimensions, of life.[1]

Wellness is made up of many dimensions, including physical, mental, social, intellectual, and spiritual (a simple model depicting these dimensions of wellness is provided in figure 5.1).

- *Physical wellness* is evidenced by the ability to carry out routine tasks of daily living and addresses fitness, body composition, nutrition, sleep, and a healthy approach to drug and alcohol use.
- *Mental wellness* is evidenced by the ability to cope with daily stressors and circumstances in a constructive and positive manner.

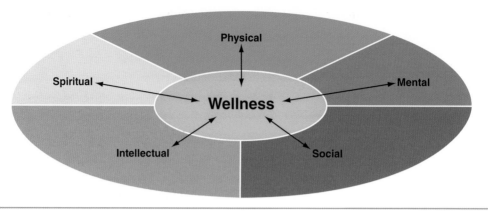

Figure 5.1 Dimensions of wellness.

- *Social wellness* is evidenced by appropriate interactions with others and relationships that provide mutual benefit.
- *Intellectual wellness* is evidenced by self-directed behavior that results in continuous learning and development.
- *Spiritual wellness* is evidenced by a pursuit of meaning and purpose that transcends self and considers the role of a higher spiritual force or being.

Wellness exists across a continuum between the presence or absence of each dimension or aspect of life. Table 5.1 provides a pair of terms for each wellness dimension. Consider where you fall on the continuum between the two indicators listed for each dimension. At any time, you may find some dimensions to be more present than others in your life. By adopting healthy behaviors, you can have greater balance in each dimension and therefore a greater sense of well-being and health.

Wellness is a multidimensional concept, and fully discussing all the aspects is beyond the scope of this book. Because the focus of this book is physical wellness, the remainder of this chapter provides insights regarding several factors that

Table 5.1 **Dimensions of Wellness Indicators**

		Indicator
Dimension	**Description**	**Absent .... Present**
Physical	Ability to carry out daily activities with vigor and relative ease	Unfit...................... Fit
Emotional	Ability to understand feelings, accept limitations, and achieve stability	Miserable.............Content
Social	Ability to relate well to others within and outside the family unit	Disengaged........Connected
Intellectual	Ability to learn and use information for personal development	Mindless...............Aware
Spiritual	Ability to find meaning and purpose in life and circumstances	Lost .... Secure

can influence your physical wellness—sleep; stress; and alcohol, tobacco, and drug use.

Influence of Sleep

One area of physical wellness that is often neglected is sleep. Obtaining adequate sleep—in terms of both quantity and quality—contributes to how you feel and function. A restful night of sleep provides the energy and alertness necessary for positively handling daily challenges. In contrast, the lack of adequate sleep negatively impacts productivity, relationships, and physical health.

Simply put, sleep is important for many reasons and significantly affects many dimensions of wellness and quality of life. The general recommendation is for adults to average seven to nine hours of sleep each night. Although many adults can function normally on less sleep, others may require significantly more. Sleepiness during the day is a simple but clear indicator that your body requires more sleep. Significant sleepiness during the day suggests the need for more or better sleep, or both. More than one third of adults get less than seven hours of sleep each weeknight, and similar numbers are so sleepy during the day that normal activities are affected.[7] Although lack of sleep and sleepiness may seem more like a nuisance than a significant health problem, inadequate sleep is linked to increased health risks including impaired immunity to the common cold, obesity, hypertension, and depression.[4]

Adequate sleep, on the other hand, can improve health outcomes. Changing behavior to obtain the sleep you need requires making a conscious health choice (see *Tips for Good Sleep*). Note that regular physical activity is associated with improved sleep. Moderately intense aerobic exercise that is completed at least three hours before bedtime is recommended to improve sleep.

Tips for Good Sleep

- *Stick to a sleep schedule.* Setting a regular time for sleeping and waking helps your body develop a healthy rhythm that improves sleep.
- *Avoid caffeine and nicotine.* Both caffeine and nicotine are stimulants that tend to increase alertness and decrease sleepiness and sleep quality.
- *Exercise regularly.* Sleep quantity and quality are positively affected by exercise, especially moderately intense aerobic exercise performed several hours before bedtime.
- *Relax before going to bed.* Being too activated mentally or physically before going to bed can result in bodily changes that promote wakefulness.
- *Don't lie in bed awake.* Experts recommend getting out of bed and doing something relaxing if you are awake, and returning to bed when sleepy.
- *Limit naps.* Although debate exists around the subject of napping, most experts recommend that naps be less than 45 minutes in length and several hours before regular sleep.
- *Talk to your physician.* Difficulty falling asleep, staying asleep, and achieving restful sleep for extended periods of time are indicators to seek the advice of a physician.

Influence of Stress

The role of stress in health is an issue that receives significant attention, and rightly so. However, there is more to stress than may be readily apparent, and even its definition can be elusive. Stress is traditionally defined as the body's response to the demands placed on it. This definition is based on the idea that a body at rest and without stress is in a state of homeostasis, which is characterized by stability and calm. Events that disrupt homeostasis are described as stressors. The psychological and physiological changes to the body are referred to as stress, or the stress response. Although some disruptions in homeostasis are viewed negatively and as distress (e.g., divorce, deadlines), some are perceived positively and are known as eustress (e.g., exercise, graduation, job promotion). The healthfulness of a stressor is influenced by your response to it, which speaks to the importance of how stressors are perceived and processed. Positive stress tends to motivate and fulfill, whereas negative stress can produce suffering and anxiety.

The outcomes associated with short-term (acute) and ongoing (chronic) stress are difficult to predict. Acute stress is linked to reduced concentration, poor self-control, decreased memory, and low self-esteem.[2] Similarly, chronic stress has been linked to many chronic conditions such as diminished immune function, sleep disorders, cardiovascular disease, obesity, and disorders of the digestive system.[8] The cost of stress and stress-related conditions is significant; it is estimated that the vast majority of physician office visits are in some way stress related.

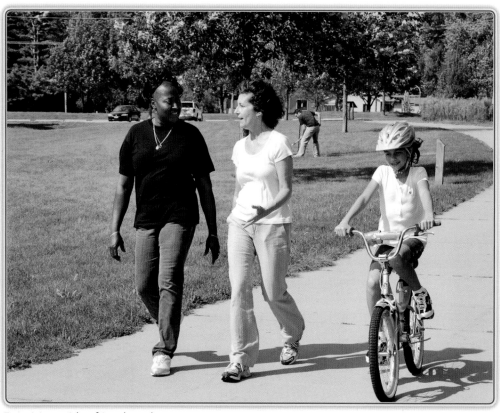

Exercising with a friend can be a great way to manage stress.

Tips for Managing Stress

- *Plan your schedule.* Being aware of and in charge of your schedule provides an empowering feeling that helps to reduce the impact of stressful situations.
- *Relax with deep breathing.* The process of consciously slowing your breathing rate as you increase the depth of each breath helps to counteract the fast and shallow breathing that is common when experiencing stress.
- *Limit alcohol consumption.* Although alcohol may reduce stress temporarily, relying on alcohol to cope with stress has the opposite effect and produces more bodily stress.
- *Get active.* Regular exercise gives the body regular practice in dealing with stress and can be helpful in treating and managing stress.
- *Eat well.* Healthy diets that meet recommendations (see chapter 4) facilitate a healthy state.
- *Talk to family and friends.* Discussing stressful events with others you trust can be beneficial both because it helps you "get it off your chest" and because you might receive helpful recommendations.
- *Get help if needed.* Stressors that cannot be managed reasonably well through basic techniques may require the involvement of health professionals.

Strategies for and approaches to stress management are numerous, and no one approach is best for everyone. *Tips for Managing Stress* offers a range of ideas that may be beneficial. One important tool used routinely to manage stress is regular participation in exercise. The role of exercise in stress reduction is not yet clear, but active people appear to be able to buffer stress more effectively than sedentary people do.

Influence of Drugs, Alcohol, and Tobacco

The appropriate use of drugs that prevent, treat, and cure health maladies has resulted in significant improvements in quality of life and life expectancy. These medicinal drugs play an important role in modern health care. In contrast, drugs that are not designed for medicinal use and abuse of prescription drugs can create many problems that interfere with wellness.

Drugs are often defined as any nonfood substance that alters the body's function. Drug misuse is the use of any drug for any purpose other than that for which it was intended. Similarly, drug abuse is characterized by excessive use of a drug that can have resulting dangerous side effects. Both drug misuse and drug abuse increase the risk for negative health outcomes. Recent research indicates that approximately one fourth of all adults use tobacco products and either binge drink or consume excessive amounts of alcohol. Additionally, almost one tenth of all adults reported the use of illicit drugs in the past month.[9]

Misuse and abuse of drugs produce specific and numerous outcomes, including both acute side effects and long-term consequences. Side effects vary greatly based on the drug but can include dizziness, memory loss, anxiety, slurred speech, and nausea. Long-term consequences also vary and may result in negative health outcomes such as cancer, heart disease, liver disease, and kidney dysfunction. Additionally, many drugs have addictive properties that can be harmful to health and well-being.

Drug use outside of medically supervised prescriptions is risky behavior. Although consumption of drugs such as caffeine and alcohol may not need to be eliminated entirely, be mindful of excessive intake of these drugs because it could interfere with a balanced approach to the many aspects of wellness. Following are recommendations related to drug use:

- Make educated and informed choices.
- Consider side effects and the possibility of addiction.
- Carefully read and follow the instructions on over-the-counter medications.
- Avoid the use of all illicit drugs for health and legal reasons.
- Limit alcohol consumption to one drink per day if you are female and two drinks per day if you are male.

In short, wellness results from a conscious choice to balance a physically active lifestyle with an approach that is natural and focuses on a healthy diet.

MOTIVATION TO BECOME PHYSICALLY ACTIVE

Developing and maintaining a physically active lifestyle involves attention to the issue of motivation. Motivation can be defined as the determination, drive, or desire with which you approach or avoid a behavior. Consider the forces that make up your motivation to embrace or withdraw from life experiences. Behaviors tend to be ingrained over time and therefore are quite difficult to modify, but change is possible, especially with the use of basic principles of behavior modification.

Self-Determination and Motivation

The idea of self-determination suggests that you develop your motivation for an activity based on whether you believe that participation in that activity meets your basic needs.[5] When your basic needs are met, your confidence level increases (i.e., you have a greater sense of control), which in turn results in enjoying the activity, giving increased effort to it, and adhering to the program. In contrast, when your needs are not met, you may feel a lack of control or lack confidence doing the activity, or you may have negative feelings connected with the activity and thus have a harder time sticking with the program. Rather than being an on and off switch, motivation slides across a continuum ranging from no or low extrinsic motivation to intrinsic motivation.

The motivation continuum is depicted in figure 5.2 and includes amotivation, other-determined extrinsic motivation, self-determined extrinsic motivation, and intrinsic motivation. Consider the four levels of motivation and where you currently are.

Amotivation

Amotivation is at the base of the model and, when applied to exercise, represents the absence of motivation to exercise. If you are at this level, you don't expect exercise to meet your needs and thus you have absolutely no interest in or intention to exercise. Amotivation often includes a "Why bother?" mind-set. This level of motivation is often the result of bad previous experiences that affect your beliefs about the purpose and benefits of exercise.

Other-Determined Extrinsic Motivation

Other-determined extrinsic motivation exists when you are motivated to exercise by outside factors such as rewards, pressure, obligation, fear, or guilt. Examples include exercising as a result of pressure from a friend or spouse, participating in a competition or incentive program at work simply to receive the reward, training only to please a coach, and exercising because you fear becoming diseased. Each of these motives has the potential to stimulate exercise initially, but because the behavior is not freely chosen, the changes are often short-lived and the chances of dropping out are high.

Self-Determined Extrinsic Motivation

Self-determined extrinsic motivation exists because of external factors, but the behavior is chosen without a sense of pressure or coercion. An example is participating to obtain an outcome you value such as improved fitness and health, relaxation, or social benefits. The differences between self-determined and other-determined motivation are subtle but important. Motives based on health improvement and fear of disease may seem similar, but they are not. Because desiring to live a healthy lifestyle is a positive motivator, it is more sustainable. In contrast, motivation based on fear creates negative stress and may eventually become exhausting and thus loses its motivation capacity. Exercising to experience companionship is much different (and more positive) than exercising to be recognized and esteemed by others. Acting on motivations to exercise that are free of pressure and evaluation by others gives you the best chance for sticking with your exercise plan.

Intrinsic Motivation

Intrinsic motivation exists when the reason for exercise is the enjoyment and satisfaction received from the exercise itself. This type of motivation is difficult to achieve because, in fact, it is not an achievement or goal at all. It is an experience. This level of motivation is not typical because many people do not have a pure love for exercise itself. Instead, they love what exercise provides. Nevertheless, it can help to keep in mind that healthy exercise motivation is related to feelings of autonomy (independence), connectedness, and competence.

Understanding the levels of motivation can help you develop an exercise program that you will continue into the future. Moving from amotivation

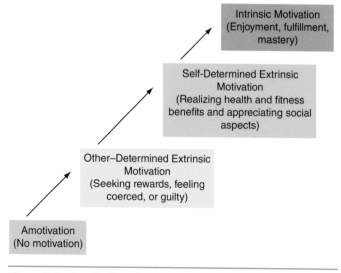

Figure 5.2 Levels of motivation.

toward intrinsic motivation is possible through education, positive encouragement, and successful experiences. Although you may not attain an intrinsic motivation for exercise, by adopting a healthy approach to exercise, you can advance to motives known to increase participation and adherence. Following are some strategies for developing a healthy motivational approach to exercise:

- Provide yourself with several exercise options to enhance perceived autonomy.
- Set goals that give you opportunities for success.
- Encourage yourself and seek out encouragement from others.
- Focus on the positive impact exercise can have on health and wellness.
- Consider participating in exercise with others to facilitate social connections.

A CLOSER LOOK
Latrell

Latrell is a 61-year-old man who works for a nonprofit agency. His employer brought in a fitness consultant to address employees' poor health, which was straining the agency's health insurance budget. Latrell is a hesitant, apparently unreceptive, participant in the educational classes and fitness assessments provided by the consultant. He appears skeptical about the benefits of exercise but does participate, although with no real enthusiasm. Latrell's motivation was other-determined at the start of the program—he participated to please his employer. For three months, the consultant worked on a weekly basis with the employees and continued to provide encouragement and suggest activities, especially to Latrell.

At some point over the three-month period, Latrell's motivation became more self-determined. As the formal aspect of the consultation was coming to an end, Latrell approached the consultant to report that he had been consistently stopping at a park on his way to work and walking for 30 minutes each morning. He actually smiled as he told the consultant that he was feeling better than he had for a long time—he said he felt as though he had "turned back the clock 10 years." The strength in his legs was improving, and he had lost some weight as well. At a community event a year later, Latrell and the consultant bumped into each other. Latrell had continued with his exercise program and was proud to report that his wife was now walking with him as well.

Self-Management Skills to Facilitate Motivation

Like motivation, self-management is a prerequisite for behavior modification and healthy living. Self-management refers to your unique capacity to exert control over your thoughts, feelings, and actions, which at least partly govern your behaviors.[3] You are not a powerless observer of the world within and around you, but rather, are actively engaged in your life. Self-management skills help you reach both short-term and long-term life goals. You may have a natural aptitude for some skills, whereas others you can learn through practice.

Wellness-related self-management skills facilitate healthy behavior change and positive outcomes. Several self-management skills are described here and summarized in table 5.2:

- *Assessment skills* allow you to assess your personal fitness level and dimensions of wellness. Simple assessments such as those outlined in chapter 2 can provide a basic picture of your current fitness level.
- *Goal-setting skills* enhance motivation and personal accountability. Goal setting—in particular, setting SMART goals—is described beginning on page 50 in chapter 3.
- *Planning skills* help you develop strategies for achieving success in behavior change programs. Effective planning considers goals, available resources, time, and social support.
- *Confidence-building skills* improve your belief in yourself with respect to your stated goals. As you achieve short-term goals, you build confidence as you continue to work toward your long-term goals. Another way to increase your confidence is to observe success in others who are relatively similar and therefore represent appropriate role models.
- *Social support skills* allow you to reach out to others. Establishing a network of people you trust can help facilitate change. Others in your network can provide encouragement or assistance as needed.
- *Barrier-busting skills* help you manage and overcome both perceived and real obstacles. Breaking down barriers often requires creativity, assistance from others, and careful planning. For example, a barrier might be getting up a bit earlier in the morning to attend a group exercise session. Planning your schedule to ensure that you are getting to bed on time in the evening as well as creating a phone-buddy system for wake-up calls are ways to deal with that barrier.

Table 5.2 **Self-Management Skills**

Skill	Description	Example
Assessment	Being able to conduct simple determinations of fitness and wellness	Use formulas related to weight and activity status to estimate fitness.
Goal setting	Learning how to set goals that are realistic and achievable	Develop and write up a set of short-term and long-term goals that facilitate success.
Planning	Developing strategies that put you in charge of schedules and activities	Practice developing a weekly plan of action for nutrition and physical activity.
Confidence building	Taking small steps that lead to success and increased motivation	Make the goals of your first week only moderately challenging.
Social support	Learning how to seek and obtain aid from significant others	Ask family members or friends to check in with you and provide encouragement each week.
Barrier busting	Having a proactive approach to potential problems that may arise with behavior change	Plan in advance how you will make healthy choices and work around less-than-healthy menu options.
Stress management	Focusing on challenges rather than impossibilities	Rehearse how you will handle a challenge at work or home that might disrupt efforts at healthy behavior.
Relapse prevention	Maintaining the plan and motivation during challenging times and lapses	Develop and use a plan for actively avoiding high-risk situations that might lead to unhealthy choices.

- *Stress management skills* help you handle challenges and difficulties without the distraction of high levels of anxiety. The outcome of effective stress management is a relaxed state that promotes clear thinking and appropriate decision making. Refer to *Tips for Managing Stress* on page 83.

- *Relapse prevention skills* help you maintain your behavior change efforts even when faced with situations that may increase the likelihood of a lapse or poor health choice. Learning to avoid situations or developing a plan for high-risk situations can help you avoid a relapse. Chapter 3 provides additional guidance on how to rebound from a relapse. Likewise, developing the mind-set that a single mistake is not the end of the world will help you rebound from setbacks.

These self-management skills can help you initiate and maintain a healthy lifestyle. Together they provide a comprehensive approach to achieving wellness.

Long-Term Approach to Motivation

One final consideration regarding behavior change and motivation relates to the development of a long-term, or lifetime, approach. In spite of advertisements that promise fitness or extreme weight loss in a week, the reality is that changes take time and require an ongoing commitment. Modern society has conditioned everyone to value things that are instant and disposable. This "now" perspective conflicts with the long-term commitment needed for building a healthy life. This mismatch in values helps explain the high dropout rate observed among new exercisers and the difficulty people have sustaining new behaviors.

The perspective that anything worth doing should provide immediate and desirable results connects very closely to the concept of hedonism and can influence health and wellness. Hedonism is the belief that motivation is based on perceptions of pleasure and pain. Pleasure includes experiences of joy and gratification, whereas pain includes feelings of suffering, discomfort, and grief. Hedonism suggests the primary goal of behavior should be enjoyment, therefore activities that cause pain, discomfort, or effort should be avoided. The hedonistic view of life reduces the desire to engage in behaviors that bring about a healthy balance in life experiences.

A wellness approach focuses on balancing as many aspects of life as possible. Immediate pleasure is not always the outcome of exercise participation. Rather, physical discomfort such as muscle aches may occur, especially in the early weeks after starting a new program. A hedonistic attitude tends to dismiss exercise as a viable option and thus can undermine a healthy lifestyle.

Behavior change does not require that you completely override the tendency to seek pleasure and avoid pain. Instead, your focus should be on becoming mindful of each choice you make. A classic human hedonistic tendency is to pursue short-term pleasures and put off or deny dealing with any negative consequences (e.g., the potential of reduced health later in life). A mindfulness of the present moment allows you to accept every moment (even the uncomfortable ones) as temporary. In this way you can experience each moment for what it is. Thus, both the enjoyment and the effort associated with the exercise experience can be balanced resulting in an overall greater feeling of well-being along with the potential of better health and fitness.

ACTIVITY PROGRAM OPTIONS

Knowing about motivation and developing self-management skills will help you increase activity and move toward a lifestyle focused on wellness. However, as you look to initiate or add to your existing exercise program, you will face a multitude of decisions that may affect your motivation, your adherence, or the benefits you receive from the exercise program. For example, should you exercise alone or participate with a partner or in a larger group? Would it be best to join a community-based fitness facility or a large commercial health club? What types of equipment should you buy? The sections that follow provide some assistance in navigating some of these decisions.

▶ *Should I Exercise Alone or in a Group?*

Exercising alone is a viable option for many people. Unless you have health issues that need to be professionally monitored, going solo with an exercise program can be very satisfying. Exercising alone can be done at home, outdoors, or even at a health club (many are now open 24 hours a day). If your schedule is busy, you may appreciate the freedom of not having to coordinate your schedule with anyone else. The time you spend exercising can be a chance to turn off your mind from the stress of the day and focus on your exercise experience.

An important consideration when exercising alone at home or outdoors is safety. Staying within a level of intensity appropriate to your current fitness level will enhance the safety of a home-based program. Exercising outdoors brings up safety issues in terms of people, traffic, and weather conditions. When exercising outdoors, always walk or run on a sidewalk, if available, and face traffic at the edge of the road when a sidewalk is not available. When cycling, ride with traffic in a designated bike lane or as far to the right as possible in the outside lane when bike lanes are absent. Avoid exercising in high heat and humidity, and always wear appropriate clothing and shoes in cold, snowy, and inclement weather. Although listening to portable music players is enjoyable, use caution when exercising in places where you will encounter motor traffic because these devices reduce the ability to attend to sounds that may be important for safety. To help prevent accidents and injuries, never assume that others around you are being diligent with respect to your safety. If you exercise in and around traffic, wear bright and reflective clothing and be vigilant and careful in every way possible.

Although exercising alone is a great choice for some, many people prefer exercising with others. Exercising in groups can take the form of organized classes in aerobics, spinning, or kickboxing at fitness facilities, or of more informal situations such as mall-walking groups. Most commercial health clubs and community fitness facilities offer a variety of group exercise classes as part of the regular membership package. These classes can be great ways to meet people with similar interests. Be sure to check what is available when deciding where to join.

Community-based programs foster group dynamics that offer support and encouragement, which can be highly beneficial regardless of your level of experience. Examples include cycling clubs, running clubs, and ballroom dance groups. Such groups form within communities either spontaneously, through the grassroots efforts of a group of individuals, or by way of local agencies hoping to promote physical activity and healthy living. Along with fitness benefits, such groups also typically provide a great social outlet.

▶ *Should I Join a Fitness Facility or Exercise at Home?*

Although there are many ways to participate in exercise and focus on health, one of the most popular is membership at a fitness facility. Options include large commercial health clubs, community fitness centers, and small storefront centers. Issues to consider when making your choice will be the services that are most important to you and the cost of membership.

One great advantage of fitness facilities is the wide range of options available for aerobic and muscular fitness training. Most facilities have a large number of treadmills, stationary bikes, and elliptical machines, and many also include a swimming pool and a variety of areas to play basketball and court-based sports. Likewise, many facilities offer a wide range of weights and resistance machines for muscular fitness training. These options, along with any number of group exercise classes and child care, make joining a fitness facility an attractive option for many individuals and families.

When deciding whether to join a fitness facility, consider location, hours of operation, equipment, supervision, shower facilities, member services, and cost (see table 5.3). One other important part of your decision relates to the environment of the facility. Some exercisers are drawn to facilities that are family-focused and more relaxed, whereas others prefer a more serious athletic environment. Before joining, tour the facility at the time of day you plan to exercise to get a clear picture. Many facilities offer short-term memberships at very low cost, allowing you to see if the facility is a good match for you. Careful consideration of each of these issues and others unique to your circumstances can help you make your decision.

Rather than joining a health club or fitness facility, you may prefer to exercise in the comfort and convenience of your own home. You can develop a very effective fitness program at home with little to no equipment, or you may choose to look into purchasing some exercise equipment. Following are examples of no-cost, equipment-free options:

Table 5.3 Considerations in Selecting a Fitness Facility

Location	• Is the facility located in a safe area? • Is the facility easily accessible from work or home?
Hours of operation	• Can you access the facility during the time of day that you plan to exercise? • How busy is the facility during this time? • Will the pool be available for open swim when you want to swim?
Equipment	• Is the equipment clean and in good repair? • Does the facility have enough equipment to accommodate members?
Shower facilities	• Are the shower and changing facilities clean and well-maintained? • Does the facility provide a towel service?
Supervision	• Are the employees properly trained and certified for their positions? • Does the facility have an emergency action plan?
Member services	• Does the facility have special incentive programs to enhance participation and motivation? • Is the cost reasonable and affordable? • Are staff members friendly and knowledgeable? • Is child care available?

- Calisthenics (such as push-ups, curl-ups, jumping jacks) and walking or jogging in place
- Flexibility exercises that require only a space on the floor
- Fitness-based programming on public television
- Exercise videos or DVDs from the local public library

With regard to the last two options, it is beyond the scope of this book to evaluate all of the available fitness programs, videos, and DVDs. If you choose these options, consider the credentials of the people associated with the materials. In addition, consider your own personal style and follow the guidelines outlined in this book when choosing a home-based program.

Although no-cost options are available, you may want more variety in your home-based program. Following are some rather inexpensive items that will broaden the scope of activities you can do:

- Exercise mat for stretching or doing yoga or Pilates
- Elastic tubing or medicine balls for resistance training
- Stability ball to work on balance and coordination

Exercise equipment is another consideration, depending on your budget and the space you have available. The starting cost for exercise equipment likely is more than a yearly membership to a local fitness facility or health club, but consider the long-term use and convenience when making your decision. If you decide to purchase your own equipment for use at home, the challenge will be to meet your personal fitness needs while simultaneously finding a good blend of price and quality. The following list of questions will help you purchase equipment that will provide years of use rather than turning into a garage sale casualty:

- *What are your fitness goals?* If you plan to focus on a walking program, you don't need a treadmill with capabilities for an Olympian! However, if you have some competitive goals in mind, be sure the equipment can withstand the rigors of your training. All types of aerobic equipment (treadmills, stationary bikes, elliptical machines) can improve fitness and help with weight management, but realize walking up a grade and jogging on a treadmill allows for greater caloric expenditure than most other types of commercially available equipment.[6] Match your use with the construction and purpose of the equipment and also the activities you most enjoy.

- *How much space do you have available?* Take time to measure your floor space. A piece of equipment always looks much smaller in a showroom than it will in your home. You will need some space around the equipment to allow for safe usage, so calculate that into your plans. Some resistance training equipment has a significant vertical component, so knowing ceiling height is also important.

- *How much money do you have to spend?* Home exercise equipment varies greatly in price. Cost is always a consideration, but keep the first question in mind, too. If a simple piece of equipment will fulfill your fitness goals, don't be pulled into purchasing more expensive equipment with options you will never use. Quality should be a major consideration. One or two high-quality pieces of equipment are better than a number of poor-quality items that do not provide the enjoyment you anticipated.

- *How does the equipment feel?* You should try out any piece of equipment you plan to purchase. You are not likely to buy a car based on a picture in a magazine. In the same way, you should take exercise equipment on a "test drive" to ensure that it matches your needs. All moving parts should be smooth and fluid, not jerky or rubbing. Also make sure the equipment fits—treadmill belts should be long enough for your stride, stationary bikes should be adjustable to allow a 5 to 10 degree bend at your knee at the bottom of the pedal stroke, and resistance training equipment should adjust to your limb lengths.

- *Is assembly provided?* When it comes to any home-based purchase, there are three dreaded words: *to be assembled.* Some items may be simple to assemble, but for others you may want to ensure that professional assembly is included in the purchase price.

If you start out with this list of questions, you will maximize the benefits of home-based exercise equipment and realize years of enjoyment.

▶ *Should I Hire a Fitness Specialist or Personal Trainer?*

One other important variable you may want to consider when planning a new or revised exercise program is hiring a fitness professional to help with assessment and prescribe appropriate exercise. Though titles vary considerably within the fitness industry, this kind of professional has typically been known as a personal trainer or a health fitness specialist. Unlike in the medical field, mandated standards are not in place for personal trainers or fitness specialists, so you should ask some specific questions to determine whether the person has appropriate qualifications. Figure 5.3 provides a list of questions you can ask; several "no" responses indicate that you may need to look elsewhere.

FIGURE 5.3

Questions for Prospective Fitness Professionals

Do you have a certification from a nationally recognized organization such as the American College of Sports Medicine* or the National Strength and Conditioning Association?	____ Yes ____ No
Do you have a college degree in the health and fitness field?	____ Yes ____ No
Do you participate in continuing education to stay current in the field?	____ Yes ____ No
Do you have certifications in CPR and first aid?	____ Yes ____ No
Do you have liability insurance?	____ Yes ____ No
Do you have experience working with people similar to me in terms of age, sex, and goals?	____ Yes ____ No
Do you use preactivity screenings and fitness assessments?	____ Yes ____ No
Do you include cardiorespiratory, muscular, and flexibility training in your program?	____ Yes ____ No

*ACSM-certified professionals can be found in your area by looking at the ACSM's Pro Finder (see www.acsm.org).
From ACSM, 2011, *ACSM's complete guide to fitness & health* (Champaign, IL: Human Kinetics).

Selecting Proper Shoes and Clothing

Whatever your preference—solo exercise or in a group, home-based or fitness facility—common considerations for safety and comfort are shoes and clothing. Attention to these basic items can optimize your enjoyment and help you avoid injury that could derail your exercise plans.

Before selecting a pair of shoes, determine your primary activity and the surface (e.g., pavement, exercise facility floor). Spend some time in an athletic shoe store consulting with an expert regarding the type of shoe that will best serve your purpose. For example, running shoes are constructed for forward motion rather than side-to-side, so if you are taking an aerobic dance class or playing tennis, you will want a shoe that is constructed to handle lateral movements. Don't fall into the trap of believing that the most expensive shoe is the best. The most important factor when selecting a shoe is good support and proper fit.

Clothing doesn't have to be high priced to provide comfort during exercise. Select clothing appropriate for the temperature and environmental conditions in which you will be exercising. Clothing that is appropriate for exercise and the season can improve your exercise experience. In warm environments, clothes that have a wicking capacity are helpful in dissipating heat from the body. In contrast, cold environments are best faced with layers so you can adjust your body temperature to avoid sweating and remain comfortable.

Until more uniform and rigorous hiring standards are in place within the fitness industry, a "buyer beware" mind-set seems to be appropriate and prudent. Your interview should help you determine whether the prospective trainer is a good match for you in terms of style and general approach to health and fitness. Some people prefer a very nurturing and encouraging style, whereas others tend to respond more positively to a trainer who has a lot of energy and is more demanding. Your task is to determine what motivational style and approach best suits your personality.

An issue to address is whether a fitness professional is a necessity or a luxury. Most experts agree that meeting recommendations for physical activity does not require a trainer, but having someone who is focused on helping you reach your health and fitness goals can be helpful. One reasonable option is to hire a trainer to conduct fitness assessments, develop a comprehensive fitness program, and provide instruction and feedback in the early stages of the program. Thereafter you may be able to consult with the trainer periodically for updates.

HEALTHY HABITS AND DIET

Although this chapter has been focused on physical activity, many of the same concepts apply to your approach to a healthy diet. As pointed out at the start of the chapter, nutrition is part of physical wellness because it also affects your ability to carry out your day-to-day tasks. The motivation continuum applies to your diet as well—amotivation (no motivation or inclination to change), other-determined motivation (e.g., eating vegetables to please a parent, or avoiding high-fat foods out

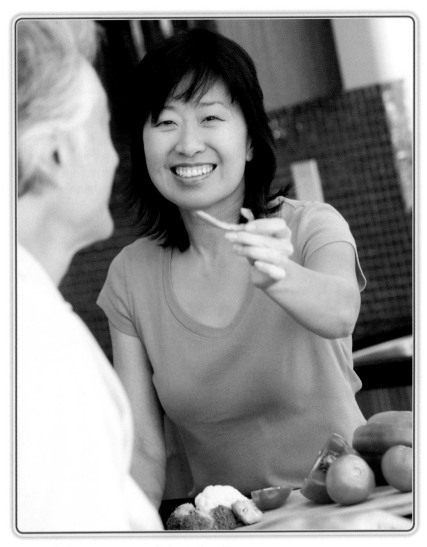

Good nutritional choices are part of physical wellness.

of fear of a heart attack), self-determination motivation (e.g., making food choices that promote good health), and intrinsic motivation (e.g., simply enjoying the taste and nourishment of a healthy meal).

If you already have healthy eating habits, keep doing what you are doing. Chapter 4 provides support for the choices you have made. On the other hand, if you see that your diet could be improved, it is time to write down goals. Short-term goals may involve individual food choices (e.g., replacing a vending machine afternoon snack with a piece of fruit that you bring from home) that, when taken together, lead to the fulfillment of your long-term goals. Long-term goals may include weight loss (if appropriate) or improving the nutritional quality of the calories you consume.

Like physical activity and exercise, a healthy nutrition plan should have a long-term perspective. As outlined in chapter 4, nutrition is vital to overall body functioning, and paying attention to what and how much you eat can have a great influence

Sasha

Sasha, a 29-year-old mother of 2-year-old twins, is struggling with regaining her pre-pregnancy body shape and is feeling constantly tired and fatigued. Her routine is to wake up with a diet cola as she prepares the twins to be dropped off at day care by her husband. Her job as an office receptionist is enjoyable but fast-paced. When she is able, she slips away to grab some fast food or otherwise snacks on vending machine candy bars at her desk. To keep her energy up, her caffeinated diet soda is never far away. She is typically the last to leave the office and then rushes home to spend time with her family. Her husband handles the evening meal preparation while Sasha feeds the twins. By the time her own dinner time arrives, she tends to overeat because it is the first "real" food she has had all day. What can Sasha do to improve her nutrition and her health?

- *Include breakfast.* Including breakfast will help Sasha start the day off on a better foot. A quick bowl of cereal with skim milk or instant oatmeal, along with a piece of fruit, is a positive change from diet cola, which has no nutritional value.

- *Prepare food ahead of time for lunches.* Rather than being at the mercy of her busy schedule to determine whether she can eat lunch, Sasha can prepare some items to take from home so she doesn't have to skip lunch if things get too busy at the office. Some cut vegetables, fruit, a turkey sandwich on whole wheat bread, and a low-fat yogurt will provide her with better nutrition than her fast-food choices or candy bars from the vending machine. To keep from getting hungry between meals, Sasha can snack on some dry-roasted nuts, low-fat microwave popcorn, vegetable sticks, or fruit. By providing nutritious food throughout the day, she can cut back her dependence on caffeine as a stimulant.

- *Eat throughout the day to avoid overeating at night.* Sasha has good nutritional choices available at dinner, but unfortunately, she falls into the trap of overconsuming calories as a result of the food choices she made earlier in the day. By including breakfast as well as a nutritious lunch and snacks at work, Sasha will be able to better portion her food throughout the day and ultimately control her calorie intake. This will help her with her two concerns—weight loss and feeling tired and fatigued.

- *Incorporate exercise.* Finally, Sasha realizes that she has not been committed to exercise the way she was before the twins were born. She and her husband agree to increase their activity by taking the twins out in their strollers in the evening for a long walk around a neighborhood park. In addition, because Sasha doesn't have to leave the office to drive to a restaurant to grab her lunch, she has time for about 15 minutes of brisk walking during her lunch break. This provides her with close to an hour of activity on most days of the week.

on your health. In the upcoming chapters, areas of concern for various age groups and health situations are highlighted. These may be helpful areas to focus your attention. Once you are meeting the dietary recommendations outlined in chapter 4, continuing those habits will provide the most favorable long-term benefits. A lifelong approach to balanced nutrition will maximize the benefits of a healthy diet.

Living a wellness lifestyle is a joyful struggle. The struggle, or challenging aspect, is rooted in the reality that making healthy choices is not always easy. The joyful aspect is the great satisfaction and feeling of well-being that accompany a health-centered life. As a reader of this book, you are choosing to reject the notion of living life passively with a limited sense of direction and instead are embracing active engagement in learning about living a healthy lifestyle. Wellness is a multi-dimensional concept that is influenced by a number of factors including sleep, stress, physical activity, and nutrition. As you have read, adopting healthy habits and maintaining them are the keys to sustaining your well-being. As you work to develop and maintain a physically activity lifestyle and healthy diet, understanding motivation and cultivating self-management skills will be critical.

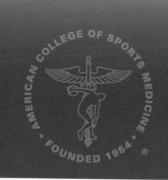

part II

Exercise and Activity for Building a Better You

Incorporating activities to improve your aerobic fitness, muscular fitness, flexibility, and balance helps you develop your fitness ID. The upcoming chapters provide you with insight into why each area is important. Knowledge is good, but having the tools to create your individualized program is even better. This section contains specific activities that you can make part of your exercise program. Your health status, fitness level, and goals are unique to you. No matter whether you are just starting out or are already a regular exerciser, these chapters guide you in taking the next step in developing your fitness.

chapter 6

Aerobic Activity

Consider how you can feel breathless when quickly going up a flight of stairs—your body is showing the need for oxygen! *Aerobic* means "with oxygen," and aerobic fitness, or cardiorespiratory endurance as it is also called, pertains to how well your body is able to take in oxygen and put it to use. Activities that involve large-muscle groups engaged in dynamic movement for prolonged periods of time are considered aerobic. Your cardiovascular system (heart and blood vessels) and your respiratory system (lungs and air passages) work together during longer-duration activities to supply working muscles and organs with the oxygen they need. Examples of aerobic activities include walking, jogging, running, cycling, swimming, dancing, hiking, and team sports such as basketball.

HEALTH AND FITNESS BENEFITS OF AEROBIC ACTIVITY

Regular and consistent aerobic activity improves your cardiorespiratory endurance. In other words, your heart, blood vessels, and lungs benefit from working harder than normal. Exercise improves your cardiorespiratory function by increasing the activity of these organ systems above what they experience at rest. Over time, your body adapts to these stresses and your fitness improves.[2]

Cardiorespiratory endurance is an important aspect of health for a number of reasons:[1]

- Better cardiorespiratory endurance typically leads to higher levels of routine physical activity as you go about your day-to-day life. This in turn provides additional health benefits.

- Low levels of cardiorespiratory fitness are associated with higher risk of premature death from all causes, and specifically from cardiovascular disease. To look at this from a more positive perspective, increases in cardiorespiratory fitness are associated with a decreased risk of death from all causes.

- Aerobic fitness is an important foundation that will allow you to engage in activities of daily living with greater ease.
- Increases in cardiorespiratory endurance allow you to more fully participate in recreational and sport activities.
- Aerobic activities that promote cardiorespiratory endurance also burn a relatively large number of calories and thus help to maintain appropriate body weight.

This is not an exhaustive list but does demonstrate the wide-ranging benefits of aerobic exercise for health as well as fitness.

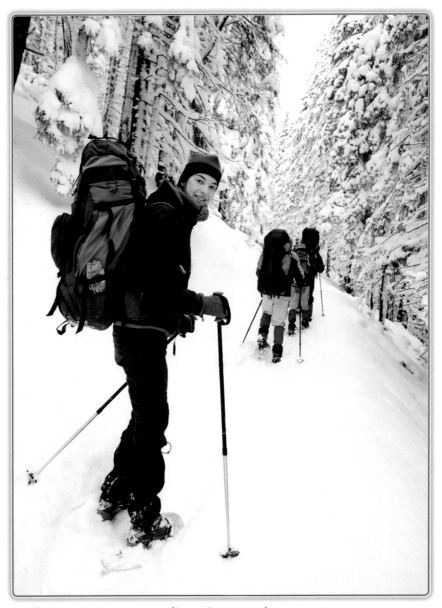

Aerobic exercise improves cardiorespiratory endurance.

AEROBIC WORKOUT COMPONENTS

An aerobic workout should follow a consistent pattern to optimize safety as well as enjoyment. You should begin with a warm-up, which is followed by the main part of the workout, called the endurance conditioning phase. The workout is then wrapped up with a cool-down. See figure 6.1 for an overview of an aerobic exercise session.

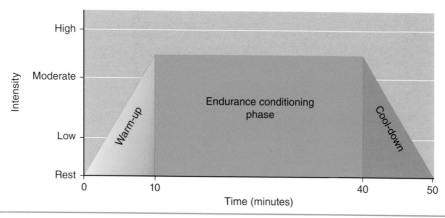

Figure 6.1 Overview of aerobic exercise session.
Reprinted by permission from Bushman and Young, 2005, p. 35.

Warm-Up

A warm-up that consists of a minimum of five to ten minutes of low- to moderate-level activity is essential.[1] The intent of the warm-up is to literally increase the temperature of the muscles, thus preparing the body for the demands of the endurance conditioning phase, or main focus, of the workout. A warm-up prepares your heart, lungs, and muscles for the endurance conditioning phase of your aerobic training session. Think of the warm-up as an on-ramp to a freeway. The on-ramp gives you time to bring your vehicle up to the speed of traffic to avoid an accident. The faster the traffic is, the longer the on-ramp should be. In the same way, your warm-up should be longer if the intensity of the conditioning phase is high.

Warm-up activities may include some light calisthenics or lower-level activities similar to what you will be including in the conditioning phase. For example, if your program includes brisk walking for the conditioning phase, then the warm-up could include slower-paced walking. If the conditioning phase includes a more intense activity such as running, then jogging would be appropriate in the warm-up. The point is to gradually increase the intensity from resting levels to the intensity you plan for the conditioning phase.

Endurance Conditioning Phase

To continue with the freeway analogy, the endurance conditioning phase is the freeway itself—the main focus of your journey. The conditioning phase for aerobic activity is guided by the FITT principle, which stands for *frequency, intensity, time, and type*.[2] Frequency refers to the number of days per week in which you set aside time for exercise. Intensity reflects how hard you are working when exercising.

Time simply refers to the duration you are active, on a daily or weekly basis. And, type, or exercise mode, focuses on activities that involve large-muscle groups to improve cardiorespiratory fitness.

Although FITT nicely summarizes the conditioning phase, some fitness professionals like FITTE better—the E stands for *enjoyment*! All the recommendations and information in the world will mean little if you do not stick with your exercise program. Understanding the benefits of an exercise program (as outlined in chapter 1) will help you adhere to it, but considering the time commitment you are making, you should also be sure you are having some fun. Suggestions for keeping exercise enjoyable are found later in this chapter. First, consider the nuts and bolts of an aerobic exercise program.

Frequency

The recommended frequency of aerobic exercise is between three and five days per week. How many days you exercise will depend on your goals and the intensity that is most appropriate for you. Although as few as a couple of days per week of activity can provide benefits, regular physical activity provides more benefits and has a lower risk of musculoskeletal injury than sporadic activity.[1, 3] You will need as few as three days per week if you are engaging in vigorous activity, but at least five days per week is recommended if you plan on moderate-intensity activity. For example, if you enjoy running (a vigorous activity), three days per week will provide you with health and fitness benefits. However, if you plan on a walking program (a moderate-intensity activity), then at least five days per week would be better. If you enjoy mixing types and intensities of activity,[3] then a weekly combination of three to five days of moderate and vigorous activity is recommended.[1] For example, you may walk a couple days per week and jog on another couple days. This would be considered at two days per week of moderate activity (i.e., walking) and two days per week of vigorous activity (i.e., jogging), allowing you to meet the recommended amount of physical activity.

Intensity

As the intensity of activity increases, so do the potential health benefits. To promote health and fitness benefits, your exercise must place some stress on your cardiorespiratory system. In other words, you should notice an increase in your heart rate and breathing. When speaking of intensity, fitness professionals generally use the terms *moderate* and *vigorous*.[3] For a quick picture, consider moderate-intensity activity to be equivalent to brisk walking and vigorous-intensity activity to be equivalent to jogging or running.[3]

A variety of simple methods are available to help you quantify the intensity of your exercise bout. One method is to monitor your perceived level of effort. Although this is subjective (i.e., you determine how easy or hard you are exercising), a numerical scale can help guide you to appropriate levels of activity. The U.S. Department of Health and Human Services' *Physical Activity Guidelines for Americans* suggests a scale of 0 to 10. Sitting at rest is 0, and your highest effort level possible is 10.[3] Moderate-intensity activity is a 5 or 6 on this effort scale. Vigorous-intensity activity is at a level of 7 or 8. This method allows you to individualize your exercise based on your current level of cardiorespiratory fitness.[3] For an example of applying this scale, see figure 6.2.

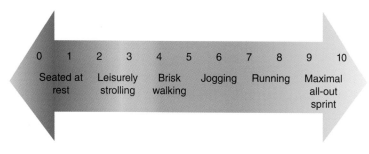

Figure 6.2   Sample scale of where activities fall within the various intensity levels.

Another method, called the talk test, can also be used to establish exercise intensity at a moderate level. If you are working at an intensity that increases breathing rate but still allows you to speak without gasping for breath between words, you are likely exercising at a moderate intensity. The goal would be to exercise to the point at which speech would start to become more difficult. The *Physical Activity Guidelines for Americans* suggests that moderate-intensity activity allows you to talk but not to sing, whereas more vigorous activity results in an inability to say more than a few words without pausing for a breath.[3]

Heart rate monitoring can also be helpful for determining your intensity level, although it is a bit more technical than the subjective measures of effort level and the talk test. The maximal heart rate for adults can be estimated by multiplying your age in years by 0.67 and then subtracting that product from 206.9 (numbers in bold are constants, or set values, in the following equation).

206.9 – (age in years × **0.67**) =   estimated maximal heart rate

You will not be exercising at maximal heart rate, but rather, at a percentage of that value; the percentage will depend on your fitness level (consider the values in table 6.1 as a starting point).[2] Multiply your estimated maximal heart rate by the activity factor from table 6.1 to determine your target heart rate.

        estimated maximal heart rate ×   activity factor

  =   target exercise heart rate in beats per minute

Note that your heart rate can also be influenced by environmental conditions (e.g., hot, humid environments) as well as medications (e.g., beta-blockers used for migraines and heart disease can lower heart rate). The calculated value should be used in conjunction with perceived exertion or the talk test. You can adjust your workload up or down depending on your perception of effort on a given day. A description of how to assess your heart rate is found on page 24 in chapter 2. Recall that during exercise you can count the number of beats in 15 seconds and then multiply that number by 4 to determine your beats per minute.

Recognize, too, that you can vary your intensity during the conditioning phase. Athletes often use interval training, which includes some time at higher intensity followed by lower-intensity exercise. This provides a unique stress on the body that translates into improved aerobic fitness. This principle can be used for general exercise programs as well. For example, if you are just beginning to exercise, you could include a few minutes at a faster walking pace within your conditioning phase. Alternating between lower and higher intensity provides variety as well as a stimulus to improve your aerobic capacity, no matter your current level of fitness.

Table 6.1 **Heart Rate Intensity Guidelines**

Fitness classification	Description	Percentage of maximal heart rate	Activity factor*
Low	Those who are currently inactive with no activity/exercise and are thus very deconditioned	~60%	0.60
Low to fair	Those who participate in minimal physical activity but have no regular exercise plan and thus are deconditioned	~65%	0.65
Fair to average	Those who are sporadically active but do not have an optimal exercise plan and thus are moderately deconditioned	~75%	0.75
Average to good	Those who are regularly engaging in moderate to vigorous exercise	~85%	0.85
Good to excellent	Those who are engaging in regular high-intensity exercise	~90%	0.90

*Multiply activity factor by maximal heart rate to determine target heart rate.
Adapted by permission from American College of Sports Medicine, 2010, pp. 166-167.

A CLOSER LOOK
Rhoda

Rhoda is a 40-year-old woman who would like to use her heart rate response to help guide her exercise intensity. She doesn't know her maximal heart rate (few people do). She can estimate her maximal heart rate by multiplying her age by 0.67 and then subtracting that product (40 × 0.67 = 26.8) from 206.9. This results in an estimated maximal heart rate of 180 beats per minute (206.9 − [40 × 0.67]). She will exercise at a percentage of that value; the percentage will depend on the fitness level that she determines using table 6.1.

Rhoda is currently doing only minimal activity and thus she places herself in the "Low to fair" fitness classification. As a result, she selects 65% of her maximal heart rate for her target. To calculate this, she takes her estimated maximal heart rate (180) and multiplies it by the activity factor of 0.65 (decimal version of 65%). This calculates to be 117 beats per minute. This is a starting point for her, and she can adjust her intensity up or down depending on how she feels. Over time, as Rhoda's fitness level improves, she will increase the intensity (e.g., 75% intensity would provide a target heart rate of 135 beats per minute).

Time

The duration of each of your exercise sessions is determined by the amount of time you are able to commit as well as your current fitness status. If you are a beginner, don't worry about some arbitrary time goal, but rather, find an activity that you can do continuously for 10 minutes. Increase the duration of the exercise session as it becomes easier to complete. Add a couple of minutes per session until you reach about 30 minutes of aerobic exercise per day. Depending on your initial fitness level, this may take a number of weeks or even a month or more. The key is to keep going and make progress!

If you have already been doing some exercise (or have now built up to 30 minutes of continuous activity) and feel comfortable with moderate-intensity activity for this length of time, decide whether you want to maintain your current intensity and go for a bit longer, or if you want to begin to increase the intensity. Time and intensity are like a teeter-totter. When you increase intensity, you generally decrease the length of the session. If you decrease intensity, you will need to increase the time you spend exercising to achieve full health benefits. A general rule of thumb from the *Physical Activity Guidelines for Americans* is that one minute of vigorous-intensity activity can be counted as the same as two minutes of moderate-intensity activity. For example, a 15-minute run would provide the same health benefit as a 30-minute walk.

Labels are difficult to apply universally, but table 6.2 provides some terminology related to activity status that was introduced in chapter 3. For the purposes of this book, beginners are those who currently have limited activity. As you can see in the table, beginners are focusing on light to moderate activity and will build up to at least 150 minutes per week. The intermediate level of activity reflects people who have not yet achieved a regular exercise pattern and thus will focus on increasing moderate-intensity aerobic activity up to at least 200 minutes per week.

Table 6.2 Activity Status and Aerobic Training Focus

Activity status	Aerobic training focus
Beginner (those who are inactive with no or minimal physical activity and thus are deconditioned)	*No prior activity:* Focus is on light- to moderate-level activity for 20–30 minutes over the course of the day. Accumulating time in 10-minute bouts is an option. Overall, your target is 60–150 minutes per week. *Minimal prior activity* (i.e., once you have met the previous target level): Focus is on light- to moderate-level activity for 30–60 minutes per day. Accumulating time in 10-minute bouts is an option. Overall, your target is 150–200 minutes per week.
Intermediate (those who are sporadically active but do not have an optimal exercise plan and thus are moderately deconditioned)	*Fair to average fitness:* Focus is on moderate activity for 30–90 minutes per day. Overall, your target is 200–300 minutes per week.
Established (those who are regularly engaging in moderate to vigorous exercise)	*Regular exerciser* (moderate to vigorous): Focus is on moderate to vigorous activity for 30–90 minutes per day. Overall, your target is 200–300 minutes per week of moderate-intensity activity or 100–150 minutes of vigorous-intensity activity or a combination of moderate- and vigorous-intensity activity.

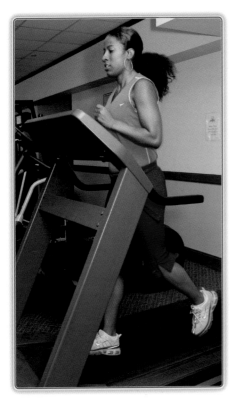

Walking and jogging are common aerobic activities.

Typically, people at this level are of fair to average fitness levels. Established exercisers are those who have been engaged in regular exercise for at least six months. As you can see, fitness levels vary according to genetic potential as well as personal fitness goals. Typically, established exercisers have average to excellent aerobic fitness.

The *Physical Activity Guidelines for Americans* recommends working toward a minimum of 150 minutes per week of moderate-intensity activity, or 75 minutes per week of vigorous-intensity activity.[3] If you are already physically active at this level, then consider increasing your activity to gain additional health and fitness benefits. For you, a new target of 300 minutes per week of moderate-intensity activity, or 150 minutes per week of vigorous-intensity activity, would be a goal.[3]

Type, or Mode

Aerobic activities are grouped into four categories along with recommendations on who would most appropriately engage in that particular activity (see table 6.3). Exercises in group A are recommended for everyone because they are relatively simple activities that can be started at a low level of effort.

Table 6.3 Aerobic Exercise Groupings

Exercise group	Group characteristics	Recommended participants	Examples
A	Endurance activities that can be done with minimal skill and with minimal fitness	Everyone	Walking, easy bicycling, slow dancing
B	Endurance activities that are more vigorous but can be done with minimal skill	Because of the higher intensity, adults who are regularly active and have at least an average level of fitness would be best suited.	Jogging, running, spinning, elliptical exercise, fast dancing
C	Endurance activities that require a certain level of skill to perform	Assuming a skill level has been achieved, people should have at least an average level of fitness to be suited for these activities.	Swimming, cross-country skiing, skating
D	Recreational sports	Because of the changing exertion level due to competition or terrain, people should have at least an average level of fitness.	Basketball, tennis, soccer, downhill skiing, hiking

Adapted by permission from American College of Sports Medicine, 2010, p. 164.

Group B activities are more vigorous and thus are most appropriate if you already have a good fitness base (i.e., you have been exercising regularly and have determined your fitness level to be at least in the fair to average range). Group C activities are those that have a definite skill component and thus may require some learning before being used as a fitness tool. Group D activities are recreational and, because intensity varies depending on the situation, are best reserved for people who are regularly active and have a good fitness base. Do not consider these groupings progressive (i.e., that group C activities are better than group B activities), but rather, as a way to classify various aerobic exercises.

Cool-Down

The cool-down should consist of a minimum of five to ten minutes of low- to moderate-level activity.[1] The cool-down provides an opportunity for body systems to gradually return to pre-exercise levels. Heart rate slows down, blood pressure decreases, and the muscles recover from the conditioning phase. Activities included in a cool-down are similar to those in the warm-up, but the intensity will need to gradually diminish toward resting levels. A cool-down is recommended to allow the heart to slow down in a controlled manner, thus avoiding negative changes in heart rhythm. In addition, if you stop your activity too abruptly, blood that was circulating to the working muscles can pool in your legs resulting in a drop in blood pressure. A cool-down will also help to gradually decrease body temperature, which naturally increased during the endurance phase.

A proper cool-down is driven by both practical issues (e.g., avoiding fainting from a drop in blood pressure) and safety issues (e.g., avoiding negative changes in heart rhythm). The cool-down is like a freeway off-ramp. When shifting from freeway speeds to those appropriate on city streets, time is needed for an adjustment. In a similar way, the cool-down allows the body to adjust back toward normal resting levels. The higher the intensity of your conditioning phase, the longer your cool-down should be.

Using METs to Estimate Calories Burned

Addressing frequency, intensity, time, and type of activity helps you create a personal aerobic exercise plan, which may include a variety of activities. One way to provide a summary of your aerobic exercise is to determine the calories you use when engaging in activity each week. A minimum recommended target is 1,000 calories per week with higher amounts potentially providing even greater health benefits.[2]

To determine how many calories you burn for a given activity, you will need more information about the activity and the intensity at which you exercised. To keep things simple, researchers have created a unit of measure called a metabolic equivalent, or MET. A MET is equal to the oxygen cost at rest (i.e., 1 MET = resting level = 3.5 ml of oxygen per kg body weight per minute). Multiples of a MET are then applied to various activities. For example, walking at 3.5 miles per hour (5.6 km/h) is equal to 4 METS. In other words, you are working four times harder when walking at 3.5 miles per hour than you are when seated in a resting position. MET values have been determined for a wide variety of activities (see table 6.4 for some examples of basic activities).

(continued)

Calculating calories burned can be helpful when you are interested in losing weight, but it is also a great way to pull together the four parts of your aerobic exercise prescription—intensity, time, frequency, and type of activity—into one number. Whether you do the same activity each day or change it up, you still can take a look at your weekly total to ensure that you are on track.

Once you know the MET value for a given exercise, you can estimate how many calories you burned per minute by inserting that value into the following formula (numbers in bold are constants—in other words, they do not change):

MET value of activity × **3.5** ×   weight in kg ÷ **200**

=   calories burned per minute

Insert the MET value for the activity and then your body weight (to convert from lb to kg, multiply your weight in lb by 0.454 to determine your weight in kg).

Table 6.4   MET Values for Selected Activities*

Activity	MET value
Bicycling outdoors, <10.0 mph (16 km/h), leisure riding	4.0
Bicycling outdoors, 10.0–11.9 mph (16–19.2 km/h)	6.0
Bicycling outdoors, 12.0–13.9 mph (19.2–22.4 km/h)	8.0
Bicycling outdoors, 14.0–15.9 mph (22.5–25.6 km/h)	10.0
Biking, stationary, 50 watts, very light effort	3.0
Biking, stationary, 100 watts, light effort	5.5
Biking, stationary, 150 watts, moderate effort	7.0
Biking, stationary, 200 watts, vigorous effort	10.5
Running, 5 mph (8 km/h)	8.0
Running, 6 mph (9.7 km/h)	10.0
Running, 7 mph (11.3 km/h)	11.5
Running, 8 mph (12.9 km/h)	13.5
Swimming laps, freestyle, moderate to light effort	8.0
Swimming laps, sidestroke	8.0
Swimming laps, backstroke	8.0
Swimming laps, breaststroke	10.0
Swimming laps, butterfly	11.0
Walking, 2.0 mph (3.2 km/h)	2.5
Walking, 2.5 mph (4 km/h)	3.0
Walking, 3.0 mph (4.8 km/h)	3.5
Walking, 3.5 mph (5.6 km/h)	4.0
Walking, 4.5 mph (7.2 km/h)	4.5

*For a comprehensive list of activities and MET values, see http://prevention.sph. sc.edu/tools/compendium.htm.

Source: Ainsworth, Haskell, Leon, et al., 1993, pp. 74-79.

Derrick is a 25-year-old graduate student who tries to fit exercise into his busy schedule. He enjoys both walking with his girlfriend and running on his own but wonders which one is better with regard to his exercise program. Taking a look at the MET values can help him examine how intensity influences the number of calories he burns. He compares walking at 3.5 miles per hour (5.6 km/h) for 50 minutes to running at 6 miles per hour (9.7 km/h) for 20 minutes (see the MET values for each in table 6.4). Which one burns more calories for Derrick, a 150-pound (68.1 kg) person?

Walking at 3.5 miles per hour (5.6 km/h) is equal to 4 METS, so using the formula provided previously, a 50-minute workout burns about 240 calories (determined by multiplying 50 minutes by 4.8 calories per minute), as follows:

$$(4 \text{ METS} \times \mathbf{3.5} \times 68.1 \text{ kg}) \div \mathbf{200} = 4.8 \text{ calories per minute}$$

Running at 6 miles per hour (9.7 km/h) is equal to 10 METS, so using the formula provided previously, a 20-minute workout would burn 238 calories (determined by multiplying 20 minutes by 11.9 calories per minute), as follows:

$$(10 \text{ METS} \times \mathbf{3.5} \times 68.1 \text{ kg}) \div \mathbf{200} = 11.9 \text{ calories per minute}$$

Both workouts burn approximately the same number of calories! If Derrick selects moderate-intensity exercise (such as brisk walking), he needs to remember that he has to exercise longer than if he engaged in more vigorous exercise (such as running). Either option provides health and fitness benefits.

YOUR AEROBIC PROGRAM

If you are just getting started with your exercise program, be sure to complete the PAR-Q and the risk stratification found in chapter 2. These simple tools can help you determine whether you should visit your health care provider before starting an exercise program. Of course, regardless of the outcome, consulting with your personal health care provider is always appropriate. In addition, you need to consider your current fitness level and begin at a point appropriate to your current status. Over time, with regular activity, you will progress and improve.

Your personal exercise prescription takes into account the frequency, intensity, time, and type of activity. Take walking, for example, which is the most commonly reported exercise and is a great activity for the start of an exercise program (walking is a group A activity as shown in table 6.3). Figure 6.3 shows an example of a progressive walking and jogging program. You can determine where to enter into the exercise progression based on your current level of fitness.

Once you feel comfortable with 30 minutes of continuous moderate-intensity activity, you may be interested in other activity options. Swimming, a group C activity, is another excellent aerobic activity if you have basic swimming skills or are willing to gain those skills. Follow the time and intensity progression described in figure 6.3, substitute swimming (using different strokes for variety) for walking and jogging.

Figure 6.4 provides a sample program for someone with a membership at a health club. Activities at the club, when done at a low intensity, would fall into group A, but as the person's fitness level improves, the intensity increase will likely result in a shift to group B exercise.

The examples in figures 6.3 and 6.4 show a progression from beginner to established exerciser. Depending on your current status, you may be at the start of the table as a beginner or already in the established, or maintenance, phase. If you are just beginning to exercise, progress slowly and base your advancement on how your body is responding to the exercise. If you are in the established, or maintenance, phase, keep tracking your activity. Also, stay focused on the FITT factors as discussed previously, and if you are becoming bored with your current activity program, consider other modes of exercise or joining an exercise group.

As you move along in your exercise journey, increase the duration (time) first; once you are comfortable with the activity at the longer session length, then consider increasing the intensity. To avoid injury, do not increase the session duration and intensity at the same time. Although placing a stress on the body is necessary for improvement, excessive overload can result in injury as well as frustration. To keep steady forward progress, refer to table 6.2 on page 105 for general guidance.

In addition, as you examine the sample programs, once again consider the FITTE factors as discussed on pages 101-102 and how each relates to your fitness goals. Don't forget about the E for enjoyment. As you create your plan of action, consider the type of activities you enjoy and also are accessible to you. Joining a health club can be a great way to increase your access to a variety of activities (equipment as well as group classes). If you don't want to join a health club, you can easily find aerobic activities at no cost. Walking and running trails are becoming more common in cities, many malls open their doors early to allow walkers to use the corridors before the stores open, and your local library has many aerobic exercise videos that you can use in the privacy of your own home. To get started, you need to pick a day and take the first step—literally as well as figuratively.

FIGURE 6.3

Sample Walking and Jogging Program

Stage	Time point	Warm-up	Workout*	Cool-down
Beginner	First week	Slow, easy walking pace for a couple of minutes	Walk at a pace that gives a light level of exertion (level 3 or 4) for 10 minutes at least twice a day for a total of 20 minutes each day (three days per week). Your weekly total should be 60 minutes.	Slow, easy walking pace for a couple of minutes
	Progression, part 1	Slow, easy walking pace for five minutes	Each week add 15 minutes to your weekly total until you reach 120 minutes of activity (e.g., 30 minutes four days per week). Stay at this duration and increase your intensity over the next couple of weeks from light (level 3 or 4) to moderate (level 5 or 6). Once you are comfortable with this time and intensity for a couple of weeks, continue to add 10–15 minutes per week until you reach 150 minutes.	Slow, easy walking pace for five minutes
	Progression, part 2	Easy walking pace for 5–10 minutes	Walk at a pace that gives a moderate level of exertion (level 5 or 6); continue to add 10–15 minutes each week to progress from 150 minutes per week to a total of 200 minutes.	Easy walking pace for 5–10 minutes
	Final week	Easy walking pace for 5–10 minutes	Walk at a pace that gives a moderate level of exertion (level 5 or 6) for 30–60 minutes (3–5 days per week). Your weekly total should be 200 minutes.	Easy walking pace for 5–10 minutes
Intermediate	Initial week	Easy walking pace for 5–10 minutes	Walk at a pace that feels moderate (level 5 or 6) for 30–60 minutes (3–5 days per week). Your weekly total should be 200 minutes.	Easy walking pace for 5–10 minutes
	Progression	Easy walking pace for 5–10 minutes	Continue to increase exercise duration by 10–15 minutes per week to approach 300 minutes of moderate activity accumulated on a weekly basis. Another option is to introduce a more vigorous activity, such as jogging, realizing that the time needed will be less (typically two minutes of moderate activity equals one minute of vigorous activity).	Easy walking pace for 5–10 minutes
	Final week	Easy walking pace for 5–10 minutes	Walk at a pace that feels moderate (level 5 or 6) for 45–90 minutes (3–5 days per week). Your weekly total should be 300 minutes (moderate intensity). *Or:* Combine moderate and vigorous walking on alternate days. Your weekly total should be equivalent amounts of moderate and vigorous activity (e.g., 200 minutes of moderate plus 50 minutes of vigorous).	Easy walking pace for 5–10 minutes

(continued)

Stage	Time point	Warm-up	Workout*	Cool-down
Established	Continue/maintain	Easy walking pace for 5–10 minutes	Walk at a pace that feels moderate (level 5 or 6). Your weekly total should be a minimum of 300 minutes (moderate intensity). *Or:* Jog (level 7 or 8). Your weekly total should be a minimum of 150 minutes (vigorous intensity). *Or:* Combine moderate and vigorous walking on alternate days. Your weekly total should be equivalent amounts of moderate and vigorous activity (e.g., 200 minutes of moderate plus 50 minutes of vigorous).	Easy walking pace for 5–10 minutes

*Level of exertion is on a scale of 0 to 10 (sitting at rest is 0 and your highest effort level is 10).

FIGURE 6.4

Sample Cross-Training Program at a Health Club

Stage	Time point	Warm-up	Workout*	Cool-down
Beginner	First week	Slow, easy walking pace for a couple of minutes	Pick one activity each day at a light level of exertion (level 3 or 4) for 10 minutes at least twice a day for a total of 20 minutes each day (three days per week). Select from walking on the treadmill or stationary biking. Your weekly total should be 60 minutes.	Slow, easy walking pace for a couple of minutes
	Progression, part 1	Slow, easy walking pace for five minutes	Each week add 15 minutes to your weekly total until you reach 120 minutes of activity (e.g., 30 minutes four days per week). Potential activities include treadmill walking, stationary biking, and using a stair climber. Stay at this duration and increase your intensity over the next couple of weeks from light (level 3 or 4) to moderate (level 5 or 6). Once you are comfortable with this time and intensity for a couple of weeks, continue to add 10–15 minutes per week until you reach 150 minutes.	Slow, easy walking pace for five minutes
	Progression, part 2	Easy walking pace for 5–10 minutes	Exercise at an intensity that gives a moderate level of exertion (level 5 or 6); continue to add 10–15 minutes each week to progress from 150 minutes per week to a total of 200 minutes.	Easy walking pace for 5–10 minutes
	Final week	Easy walking pace for 5–10 minutes	Exercise at an intensity that gives a moderate level of exertion (level 5 or 6) for 30–60 minutes (3–5 days per week). Activities may include treadmill walking; stationary biking; or using a stair climber, elliptical trainer, rowing machine, or Nordic ski machine. Your weekly total should be 200 minutes.	Easy walking pace for 5–10 minutes
Inter-mediate	Initial week	Easy walking pace for 5–10 minutes	Exercise at a level that feels moderate (level 5 or 6) for 30–60 minutes (3–5 days per week) using a treadmill, stationary bike, stair climber, elliptical trainer, or Nordic ski machine. Your weekly total should be 200 minutes.	Easy walking pace for 5–10 minutes
	Progression	Easy walking pace for 5–10 minutes	Continue to increase exercise duration by 10–15 minutes per week to approach 300 minutes of moderate activity accumulated on a weekly basis. Another option is to introduce more vigorous activity a couple of days per week, such as jogging on the treadmill, taking a spinning class, or joining a step aerobics class, realizing that the time needed will be less (typically, two minutes of moderate activity equals one minute of vigorous activity).	Easy walking pace for 5–10 minutes

(continued)

Stage	Time point	Warm-up	Workout*	Cool-down
Inter-mediate *(continued)*	Final week	Easy walking pace for 5–10 minutes	Exercise at a level that feels moderate (level 5 or 6) for 45–90 minutes (3–5 days per week). Your weekly total should be 300 minutes (moderate intensity). *Or:* Combine moderate and vigorous walking on alternate days. Your weekly total should be equivalent amounts of moderate and vigorous activity (e.g., 200 minutes of moderate plus 50 minutes of vigorous).	Easy walking pace for 5–10 minutes
Esta-blished	Continue/ maintain	Easy walking pace for 5–10 minutes	Exercise at an intensity that feels moderate (level 5 or 6). Your weekly total should be a minimum of 300 minutes (moderate intensity). *Or:* Exercise at a higher intensity (level 7 or 8). Your weekly total should be a minimum of 150 minutes (vigorous intensity). *Or:* Combine moderate and vigorous walking on alternate days. Your weekly total should be equivalent amounts of moderate and vigorous activity (e.g., 200 minutes of moderate plus 50 minutes of vigorous).	Easy walking pace for 5–10 minutes

*Level of exertion is on a scale of 0 to 10 (sitting at rest is 0 and your highest effort level is 10).

Cardiorespiratory (or aerobic) fitness is important for promoting health and, in particular, is associated with a reduced risk of cardiovascular disease. An aerobic exercise session includes a warm-up, a conditioning phase, and a cool-down. The warm-up and cool-down are links between the resting state and the exercise portion of your workout. The main focus, the endurance conditioning phase, is guided by the FITT principle: frequency, intensity, time, and type. General recommendations are as follows: three to five days per week (frequency), moderate to vigorous level of exertion (intensity), 20 to 30 minutes or more per session (time), and large-muscle group activity (type of activity).

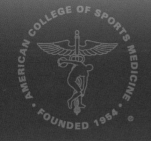

chapter 7

Resistance Training

Muscle-strengthening activities that involve all the major muscle groups are recognized as an essential component of an overall fitness program for adults[15] as well as youth.[1] Muscular fitness includes both muscular strength and muscular endurance. Just as aerobic fitness is improved by stressing the heart and lungs, muscular fitness requires a stress, or resistance, to be placed on the muscles. Resistance training involves the use of a variety of activities that include free weights (barbells and dumbbells), weight machines, elastic tubing, medicine balls, stability balls, and body weight. Resistance training does not refer to one specific mode of conditioning, but rather, is an organized process of exercising with various types of resistance to enhance muscular fitness.

Resistance Training Terminology

Following are definitions of some common terms used in the design of a resistance training workout:

Atrophy—A reduction in muscle fiber size.

Concentric—A type of muscle action that occurs when the muscle shortens.

Eccentric—A type of muscle action that occurs when the muscle lengthens.

Hypertrophy—An enlargement in muscle fiber size.

Muscular strength—The ability to exert maximal force in a single effort.

Muscular endurance—The ability to repeat or maintain muscle contraction.

Repetition—One complete movement of an exercise.

Repetition maximum (RM)—The maximum amount of weight that can be lifted for a predetermined number of repetitions with proper exercise technique.

Set—A group of repetitions performed without stopping.

Spotter—A training partner or coach who can provide assistance in case of a failed repetition.

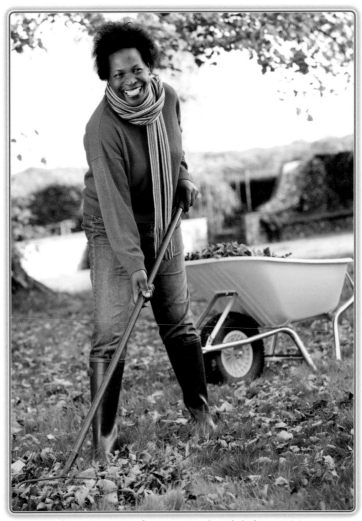

Muscular fitness is part of recreational and daily activities.

When correctly performed and sensibly progressed over time, resistance training can be a safe, effective and enjoyable method of exercise for people of a wide range of ages, fitness levels, and health conditions.[1]

HEALTH AND FITNESS BENEFITS OF RESISTANCE TRAINING

To maintain your physical capacity, you must make a lifestyle choice to include resistance training on a regular basis. Unfortunately, physical capacity and muscle strength decrease dramatically with age in adults who do not engage in resistance training.[3] Resistance training results in stronger muscles and therefore an increased capacity for force production, which is not achievable with solely aerobic-based training. Because muscles function as the engine of your body, they must be used regularly to avoid disuse atrophy (i.e., a reduction in muscle size).

You don't need to be a competitive athlete to benefit from resistance training; it is equally important from a health and fitness perspective. The benefits of resistance training include favorable changes in body composition, metabolic health, and quality of life. Resistance training activities can increase lean muscle mass, reduce body fat, fortify bone, lower blood pressure, improve blood lipid and cholesterol levels, and enhance your body's ability to use glucose.[6, 17] These benefits can optimize your day-to-day functioning while limiting the development of chronic diseases such as diabetes, heart disease, and osteoporosis.[2, 17]

The increase in muscle tissue that results from resistance exercise is accompanied by an increase in resting metabolic rate; in contrast, the decrease in muscle tissue that results from a sedentary lifestyle is accompanied by a decrease in resting metabolic rate. This gradual decrease in metabolism is associated with the gradual increase in body fat that typically occurs with age. Calories that were previously used by muscle tissue (now smaller as a result of disuse) are stored as fat. On the other hand, resistance training raises resting metabolic rate and results in more calories burned on a daily basis. In theory, if you gain 2 pounds (1 kg) of muscle mass, your resting metabolic rate should increase by about 21 calories per day.[16] Thus, performing resistance training throughout your life can help you maintain your health and physical function.

In addition to the effect of muscle on metabolism, one of the most direct benefits of regular resistance training is an increase in bone mineral density that may reduce the risk of osteoporosis.[4] On top of the direct effect of strength-building (and weight-bearing) exercises on bone, the act of muscles pulling on bones during resistance exercises may also be a potent stimulus for new bone formation in certain people. This potential benefit is of particular importance to women who are at increased risk of functional limitations as a result of age-related losses of bone mass.

Strong muscles serve as shock absorbers and balancing agents that help dissipate the repetitive landing forces from weight-bearing activities for active people and also reduce the risk of falling in older adults.[3, 6] As such, a resistance training program that requires agility and balance may be the most effective way to avoid injury as well as reduce the risk of many degenerative diseases.[1, 14] Moreover, strength-building activities are particularly important for low back health, which is a growing health care concern.

Regular participation in resistance training activities that are consistent with your needs, goals, and abilities can improve muscle function, enhance quality of life, and lower the risk of premature all-cause mortality.[2, 13] The health and fitness benefits are clear. You can also realize benefits linked to personal appearance. Firm, toned muscles are possible with regular resistance training. Whether you are looking to improve in recreational or sport activities or just to look and feel better, resistance training should be part of your plan.

FUNDAMENTAL PRINCIPLES OF RESISTANCE TRAINING

Improvements in muscular fitness will only occur if the resistance training program is based on sound training principles and is prudently progressed over time.[5, 10] Although factors such as your initial level of fitness, genetics, nutrition, and motivation will influence the rate and magnitude of adaptation that occurs, you can maximize the effectiveness of your resistance training by addressing three fundamental principles: progressive overload, regularity, and specificity.

Progressive Overload

The progressive overload principle states that to enhance muscular fitness, you must exercise at a level beyond the point to which your muscles are accustomed. This goes back to the idea of having to stress the muscle to get a positive response. Doing the same workout month after month will not maximize benefits. The principle of progression refers to consistently boosting the training stimulus or load at a rate that is compatible with the training-induced adaptations that are occurring.[10] Following the principle of progressive overload requires that you provide your muscles with a new stimulus when they have adapted to the current overload. You can do this in a variety of ways:

- *Increase the number of repetitions.* Typically, 8 to 12 repetitions are recommended for muscular fitness (for older adults, 10 to 15 repetitions are recommended). People focusing on strength development may select fewer repetitions, whereas those focusing on endurance may include up to 15 to 25 repetitions.[1]

- *Increase the number of sets for a given muscle group.* You could do additional sets of the same exercise, or you could add another exercise that targets the same muscle group.

- *Increase the resistance.* The increase in weight needed will vary depending on the exercise but is often prescribed by the increments available (e.g., next weight dumbbell, increasing by one plate on a weight machine).

When providing an overload, select one of the preceding options at a time. Although you want to provide a new stress on the muscle, you do not want to overtax the muscle to the point of injury.

Although every training session does not have to be more intense than the last session, the principle of progressive overload states that the training program needs to be increased gradually over time to realize gains. For example, if you have been

Megan

Megan is a 25-year-old health care worker. She has been doing resistance training for almost two months with a focus on improving her muscular fitness and toning her muscles. Initially, she was able to complete only 8 repetitions with 20 pounds (9 kg) while performing a barbell curl. Over the past two months, she was able to increase the number of repetitions from 8 to 12 before she become fatigued (i.e., repetitions number 11 and 12 were a bit of a struggle to complete). Increasing the repetitions is one way to overload the muscle. She is now able to easily complete 12 repetitions with 20 pounds (9 kg). This is evidence that her muscles have adapted to the overload and now it is time for her to progress to a higher weight to provide greater resistance. Megan selects a weight of 25 pounds (11.4 kg), which she can lift only 8 times. By doing so, she is once again providing an overload on her muscles, which will allow her to continue to improve.

able to easily complete a given workout for a couple of weeks, it may be time to make changes to provide an overload once again.

Regularity

The principle of regularity states that exercise must be performed several times per week on a habitual basis to enhance physical fitness. Although training once per week may maintain training-induced gains, more frequent workouts are needed to optimize gains in health and fitness.[5] In short, the adage "Use it or lose it" is true because you will lose strength gains if you do not progress your program over time and perform it on a regular basis.[10] Although consecutive days of heavy strength training for the same muscle groups are not recommended, regularly training each major muscle group two or three times per week with at least 48 hours separating training sessions for the same muscle group is needed to enhance muscular fitness.

Specificity

The principle of specificity refers to the distinct adaptations that take place as a result of the training program. In essence, every muscle or muscle group must be trained to make gains in muscular fitness (see figure 7.1 for the location of the major muscle groups in the body). Exercises such as the squat and leg press can be used to enhance lower-body strength, but these exercises will not affect upper-body strength. What's more, the adaptations that take place in a given muscle or muscle group will be as simple or as complex as the stress placed on them. For example, because tennis requires multijoint and multidirectional movements, it seems prudent for tennis players to perform resistance exercises that mimic the movements of the sport. For tennis players who need strong leg muscles to move across the court, lunges are unbeatable exercises to improve lower-body performance. Lunges performed in different directions actually simulate steps used in game situations.

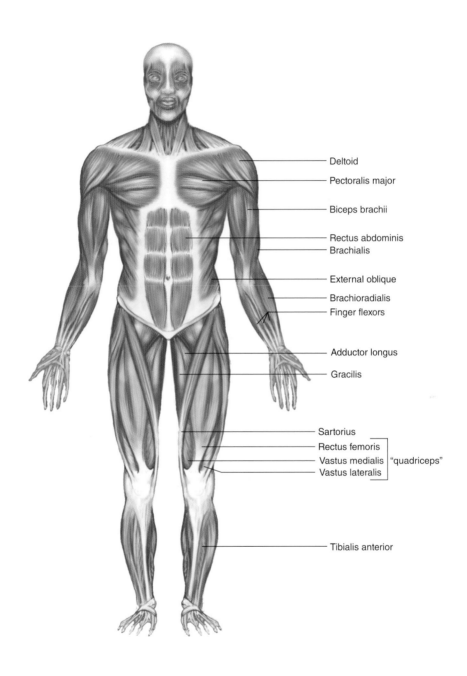

Deltoid

Pectoralis major

Biceps brachii

Rectus abdominis
Brachialis

External oblique

Brachioradialis
Finger flexors

Adductor longus

Gracilis

Sartorius
Rectus femoris
Vastus medialis } "quadriceps"
Vastus lateralis

Tibialis anterior

Figure 7.1a Major muscle groups in the body: front view.

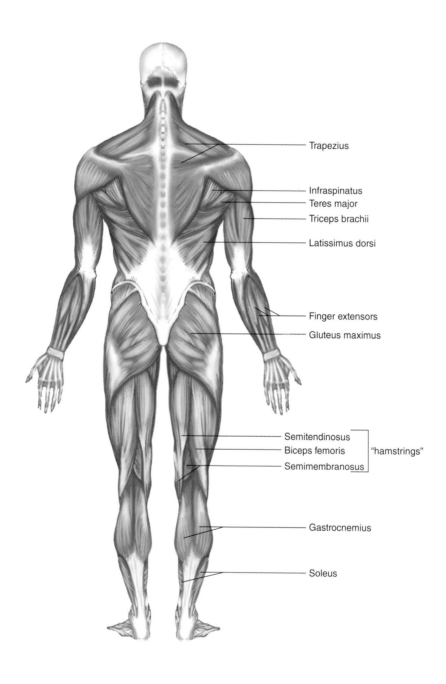

Trapezius

Infraspinatus
Teres major
Triceps brachii

Latissimus dorsi

Finger extensors
Gluteus maximus

Semitendinosus
Biceps femoris   "hamstrings"
Semimembranosus

Gastrocnemius

Soleus

Figure 7.1b Major muscle groups in the body: back view.

The specificity principle can also be applied to the design of resistance training programs for adults who want to enhance their abilities to perform activities of daily life such as stair climbing and household chores, which also require multijoint and multidirectional movements. For example, climbing stairs may be difficult as a result of poor lower-body strength. By sensibly progressing from single-joint exercises such as leg extensions to multijoint exercises such as leg presses and dumbbell squats, you can improve your stair-climbing ability. These multijoint exercises specifically strengthen the quadriceps and gluteals, which are used in stair climbing.

RESISTANCE TRAINING WORKOUT COMPONENTS

The general format of an aerobic training session (as described in chapter 6) can be applied to resistance training as well. Before beginning a session, you should perform a warm-up to prepare your muscles for the conditioning phase of the workout. The conditioning phase is the main focus, and you should follow it with a cool-down.

Warm-Up

The warm-up for resistance training should include 5 to 10 minutes of low- to moderate-intensity aerobic activities and muscular endurance activities (lower resistance with a higher number of repetitions, such as 15 to 20 reps). These activities will increase your body temperature and help reduce the potential for postexercise muscle soreness.[1]

Muscle Conditioning Phase

Despite various claims about what constitutes the best resistance training program, it does not appear that one optimal combination of sets, repetitions, and exercises will promote long-term adaptations in muscular fitness in everyone. Rather, you can alter many program variables to achieve desirable outcomes provided that you follow the fundamental training principles, as discussed in this chapter. The program variables to consider are choice of exercise, order of exercise, training weight (which determines the number of repetitions), number of sets, repetition velocity, and rest periods between sets and exercises (see *Resistance Training Guidelines for Healthy Adults*).

Exercise Choice

A limitless number of exercises can be used to enhance muscular fitness. Exercises can generally be classified as single-joint (i.e., body part specific) or multijoint (i.e., structural). The dumbbell biceps curl and leg extension are examples of single-joint exercises that isolate a specific body part (biceps and quadriceps, respectively), whereas the chest press and squat are multijoint exercises that involve two or more joints. Although it is important to incorporate multijoint exercises into a resistance training program, it is equally important to select exercises that are appropriate for your exercise technique experience and training goals. When learning any new exercise, start with a light weight to master the technique of the exercise before increasing the weight.

Your choice of exercise should also promote muscle balance across joints and between opposing muscle groups (e.g., quadriceps and hamstrings). Of particular importance is the inclusion of exercises for the abdominal and low back musculature. It is not uncommon for beginners to focus on strengthening the chest and biceps, and not spend adequate time strengthening the abdominals and low back. Strengthening the midsection, or trunk area, may not only enhance body control when performing free weight exercises such as the squat, but also reduce the risk of injury. The resistance training program suggestions in this chapter promote muscle balance by including the appropriate muscle groups (see table 7.2 on page 133 and figure 7.2 on page 131).

Exercise Order

There are many ways to arrange the sequence of exercises in a resistance training session. Traditionally, large-muscle group exercises are performed before smaller-muscle group exercises, and multijoint exercises are performed before single-joint exercises. Following this exercise order will allow you to use heavier weights on the multijoint exercises because fatigue will be less of a factor.

It is also helpful to perform more challenging exercises earlier in the workout when your neuromuscular system is less fatigued. In general, it seems reasonable to follow the priority system of training in which exercises that will most likely contribute to enhanced muscular fitness are performed early in the training session. The sample resistance training programs presented in this chapter include exercises that reflect this sequence (see table 7.2 on page 133 and figure 7.2 on page 131).

Number of Repetitions

One of the most important variables in the design of a resistance training program is the amount of weight used for an exercise.[5] Gains in muscular fitness are influenced by the amount of weight lifted, which is inversely related to the number of repetitions you can perform. As the weight increases, the number of repetitions you can perform decreases. Although you should never sacrifice proper form, the training weight should be challenging enough to result in at least a modest degree of muscle fatigue during the last few repetitions of a set. If this does not occur, you will not achieve the desired gains from your resistance training program.

Because heavy weights are not required to increase the muscular strength of beginners, weights corresponding to about 60% to 80% of the 1-repetition maximum (1RM) for 8 to 12 repetitions are recommended for untrained adults (10 to 15 repetitions for older adults) with limited resistance training experience.[1] Although weights that can be lifted for more than 15 times are effective for increasing local muscular endurance, light weights rarely result in meaningful gains in muscular strength. If you are a beginner, the best approach is to first establish a target repetition range (e.g., 8 to 12), and then by trial and error determine the maximum load you can handle for the prescribed number of repetitions.

Although it may take two or three workouts to find your desired training weight on all exercises, keep in mind that the magnitude of your effort will determine the outcome of your strength training program. For example, training within an 8RM to 12RM zone means that you should be able to perform no more than 12 repetitions with a given weight using proper exercise technique. Simply performing an exercise for 8, 9, 10, 11, or 12 repetitions does not necessarily mean you are training within the 8RM to 12RM zone. You should be stopping because of the onset of muscle fatigue, not just because you have reached a predetermined number.

Number of Sets

The number of sets performed in a workout is directly related to the overall training volume, which reflects the amount of time the muscles are being exercised. For beginners, even one set can provide benefits. Healthy adults should perform two to four sets for each muscle group to achieve muscular fitness goals.[1] Although single-set protocols can enhance your muscular strength if you are a beginner, multiple-set protocols have proven more effective in the long term.[7, 12] What's more, you do not need to perform every exercise for the same number of sets. As a general recommendation, perform more sets of large-muscle group exercises than of smaller-muscle group exercises.

It is also important to remember that using different combinations of sets and exercises varies the training stimulus, which is vital for long-term gains. For example, if you complete one set of two different exercises for the same muscle group (e.g., chest press and push-up), the pectoral muscles of the chest have performed two sets. From a practical standpoint, your personal goals and time demands should determine the number of sets you perform per muscle group.

Repetition Velocity

All exercises should be performed at a controlled, or moderate, velocity during the lifting and lowering phases. Movement control can be defined as the ability to stop any lifting or lowering action at will without momentum carrying the movement to completion. Uncontrolled, jerky movements not only are ineffective, but also may result in injury. Also, intentionally slow velocities with a relatively light weight (e.g., a five-second lifting phase and a five-second lowering phase) are not recommended because they provide a training stimulus that is less than optimal for enhancing muscle strength.[5] Strength exercises should be performed at a controlled velocity. Although different movement speeds have proven to be effective, if you are a beginner, you should perform each repetition at a moderate speed with about two seconds for the lifting phase and three seconds for the lowering phase. A longer lowering phase places more emphasis on the eccentric muscle action, which is important for strength development.

Rest Periods Between Sets and Exercises

The length of the rest period between sets and exercises is an important but often overlooked training variable. In general, the length of the rest period influences energy recovery and training adaptation. For example, if your primary goal is muscular strength, heavier weights and longer rest periods of two to three minutes are needed, whereas if your goal is muscular endurance, lighter weights and shorter rest periods of 30 to 60 seconds are required.[1] Obviously, the heavier the weight is, the longer the rest period should be if the training goal is to maximize strength gains.

Cool-Down

The cool-down brings the body systems back to resting levels. Just as the warm-up led into the conditioning phase, the cool-down helps to transition the body from the higher demands of the conditioning phase to the lower levels of physiological demand seen at rest. Shifting to moderate-intensity and then low-intensity aerobic and muscular endurance activity will lower your heart rate and blood pressure gradually and safely.[1]

Safety First

Your resistance training program should be based on your health status, fitness training experience, and goals. As discussed in chapter 2, you should assess your health status before participating in strength-building activities. In some cases, specialized exercise programs are needed for those with pre-existing medical conditions such as high blood pressure, heart disease, and diabetes. Thus, if you have a medical concern or issue, you should consult with your health care provider before resistance training.

Recognizing that resistance training to improve general fitness is different from training to enhance sport performance will further promote the development of and adherence to safe, effective, and enjoyable programs. If you have little experience with resistance training, you are strongly encouraged to seek instruction from a qualified fitness professional because most injuries are the result of improper exercise technique or excessive loading.[9] Qualified fitness professionals can provide instruction on proper warm-up procedures, offer advice on specific methods of progression, and monitor the magnitude of your effort, which, in turn, can have a positive impact on training adaptations.[8, 11]

(continued)

Knowing proper breathing techniques will help you avoid the Valsalva maneuver, which can occur if you hold your breath while lifting. Not exhaling can increase pressure in the chest cavity, which can increase blood pressure to harmful levels. To avoid this effect, continue to breathe normally by inhaling before you start the lift, exhaling during the lifting/exertion phase (as you lift against gravity), and then inhaling again as you return to the starting position. Using this technique will allow you to lift weight correctly and safely.

Following are general safety recommendations for designing and performing a resistance training program:

- *Maintain a regular breathing pattern when lifting and lowering weights.* Do not hold your breath; but rather, inhale before you start the lift, exhale during the lift, and inhale as you return to the starting position.

- *Make sure the exercise environment is well lit, clean, and free of clutter.* Tripping or falling over resistance training equipment can be avoided by following this guideline.

- *Learn proper exercise technique from a qualified fitness professional.* If you have little experience with resistance training, have someone with appropriate qualifications show you how to do resistance training exercises and to assist you with making any needed adjustments.

- *Perform warm-up and cool-down activities.* Taking time for warming up and cooling down helps your body to transition safely into and out of your workout.

- *Move carefully around the strength training area.* Resistance training by its nature is equipment intensive. Dumbbells, barbells, and weight plates are all potential tripping hazards.

- *Do not use broken or malfunctioning equipment.* Check for frayed belts or cables before using any resistance training machine. Fittings should be tight, and all belts and cables should be in good condition.

- *Use collars on all plate-loaded barbells and dumbbells.* Collars are devices placed on the ends of barbells and dumbbells to hold the individual weight plates in position. Without these fasteners in place, the weight plates could shift or even fall off, causing injury.

- *Be aware of proper spotting procedures when using free weights.* A spotter is a person who is in a position to assist you when you are using free weights. Because free weights are not supported by cables or any other devices, a spotter's role is to help guide or lift a weight if you have difficulty with the resistance.

- *Avoid jerky, uncontrolled movements while resistance training.* Maintaining controlled movements will maximize the benefits of your workout and also will help you avoid injury.

- *Periodically check all training equipment.* Checking equipment for cleanliness as well as any signs of wear-and-tear (e.g., frayed cables or belts) and making needed corrections will help keep your resistance training sessions safe and enjoyable.

- *Regularly clean equipment pads that come in contact with the skin.* Pads become soiled with sweat; maintaining a routine of wiping off contacted surfaces promotes good hygiene.

TYPES OF RESISTANCE TRAINING

Provided you adhere to the fundamental principles of training, you can use almost any type of resistance training to enhance muscular fitness. Some equipment is relatively easy to use; other equipment requires balance, coordination, and high levels of skill. A decision to use a certain type of resistance training should be based on your needs, goals, and training experience. Common types of resistance training involve the use of weight machines, free weights, body weight exercises, and a broadly defined category that involves the use balls, bands, and elastic tubing (table 7.1 summarizes the advantages and disadvantages of various types of resistance training). These types of resistance training typically include dynamic movements that involve a lifting (concentric) and lowering (eccentric) phase through a predetermined range of motion.

Weight machines train all the major muscle groups and can be found in most fitness centers. They are relatively easy to use because the exercise motion is controlled by the machine. For this reason, weight machines are a good option if you have not done resistance training before, are relatively new to this type of training, or are out of shape or deconditioned. Also, weight machines are ideal for isolating muscle groups. As a result, they often do not mimic sport activities as well as some free weight exercises do. For general health and convenience, however, they are outstanding. Although weight machines fit the typical male or female, smaller people may need a seat pad or back pad to adjust their body position to create a better fit.

Free weights, such as barbells and dumbbells, are inexpensive and can be used for a wide variety of exercises that require greater balance and coordination. Although it may take longer to master proper exercise technique using free weights compared to weight machines, proper fit is not an issue because one size fits all. Free weights also offer a greater variety of exercises than weight machines because they can be moved in many directions. Another important benefit of free weights is that they require the use of additional stabilizing and assisting muscles to hold the correct body position to perform an exercise correctly. As such, free weight training can occur in different planes of motion and is ideal for enhancing performance during activities of daily life. This is particularly true when using dumbbells because they train each side of the body independently. However, unlike weight machines, several

Table 7.1 Comparison of Various Types of Resistance Training

Type	Cost	Portability	Ease of use	Muscle isolation	Functionality	Exercise variety	Space requirement
Weight machines	High	Limited	Excellent	Excellent	Limited	Limited	High
Free weights	Low	Variable	Variable	Variable	Excellent	Excellent	Variable
Body weight	None	Excellent	Variable	Variable	Excellent	Excellent	Low
Balls and cords, or bands*	Very low	Excellent	Variable	Variable	Excellent	Excellent	Low

*Medicine balls, stability balls, and elastic cords, or bands

free weight exercises, such as the bench press, require the aid of a spotter who can assist the lifter in case of a failed repetition.

Body weight exercises such as push-ups, pull-ups, and curl-ups are some of the oldest modes of strength training. Obviously, a major advantage of body weight training is that equipment is not needed and a variety of exercises can be performed.

A CLOSER LOOK
Suzie and John

Suzie, the 55-year-old elementary school teacher who was first introduced in chapter 3, realized the benefit of resistance training as she was preparing for her 5K walk for charity. Because she doesn't have access to a fitness center, she purchased some resistance bands and ankle weights. With these relatively inexpensive purchases, in addition to exercises that just use her body weight, she is able to target the major muscle groups. As a beginner, she selected six exercises that she could do in the comfort of her home. After doing these exercises on a regular basis for a couple of months (typically on Tuesdays and Thursdays), she is feeling and looking better. She is now completing two sets of each exercise with 8 to 12 repetitions each. Her exercise program looks like this (descriptions and photos of these exercises can be found beginning on page 133):

- *Hips and legs:* Ankle weight hip flexion and extension or band leg lunge
- *Chest:* Band seated chest press or modified push-up
- *Back:* Band seated row
- *Shoulders:* Band upright row
- *Low back:* Prone plank or kneeling hip extension
- *Abdominals:* Curl-up

John, a 32-year-old accountant, who was also first introduced in chapter 3, has a membership at a local fitness center. He does his resistance training program two days per week and completes two sets of exercises with 8 to 12 repetitions. His program includes the use of resistance machines and free weights (dumbbells). Because he has been including resistance training consistently for about two years, he is maintaining his strength using the first option under the established level in the resistance training program from figure 7.2 (descriptions and photos of these exercises can be found beginning on page 133):

- *Hips and legs:* Machine leg press or dumbbell squat
- *Quadriceps:* Machine leg extension
- *Hamstrings:* Machine leg curl
- *Chest:* Machine or dumbbell chest press
- *Back:* Machine lat pull-down or machine seated row
- *Shoulders:* Machine overhead press or dumbbell lateral raise
- *Biceps:* Machine biceps curl or dumbbell biceps curl
- *Triceps:* Machine triceps press or dumbbell lying triceps extension
- *Low back:* Machine back extension
- *Abdominals:* Machine abdominal curl

Conversely, a limitation of body weight training is the difficulty in adjusting the body weight to the strength level of the person. Exercise machines that allow you to perform body weight exercises such as pull-ups and dips using a predetermined percentage of your body weight are available. Even if you do not have the strength to lift your entire body weight, these machines provide assistance allowing participants of all abilities to incorporate body weight exercises into their strength training programs and feel good about their accomplishments.

Stability balls, medicine balls, and elastic tubing are inexpensive, safe, and effective alternatives to weight machines and free weights. Stability balls are lightweight, inflatable balls (about 45 to 75 cm in diameter) that add the elements of balance and coordination to any exercise. Medicine balls come in a variety of shapes and sizes (about 2 lb to over 20 lb, or 1 kg to over 9 kg) and stress muscles as you hold, catch, and throw them.

Resistance Training That Works for You

A total-body resistance training workout is an effective way to improve muscular fitness and physical performance. Although resistance training programs that split the body into selected muscle groups are popular, a total-body workout performed two or three days per week on nonconsecutive days is appropriate for most people. Such a program gives you time to learn proper exercise technique and develop a fitness base for more advanced training. The idea is to start with a general resistance training program and gradually make it more specific as your strength and confidence improve.

Because the ultimate goal is the adoption of strength exercise as a lifestyle choice, your resistance training program should be consistent with your current fitness status and personal goals. In addition, you need to consider the time you have available for training, the equipment you can access, and your strength training experience. Consider the following questions before beginning a resistance training program:

- Do you have health concerns that may limit your participation in a resistance training program?
- Do you currently participate in an exercise program?
- How much resistance training experience do you have?
- What type of resistance training equipment is available at home or at your gym?
- How much time do you have for resistance training during the week?
- What are your specific training goals?
- Would individualized instruction from a qualified fitness profession be beneficial?

Once you have answered these questions, you are ready to design a safe, effective, and enjoyable resistance training program that is consistent with your goals. This chapter provides guidance whether you are just starting resistance training or are already doing resistance training and are looking for ways to continue to improve. To make continual gains in health and fitness, you must continue, progress, and modify your resistance training program.

Using a workout card to monitor your training progress can be very helpful. On the card, record the exercises, weight lifted, and number of repetitions and sets. It is also a good idea to exercise with a training partner or fitness instructor who can serve as a spotter on selected exercises and provide assistance when needed.

Training with elastic rubber cords, or bands, involves generating force to stretch the cord and then returning the cord in a controlled manner to its unstretched state. The more the cord is stretched, the greater the force needed to move through the range of motion. Different colors of cords reflect different amounts of resistance.

YOUR RESISTANCE TRAINING PROGRAM

Your resistance training program needs to take into account your current muscular fitness level. Beginner, intermediate, and more advanced sample programs are outlined in figure 7.2 (see page 133 for table 7.2, a workout guide that groups exercises into the appropriate body areas, as well as exercise descriptions and photos starting on page 134). If you have no resistance training experience or have not trained for several months or years, you should begin resistance training by following a general program in which weights are light to moderate and the focus is on learning proper exercise technique.

Avoid the common mistake of doing too much too soon. It is important to give your body a chance to adapt gradually to the physical stress of resistance training while making fitness gains. Use the initial months to increase your body's ability to tolerate the stress of resistance training gradually to minimize muscle soreness. The idea is to develop healthy habits early on so that resistance training becomes an enjoyable, meaningful, and long-lasting experience. Regardless of how much weight others can lift, go slowly during the first few weeks and months of resistance training as you build a foundation for more advanced training programs in the future.

As indicated in the sample programs in figure 7.2, if you are a beginner, you should perform one or two sets of six exercises with a moderate weight. Of course, regardless of your level of experience, you should use lighter loads when you are learning a new exercise or attempting to correct any flaws in your exercise technique. Also, keep in mind that you do not have to perform every exercise for the same number of sets. This preparatory period is designed to gradually enhance your physical abilities as you start the process of resistance training. If you have a very low level of fitness, you may need a longer period of time before you can participate in a resistance training program designed to maximize gains in muscular fitness. A major goal of this training phase is to learn correct form and technique for a variety of upper-body, lower-body, and midsection exercises while practicing proper training procedures. Table 7.2 outlines resistance training exercises that use weight machines, free weights (dumbbells), and your own body weight.

Once you are comfortable with the level of exercise at the beginner level, you are ready to move to the intermediate level. Typically, this takes around two to three months, although this time may be shorter or longer depending on your initial fitness level. The intermediate level begins once you have progressed through the beginner level, or you can start at this level if you are already engaging in some resistance training. The intermediate activities are broader in scope than the beginner activities and also increase the overall volume (increasing the number of exercises and sets). Depending on the consistency of your training, you may spend three months to a year or more at the intermediate level.

After a year of consistent training, you may appropriately be classified as "established." At this point you can continue with the intermediate-level exercise format but increase the weight, or resistance, over time (recall the concept of progressive overload). Figure 7.2 includes a "More advanced" category for those looking to increase their focus beyond health-related levels of resistance training. More advanced resistance training can provide additional muscular fitness benefits and includes exercises for different body parts on separate days of the week (thus increasing the overall training volume, and the time you spend training).

By varying the program variables such as the choice of exercise and number of sets, you will start to achieve specific goals in health and fitness. Although every workout does not need to be more intense than the previous one, varying your program helps to prevent boredom and training plateaus that eventually lead to a lack of adherence and dropout. As you perform additional sets, keep in mind that your effort determines your training outcomes. Thus, feelings related to exercise exertion should be an expected and welcome part of the training process. A major goal is to gain confidence in your ability to perform strength-building exercises while maximizing training adaptations.

FIGURE 7.2

Sample Resistance Training Programs

Stage*	Exercises**	Number of sets	Number of repetitions	Number of days per week***
Beginner	*Moving through this level typically takes about two to three months, although you should remain at this level until you feel comfortable enough to advance.*			
	Do a total of six exercises. Select *one* exercise from each of the following body areas: hips and legs, chest, back, shoulders, low back, and abdominals.	1–2	8–12 (10–15 for older adults)	2-3
Intermediate to established	*Moving through the intermediate to the established level typically takes 3 to 12 months depending on your level of consistency.*			
	Do a total of 10 exercises. Select *one* exercise from each of the following body areas: hips and legs, quadriceps, hamstrings, chest, back, shoulders, biceps, triceps, low back, and abdominals.	2	8–12 (10–15 for older adults)	2-3
More advanced (complete all 15 exercises)	Do a total of 10 exercises. Select *two* exercises from each of these larger muscle group areas: hips and legs, quadriceps, hamstrings, chest, and back.	2-3	8–12	2-3
	Do a total of 5 exercises. Select *one* exercise from each of these smaller-muscle group and trunk areas: shoulders, biceps, triceps, low back, and abdominals.	2	8–12	2-3

*The time spent at each stage will depend on your muscular fitness level. Transition slowly between the stages (e.g., over time a beginner can add additional exercises or increase the number of sets to move toward the intermediate level of resistance training).

** Different exercises can be performed on different days.

***Schedule your training days so that at least 48 hours separate training sessions that target the same muscle group.

After the first few months of resistance training, improvements in muscular fitness occur at a slower rate. People who started resistance training with great enthusiasm sometimes become disappointed when gains in muscle strength are less dramatic during the third month of training. You need to understand that a workout that was effective during the first few months of training may not be effective in the long term. In short, to make continual gains in muscular fitness and achieve specific health and fitness goals, you will need to work harder and engage in a more challenging training program. This is particularly important if you want to maximize gains in muscular fitness.

Because of the demands of training, you need to allow time for adequate recovery between workouts for the same muscle group. For example, more advanced lifters may perform a whole-body workout only twice per week or a greater number of sessions per week using a split routine in which only certain body areas are selected on a given day. In any case, all lifters should value the importance of adequate recovery between demanding resistance training workouts.

For continued gains in muscular fitness, you must sensibly alter your resistance training program over time so your body is continually challenged to adapt to the new demands.[10] To clarify, *every* workout does not need to be harder than the previous workout; rather, a systematic progression of the exercise program is needed for long-term gains in muscular fitness. Even though beginners will improve at a faster rate than more experienced lifters, manipulating the program variables every couple of weeks will limit training plateaus and reduce the likelihood that you become bored with your training program and lose your enthusiasm for resistance training.

Although improving at the same rate over the long term is not possible, you have to place greater demands on the musculoskeletal system gradually if you want to make steady gains in muscular fitness. In addition to increasing the amount of weight you lift, you can also progress your training program in other ways. You can perform additional repetitions with the current weight, add more sets to your program, and incorporate different types of equipment into the program to provide progressive overload. The key to long-term training success is to make gradual changes in the program to keep it effective, challenging, and fun.

Resistance training is an essential component of adult fitness programs and can offer observable health and fitness gains when properly performed and sensibly progressed over time. The importance of the training-induced changes from resistance training should not be underestimated because they can have a meaningful impact on your physical function and quality of life. Although many exercise options are available, resistance training programs based on sound training principles and consistent with your needs, goals, and abilities are most likely to result in favorable adaptations. In general, include resistance training two or three days per week (with 48 hours between sessions), do two to four sets of 8 to 12 repetitions of each exercise (10 to 15 repetitions for older adults), and target each of the major muscle groups.

RESISTANCE TRAINING EXERCISES

Descriptions and photos for each of the exercises in the sample programs are included here (see table 7.2 for a guide showing you which exercises work specific body areas). In general, the photos depict the two ends of the range of motion for each exercise. Be sure to control your movement to reap the full benefits from each exercise.

Table 7.2   Resistance Training Workout Guide

Body area	Exercise
Hips and legs (gluteals, quadriceps, hamstrings)	Machine leg press Dumbbell squat Ankle weight hip flexion and extension Band leg lunge
Legs (quadriceps)	Machine leg extension Ankle weight knee extension
Legs (hamstring)	Machine leg curl Ankle weight knee flexion
Chest (pectoralis)	Machine chest press Dumbbell chest press Band seated chest press Modified push-up Push-up
Back (latissiumus dorsi)	Machine lat pull-down Machine seated row Dumbbell one-arm row Band seated row
Shoulders (deltoid)	Machine overhead press Dumbbell lateral raise Dumbbell or band upright row
Arms (biceps)	Machine biceps curl Dumbbell or band biceps curl
Arms (triceps)	Machine triceps press Dumbbell lying triceps extension Band triceps extension
Low back (erector spinae)	Machine back extension Prone plank Kneeling hip extension
Abdominals	Machine abdominal curl Curl-up Diagonal curl-up

Machine Leg Press

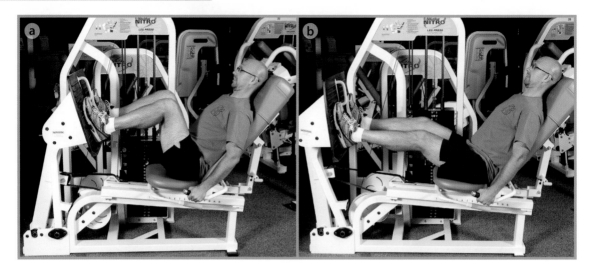

Adjust the machine so your knees are bent about 90 degrees, with feet flat on the foot pads (*a*). Your knees and feet should be in line with your hips. Exhale and push your feet and legs forward by pushing through your heels until your knees are nearly straight (*b*). Do not lock your knees.

Dumbbell Squat

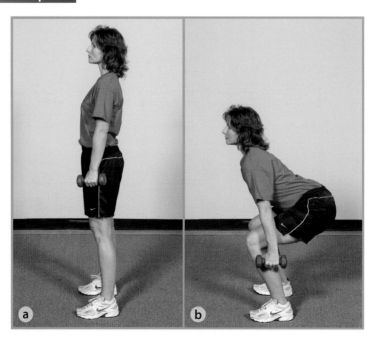

Choose your desired or appropriate dumbbell weights. Spread your feet about shoulder-width apart; your knees and feet should be in line with your hips (*a*). Bend slightly at the hips and then bend your knees until your thighs are parallel to the floor (*b*). Your knees should not go beyond your toes. Pause briefly; then return to the starting position. Keep your chest up throughout the movement to avoid excessive forward lean.

Ankle Weight Hip Flexion

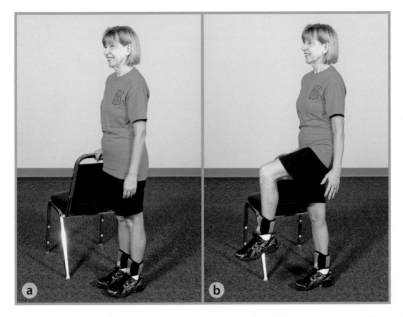

Ankle weights are needed for this exercise. Stand tall with one hand on the back of a chair for balance (*a*). Without leaning forward, lift one knee toward your chest in a marching motion (*b*), pause briefly, and then return your knee to the starting position and repeat on the opposite side.

Ankle Weight Hip Extension

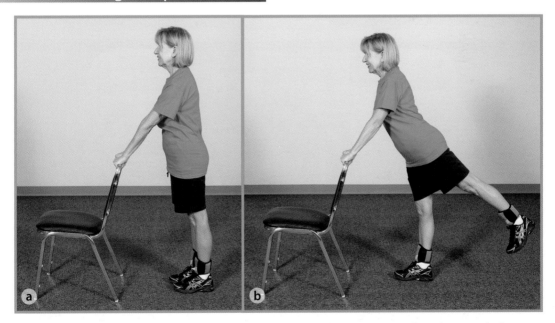

Ankle weights are needed for this exercise. Stand about 12 inches (30.5 cm) from a chair with your feet slightly apart. Bend forward slightly and hold on to the back of the chair for balance (*a*). Lift one leg backward without moving your upper body forward or bending your knee (*b*). Pause briefly; then return to the starting position and repeat on the opposite side.

Band Leg Lunge

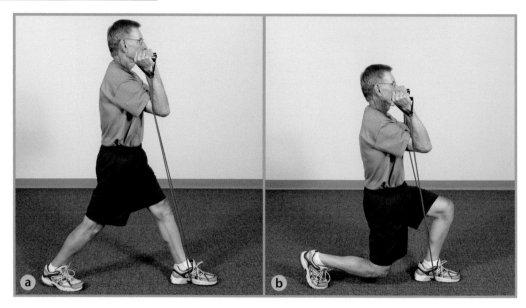

Start in a stride position with one foot in the middle of the band and the other foot extended behind your body. Pull the band tight by bending your elbows to allow your hands to be at shoulder height (*a*). Lower your body toward the floor while keeping your shoulders over your hips and your front knee over the ankle of your front foot (*b*). Return to the starting position and perform the desired number of repetitions. Repeat on the opposite side.

Machine Leg Extension

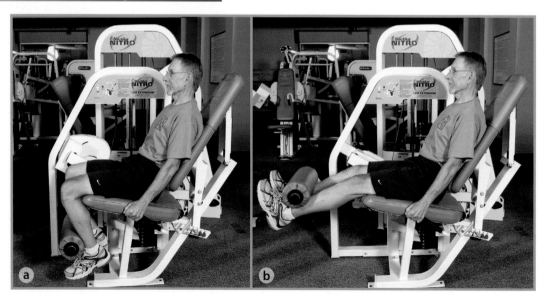

Adjust the machine so your knee joints are in line with the machine's axis of rotation and the leg pads are just above your ankles (*a*). Straighten both knees until they are fully extended (*b*), pause briefly, and then return to the starting position and repeat.

Ankle Weight Knee Extension

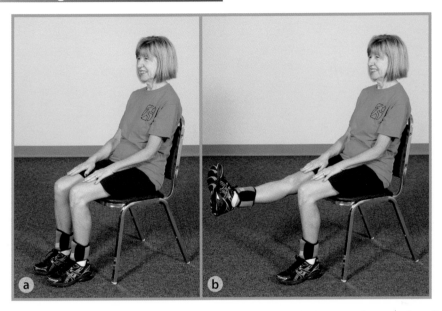

Ankle weights are needed for this exercise. Sit tall in a chair with your feet flat on the floor (*a*). Lift one leg by straightening your knee until the leg is parallel to the floor (*b*). Pause briefly; then return your leg to the starting position and repeat on the opposite side.

Machine Leg Curl

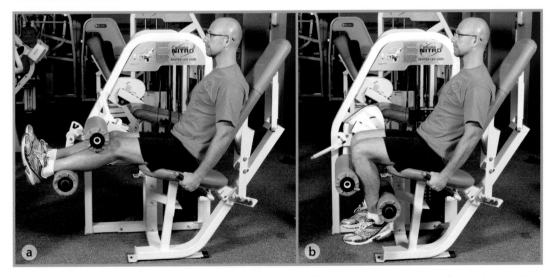

Adjust the machine so your knees are in line with the machine's axis of rotation and the roller pads are under your ankles (*a*). Grasp both handles. Pull the roller pad toward your hips until both knees are bent at least 90 degrees (*b*). Pause briefly; then return to the starting position and repeat.

Ankle Weight Knee Flexion

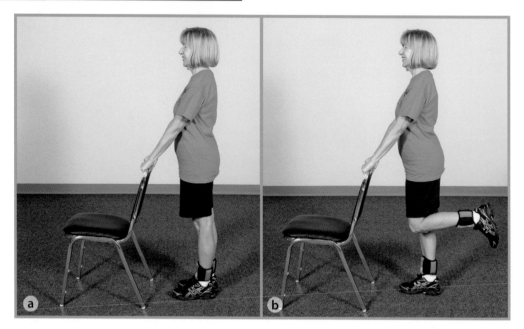

Ankle weights are needed for this exercise. While wearing ankle weights, stand tall behind a chair and grasp the chair back (*a*). Bend one knee and raise your foot toward your buttocks without moving your thigh (*b*). Pause briefly; then return to the starting position. Repeat on the other side.

Machine Chest Press

Adjust the seat so that the handles are aligned at midchest level. Sit with your back against the seat pads and grasp the bar handles with an overhand grip (*a*). Push the handles forward until your elbows are straight and fully extended but not locked (*b*). Pause briefly; then return the handles to the starting position and repeat.

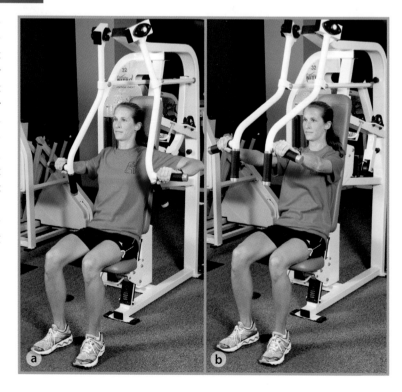

Dumbbell Chest Press

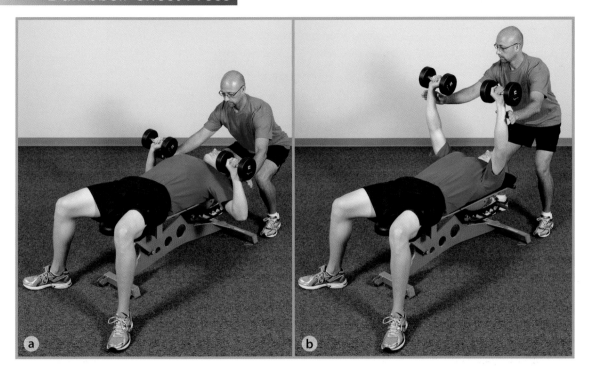

Choose your desired or appropriate dumbbell weight. Lie on a bench with your knees bent and your feet flat on the floor. Your head, shoulders, back, and buttocks must maintain contact with the bench during the exercise. Hold the dumbbells at the side of your chest with your thumbs wrapped around the handles and your elbows bent about 90 degrees (*a*). Press the dumbbells upward over your chest until your arms are straight (*b*). Return to the starting position and repeat. A spotter should be nearby to assist you if needed.

Band Seated Chest Press

Choose a band color or thickness. Sit in a chair and wrap the band around the back of the chair. Hold the ends of the band at chest level with your elbows bent (*a*). The band tension should be tight. Press both arms straight out in front of your body (*b*). Pause briefly; then return to the starting position and repeat.

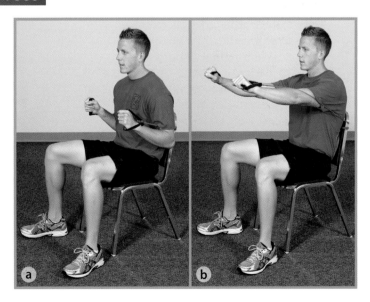

Modified Push-Up

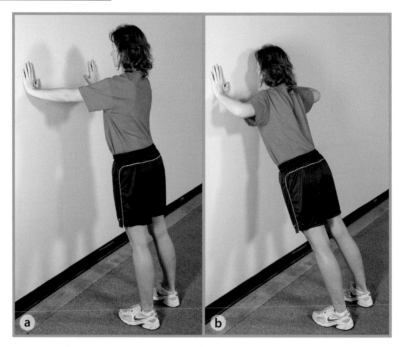

Stand 2 to 3 feet (61–91 cm) from a wall and place your palms on the wall at shoulder height (*a*). Your palms should be placed slightly wider than your shoulders. Keeping your back straight, bend your elbows until your nose almost touches the wall (*b*). Pause briefly; then press away from the wall and return to the starting position. Moving your feet farther away from the wall increases the difficulty of this exercise. As you gain more strength in your upper body, progress to bent-knee push-ups on the floor (see figure 2.10 on page 37 of chapter 2), and finally to full push-ups (see figure 2.9 on page 37 of chapter 2).

Machine Lat Pull-Down

Adjust the seat height and extend your arms overhead to grasp the bar (*a*). Your palms should face forward with your hands slightly wider than shoulder width. Lean back slightly, and pull the bar downward to the top of your chest (*b*). Tuck your chin to allow the bar to freely pass in front of your face. Focus on pulling your elbows in toward your body. Return to the starting position and repeat.

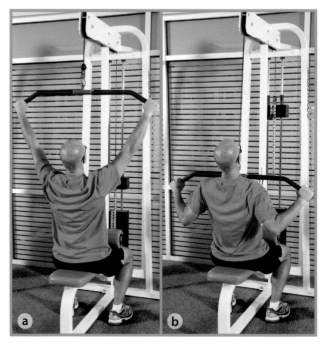

Machine Seated Row

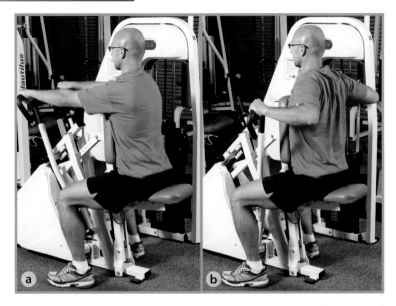

Move the seat so your shoulders are level with the machine handles and your chest is against the chest pad. Grasp the handles and sit tall with your chest up (*a*). Pull the handles backward while moving your shoulder blades together (*b*). Return to the starting position and repeat.

Dumbbell One-Arm Row

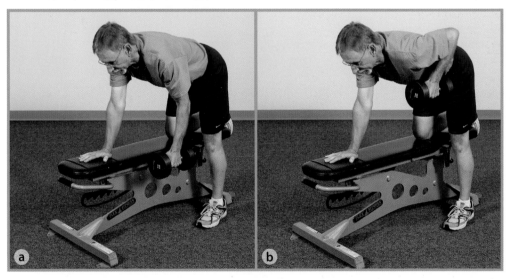

Choose your appropriate or desired dumbbell weight. Stand near the left side of the bench and place your right knee and the palm of your right hand on the bench, keeping your right arm straight and your torso almost horizontal. Hold the dumbbell in your left hand with your palm toward the bench (*a*). Pull the dumbbell toward the side of your chest by bending at the elbow and the shoulder (*b*). Return to the starting position and perform the desired number of repetitions. Repeat on the opposite side.

Band Seated Row

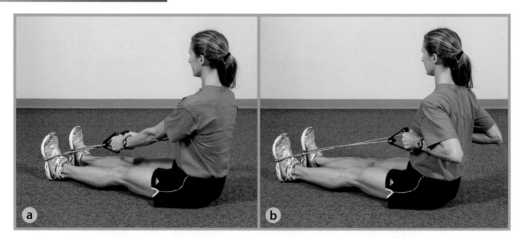

Choose a band color or thickness. Sit on the floor and wrap the band securely around both feet. The middle of the band should be placed at the center of your feet. Fully straighten your elbows with your palms facing each other (*a*). The band tension should be tight in both your hands. Pull the band toward the side of your body while keeping your back straight (*b*). Pause briefly; then return to the starting position and repeat.

Machine Overhead Press

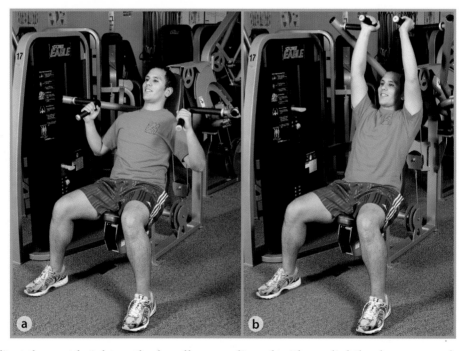

Adjust the seat height so the handles are aligned with or slightly above your shoulders. Grasp the handles and sit up straight with your head, shoulders, and back against the pad and your feet flat on the floor (*a*). Push the weight up over your head until your arms are fully extended but not locked (*b*). Pause briefly and return to the starting position.

Dumbbell Lateral Raise

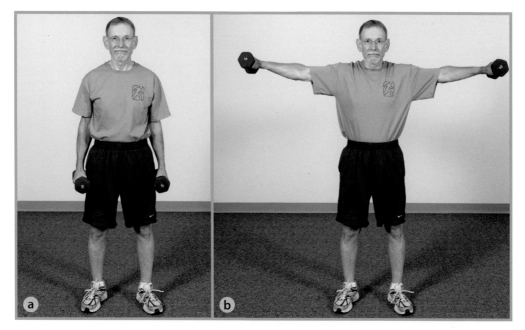

Choose your appropriate or desired dumbbell weight. Stand with your feet shoulder-width apart. Hold a dumbbell at the side of your body with your palms facing in and your elbows slightly bent (*a*). Raise both arms out to the sides until they are horizontal (*b*). Pause briefly; then return to the starting position and repeat.

Dumbbell Upright Row

Stand tall with your feet shoulder-width apart. Hold a dumbbell in each hand with your palms facing your thighs and your elbows pointing outward (*a*). Bend at the elbows and lift both dumbbells to shoulder level (*b*). Keep your elbows pointed outward during the upward movement. Pause briefly; then lower the weights to the starting position and repeat.

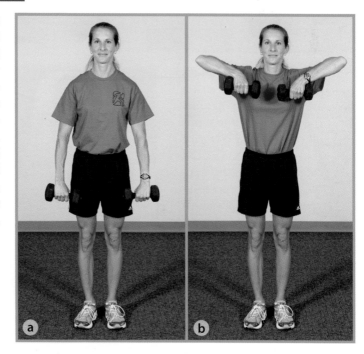

Band Upright Row

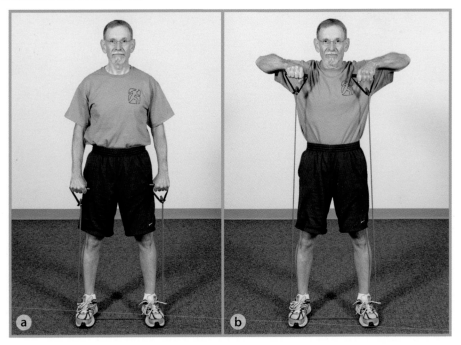

Choose your appropriate or desired band. Stand with both feet placed about shoulder-width apart on top of the band. Grasp one end of the band in each hand and stand erect (*a*). Your palms should be facing your thighs, and the band tension should be tight. Bend at the elbows and pull the band to shoulder level (*b*). Keep your elbows pointed outward during the upward movement. Pause briefly; then lower your arms to the starting position and repeat.

Machine Biceps Curl

Adjust the seat height so your upper arms are resting flat against the arm pad and your elbow is aligned with the machine's axis of rotation. Grasp the handles firmly and position your body so your chest is up and your shoulders are back (*a*). Curl your hands toward your shoulders until your elbows are fully flexed (*b*). Return to the starting position and repeat.

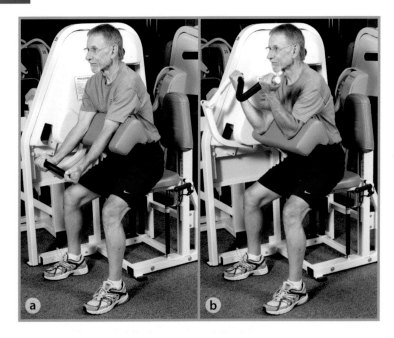

Dumbbell Biceps Curl

Choose your appropriate or desired dumbbell weights. Stand tall with your feet shoulder-width apart. Hold the dumbbells with your palms facing forward and your elbows at the sides of your body (*a*). Raise both dumbbells by bending your elbows until they are fully flexed (*b*). Keep your elbows at your sides during the entire movement. Lower the dumbbells to the starting position and repeat. This exercise can also be performed in a seated position with alternating arms.

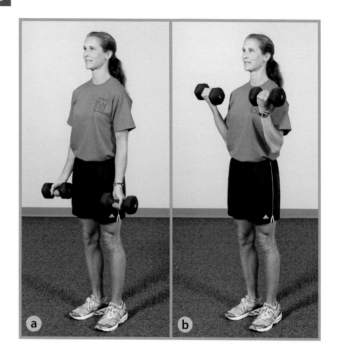

Band Biceps Curl

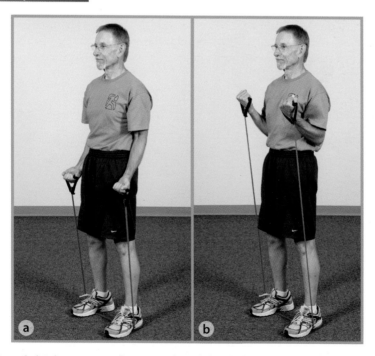

Choose a band thickness or color. Stand with both feet placed about shoulder-width apart on top of the band. Grasp one end of the band in each hand and stand erect (*a*). Your palms should be facing forward, and the band tension should be tight. Bend your elbows until they are fully flexed (*b*). Keep your elbows at your sides during the entire lift. Lower your arms to the starting position and repeat. This exercise can also be performed in a seated position with alternating arms.

Machine Triceps Press

Adjust the seat height so your upper arms are resting flat against the arm pad and your elbows are aligned with the machine's axis of rotation. Grasp the handles and position your body so your chest is up and your shoulders are back (*a*). Move the handles until your elbows are fully extended but not locked (*b*). Return to the starting position and repeat.

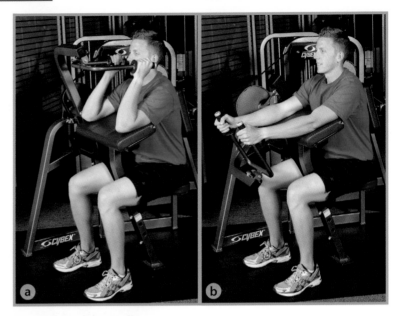

Dumbbell Lying Triceps Extension

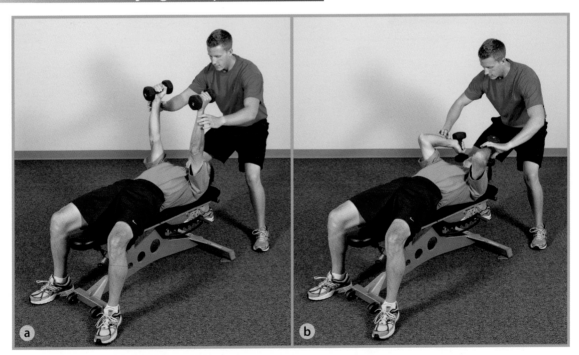

Choose an appropriate or desired dumbbell weight. Lie on a bench with your knees bent and your feet flat on the floor. Your head, shoulders, back, and buttocks must maintain contact with the bench during this exercise. Hold a dumbbell in each hand with your thumb wrapped around the dumbbell and both arms fully extended above your shoulders (*a*). Bend your elbows and slowly lower the dumbbells toward (but not touching) the side of your head (*b*). Return to the starting position and repeat. A spotter should be nearby to assist you if needed.

Band Triceps Extension

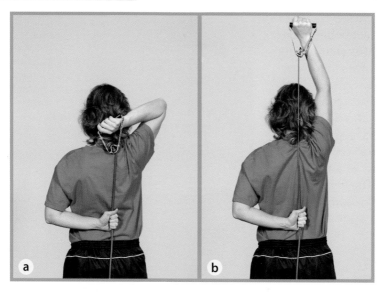

Choose a band thickness or color. Stand straight with your feet about shoulder-width apart. Hold one end of the band in your left hand placed near your low back and the other end in your right hand placed behind your neck (*a*). Move your arm up so the right elbow straightens overhead without moving your left arm (*b*). Pause briefly; then slowly return your right hand to the starting position and perform the desired number of repetitions. Repeat on the opposite side.

Machine Back Extension

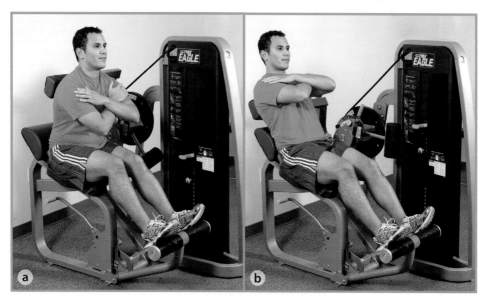

Adjust the seat so your navel is aligned with the machine's axis of rotation. Sit with your back against the pad, your feet on the foot pad, and your arms folded across your chest (*a*). Slowly extend your torso until your back is nearly straight (*b*). Pause briefly; then return to the starting position and repeat.

Prone Plank

Lie facedown on the floor with your feet behind your body. Support your weight on your knees and forearms (*a*). Keep your back flat and your head in line with your torso. Breathe normally as you hold the position for the desired number of seconds. To increase difficulty, lift your knees and support your weight on your toes and forearms (*b*).

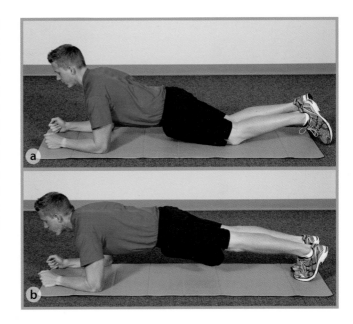

Kneeling Hip Extension

Kneel down in the crawl position with your arms directly below your shoulders (*a*). Extend your right leg backward until it is parallel to the floor while keeping your shoulders and hips level (*b*). Pause briefly; then return to the starting position and repeat on the opposite side.

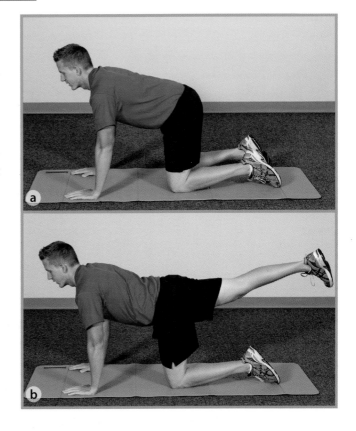

Machine Abdominal Curl

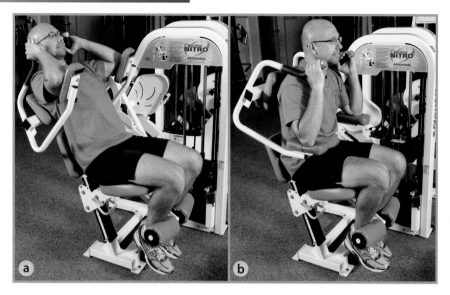

Adjust the seat so your navel is aligned with the machine's axis of rotation (*a*). Curl your torso forward while fully flexing your trunk (*b*). Pause briefly; then return to the starting position and repeat.

Curl-Up

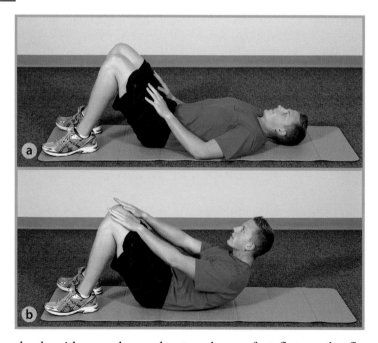

Lie on your back with your knees bent and your feet flat on the floor (*a*). Place your hands on your thighs. Curl your shoulders and upper back off the floor while sliding your hands up your thighs toward your kneecaps (*b*). Your low back should remain in contact with the floor. Pause briefly; then return to the starting position and repeat.

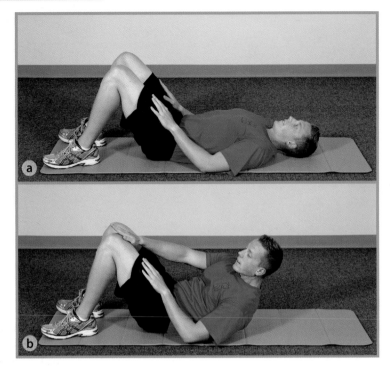

Lie on your back with your knees bent and your feet flat on the floor (*a*). Place your hands on your thighs. Curl your shoulders and upper back off the floor while sliding your right hand toward your left kneecap (*b*). Your low back should remain in contact with the floor. Pause briefly; then return to the starting position and repeat on the opposite side.

chapter 8

Flexibility and Balance

Flexibility may not have the same health benefits as aerobic or muscular fitness, but it *is* an important part of your overall physical fitness. Many activities require flexibility (e.g., golfing, swimming, dancing), and daily activities are also affected by flexibility (e.g., reaching, bending, twisting). Although distinct from flexibility, balance also plays a role in daily functioning and, in addition to the value in various sport activities, is specifically recommended for anyone at an increased risk of falls.

FLEXIBILITY

Flexibility is the ability of a joint and surrounding muscle to move through its full or optimal range of motion.[5] Improving range of motion at a joint eliminates awkward and inefficient movements, allowing you to move more fluidly.[4] You can appreciate this throughout your day-to-day activities and in any recreation or sports you may do. Maintaining or improving your range of motion through flexibility exercises will help you move more efficiently. For example, if you improve range of motion in your hips and hamstring muscle groups, which are located at the back of your thighs, you can ease the task of reaching down to pick up a grocery bag or bending over to tie your shoes as well as increase your stride when jogging or running.

Several factors influence flexibility, including age, sex, joint structure, and physical activity level.[4] Females tend to have a slightly greater range of motion at most joints than males do throughout life. This is usually explained by differences in joint structure and is often observed in joints in the upper body (e.g., shoulders, elbows, wrists, neck), with the exception of the trunk, in which males tend to have a greater range of motion than females.[7] Flexibility typically decreases with age, resulting in many significant changes in the neck, shoulder, and trunk region.[7] You can minimize these changes by adhering to a regular stretching program. Specific activities you can incorporate into your stretching routine are outlined in this chapter.

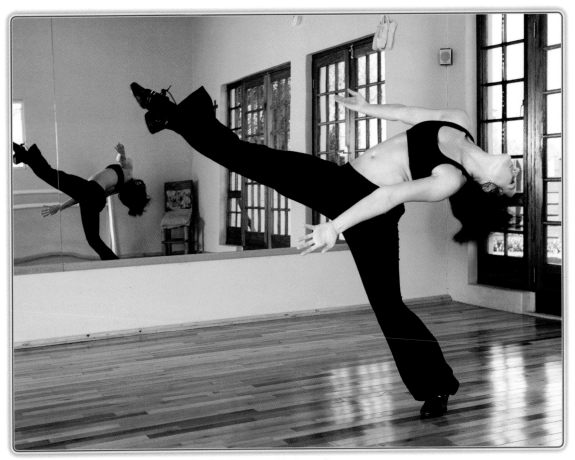

Flexibility does not have to reach this level to provide benefits.

Health and Fitness Benefits of Flexibility

Compared to less active people, active people have greater flexibility in the joints they use.[8] For example, people who walk more tend to have greater flexibility in their hips and spine than people who walk less. On the contrary, limited motion of a specific joint can lead to a loss in flexibility. If you spend several hours per day driving or sitting at a computer, you may find that your shoulders round forward as a result of decreased range of motion at your shoulder joints. A focus on stretching and body position can help you avoid such losses in flexibility and allow you to keep a strong upright posture.

In addition, improvements in flexibility may enhance performance in certain skills that require greater flexibility (e.g., dancing, golf).[6] However, unless you have poor flexibility at a specific joint, increasing flexibility beyond a normal range of motion does not benefit performance or decrease the risk of injury. Contrary to popular belief, there is not sufficient evidence to support the contention that pre-exercise stretching prevents injury or that pre- and postexercise stretching prevents muscle soreness.[8] However, you may experience relaxation or stress relief from participating in flexibility-focused exercises.

Flexibility Program Components

Flexibility, like resistance training, is specific to the muscle groups and joints that are stretched. Thus, it is important to target all the major muscle groups (see figure 7.1 on pages 120-121 for the location of the major muscle groups in the body).

   A flexibility routine should be completed after a thorough warm-up of at least five minutes or after a cardiorespiratory or resistance training session. Increasing the temperature of the muscle increases its ability to stretch. As a simple analogy, compare a rubber band you have held in your hand (warm) compared to one taken from your refrigerator (cold and stiff). In a similar way, warm muscles have a greater elastic response than cold muscles do.[2] The FITT principle can be applied to your flexibility program, including the frequency, intensity, time, and type of stretching activities.

Frequency

To improve flexibility, perform flexibility exercises at least two to three days per week for a minimum of 10 minutes.[2] Note that this is considered a minimum; stretching on a daily basis as part of a warm-up or cool-down would also be appropriate.

Intensity

The question of how far to stretch (i.e., the intensity of the stretch) is a common one. Typically, stretching exercises are done to the point of mild tightness without discomfort within the range of motion of the joint(s).[2] If a given stretch creates discomfort, release slightly—a stretch should not be painful. Over time, you may be able to move the joint farther as your flexibility improves, but the stretch should never cause pain. If it does, back off slightly.

Time

The time spent in each stretching session should be at least 10 minutes.[2] This will allow you to target the major muscle groups in the body with at least four repetitions of each stretch.

Type

Two of the most common methods of stretching to improve flexibility are static and dynamic. Both methods involve moving a joint or joints to the end of the range of motion. With static stretching, the position is held, whereas dynamic stretching involves continuous movement of the joint(s). Static stretching is more commonly used after an activity because some activities requiring strength, power, or endurance may be impaired by static stretching before the activity.[2] Dynamic stretching can be done before activity, following a general warm-up of the muscles.

Static   Static stretching is undoubtedly the most common method used to improve flexibility. Static stretching consists of slowly moving a joint to the point at which you feel tension and then holding that stretch for 15 to 60 seconds.[2] Remember, do not place your joints in any position that causes pain. As you hold the stretch, the tension should lessen as the muscle lengthens. Each static stretch should be repeated four times.

Dynamic   Dynamic stretching involves moving parts of your body through a full range of motion while gradually increasing the reach and speed of the movement in a controlled manner. An example of this is arm circles; you begin with small, slow circles and gradually progress to larger and faster circles until you reach the full range of motion of the shoulder joint. Many people think dynamic stretching involves bouncing or jerking motions—it does not! The goal is to move the joint in a controlled manner within a normal range of motion in order to minimize the risk of injury.[4] To avoid the muscle soreness that often results from novel movements, introduce dynamic stretches into your stretching program gradually, particularly if you are not accustomed to this type of stretching. Dynamic movements are typically repeated 5 to 12 times with a time frame that varies depending on the motion (approximately 30 to 60 seconds).

A CLOSER LOOK
Lydia

Lydia, a 53-year-old office manager, caught her reflection in a storefront window and was dismayed to see how her shoulders were slumped forward and her walking gait was choppy. As a child, she had participated in gymnastics on a recreational level and had always been proud of her strong upright posture and confident stride. Years of work at her computer terminal, leaning forward to review detailed accounting files, and lack of attention to flexibility had resulted in this unwanted transformation. Lydia already does five days per week of stationary biking and also includes resistance training at least two mornings per week in her family's small home gym. She now realizes the importance of also including stretching in her activity program. She includes stretches for all the major muscle groups with some extra focus on stretches for her neck, shoulders, and hips.

Your Flexibility Program

Stretching can be done anytime a muscle is warmed up and should be included before sports or activities requiring a high degree of flexibility. Stretching can be included before or after the conditioning phase of general fitness activities. Although not conclusive, some research suggests that static stretching could interfere with sports that require muscular strength, power, or endurance.[2] Thus, in the following sample programs, dynamic stretching follows the warm-up (before the conditioning phase of the workout) and static stretching is part of the cool-down.

Sample Stretching Program After a Warm-Up

After a thorough warm-up, dynamic stretches can be performed to improve the efficiency of the movements you will do during your conditioning period of cardiorespiratory or resistance training. Dynamic stretches should begin with small ranges of motion and progress to larger ranges of motion. You should repeat each movement 5 to 12 times or move continuously for 30 to 60 seconds. Figure 8.1 on page 156 outlines a dynamic stretching program you can use after a warm-up.

Flexibility Stretches to Avoid

Many stretches that have been accepted in the past have been found to cause unnecessary strain on the joints and muscles.[1] Although not everyone engaging in these activities will incur injury, it is sensible to avoid certain stretches and focus on those included at the end of this chapter beginning on page 161. Table 8.1 lists a few stretches to avoid and suggested alternatives.

Table 8.1 Stretches to Avoid and Suggested Alternatives

Stretch to Avoid		Reason to avoid	Alternative Stretch
Standing toe touch		May strain the lower back	Seated hamstring stretch, page 168
Hurdler stretch		May put strain on the bent knee	Prone quadriceps stretch, page 169
Overrounding of the back		May stress the neck and low back	Pillar/overhead reach (with slight torso rotation to involve trunk muscles), page 162
Hyperextension of the back		Ineffective at stretching the abdominal muscles and may put stress on the back	
Full neck circle		Hyperextends the neck	Forward and lateral flexion, page 161

In some situations, stretching a muscle may not be appropriate. For example, if a muscle or joint has been injured, stretching exercises would typically be postponed unless prescribed as part of a treatment plan by a health care provider.

FIGURE 8.1

Sample Dynamic Stretching Program

Body part	Stretch*
Arms and shoulders	Arm circle Shoulder shrug
Hips and buttocks	Pendulum leg swing (front/back, side/side) Hip internal and external rotation Side shuffle
Quadriceps	Butt kick
Hamstrings	High knee
Ankles	Dynamic foot range of motion
Full body	Soldier walk Wood chop

*The description and photos of these stretches can be found at the end of the chapter, beginning on page 161.

Stretching Program After a Conditioning Period

After a conditioning period, use static stretching to improve your flexibility. Figure 8.2 outlines a sample progressive static stretching program. When you begin a flexibility program, start with level 1 stretches, which are the most basic. Begin by holding static stretches for 15 seconds and slowly progress to holding the final position for up to 60 seconds, repeating each stretch two to four times. Once you are comfortable with level 1 stretches, progress to level 2 and then to level 3 stretches. The progression of certain stretching exercises (e.g., quadriceps) moves from a lying to seated to standing position. As you move through these levels, you will need more balance to perform the exercise.

If you are having trouble placing your body in the required positions, you can use a towel to provide some extension. For example, when doing the triceps stretch with the elbow behind the head (see page 165), you could hold a towel in the hand of the arm you are stretching and provide assistance with the stretch by gently pulling on the towel with the other hand placed behind your back rather than on the elbow. When using a stretching aid, be careful not to jerk or pull your limb into an awkward or painful position.

BALANCE

Balance is the ability to control your body's movement, or equilibrium, whether it is stationary (static balance) or moving (dynamic balance). Your ability to control your movement is based on input from your ears, eyes, skin pressure receptors (e.g., the ability of your feet to feel the ground), muscle and joint receptors, and brain.[3] A balance activity is any activity that increases your ability to maintain a controlled body position when your stability is challenged. Picture a skateboarder executing a complex spinning move and maintaining his body position on the skateboard as he continues down the sidewalk. A simple exercise that challenges stability is walking on your heels instead of your entire foot.

FIGURE 8.2

Sample Progressive Static Stretching Program

Body part	Stretches by level of progression*		
	Level 1	Level 2	Level 3
Neck	Forward flexion Lateral flexion	Forward flexion Lateral flexion	Forward flexion Lateral flexion
Shoulders	Arms across chest	Arms across chest	Arms across chest
Upper back	Arm hug	Kneeling cat	Pillar/overhead reach
Low back	Supine rotational stretch	Supine rotational stretch	Supine rotational stretch
Chest	Chest stretch	Chest stretch (progression)	Chest stretch (progression)
Triceps	Elbow behind the head	Elbow behind the head	Elbow behind the head
Biceps	Wall stretch	Wall stretch	Wall stretch
Hips and glutes	Seated hip rotator stretch Butterfly stretch Kneeling hip flexor stretch	Supine hip rotator stretch Butterfly stretch Standing hip flexor stretch	Supine hip rotator stretch Butterfly stretch Standing hip flexor stretch
Hamstrings	Seated hamstring stretch	Standing hamstring stretch	Standing hamstring stretch
Quadriceps	Prone quadriceps stretch	Side-lying quadriceps stretch	Standing quadriceps stretch
Calves	Seated calf stretch	Standing calf step stretch	Standing calf step stretch

*The descriptions and photos of these stretches can be found at the end of the chapter, beginning on page 161.

Health and Fitness Benefits of Good Balance

Athletes benefit from greater balance in sporting endeavors, and so can you. Through the day you are constantly responding to changing environmental conditions around you, such as uneven sidewalks, jostling crowds, or a fast-approaching tennis ball. For older adults, balance training has been shown to improve balance and stability, decrease the fear of falling, decrease the incidence of falls, and increase the ability to participate in activities of daily living.[9] Thus. the U.S. government's *Physical Activity Guidelines for Americans* recommends balance training three or more days per week for older adults.[10] The ultimate benefit, regardless of your age, is feeling confident in your ability to move throughout your day without the risk of injury. Such a feeling leads to a greater involvement in daily physical activity and mobility.

Balance Workout Components

To improve your balance, you need to be challenged. As with aerobic exercise, resistance training, and flexibility, you need to consider frequency, intensity, time, and type (FITT).

George, a 65-year-old man who was first introduced in chapter 2, found that his flexibility was lower than he hoped after completing the sit-and-reach test. He hopes to improve in this area and thus has begun a stretching program after his bike ride home from work on Mondays, Wednesdays, and Fridays. He started out following the level 1 stretches outlined in figure 8.2. He finds the time he spends stretching to be a great way to relax after a long day at work. In addition, over the past month he has found that his movements while biking as well as when just moving around during the day seem easier.

Because George is older, he also has included some balance exercises on Tuesdays and Thursdays. He completes level 2 activities from figure 8.3, such as the seated chair lean with arm and leg movements, the standing stance with forward and backward sway and lateral sway, the forward and backward walking with wide and narrow stance, and the side step on heels and toes. As with his stretching program, he finds that these activities not only help him with his physical balance but also serve as a time to clear his mind from the pressures of the workday.

Frequency

Balance and stability exercises should be performed at least two to three days per week to help prevent falls and improve mobility.[2]

Intensity

When beginning a balance and stability program, start with seated activities before progressing to standing or moving activities. The less stable your body position is, the greater the challenge is to your ability to balance. Seated activities have the most support and thus provide less challenge than do activities in which you are standing or moving. Once you have successfully performed an exercise for several sessions, you can increase the difficulty, or challenge, by narrowing your stance, closing one or both eyes, or engaging in an additional task (e.g., reading, turning your head, catching a ball). When progressing to a more difficult level of an exercise, make sure to add only one extra challenge at a time to ensure safety and success.

Time

The time required for balance training will vary, but plan for about 10 to 15 minutes per session to allow you to include a variety of balance exercises. In general, each activity should be done for 10 to 30 seconds as a starting point. If you cannot maintain a particular position for that long, just hold the position as long as you can.

Type

Balance activities can be subdivided into activities that challenge your stability in a forward and backward motion and activities that challenge your stability in a side-to-side, or lateral, motion. The necessity of stability in multiple directions is obvious in sports and recreational activities. Basketball, baseball, and soccer are competitive sports in which the body must constantly respond to changing directions and even contact from other players. In a similar way, other sports such as bowling and golf also require balance as the body moves and twists. Of course, even daily tasks such as household chores and yardwork also call on your body to be in a constant state of balance. For example, a simple task such as vacuuming includes both forward and backward movement as well as side-to-side movements as you move across a room. Because of the many directions in which your body moves, you should choose exercises from both categories to enhance stability and improve balance.

Your Balance Program

Figure 8.3 outlines a sample balance and stability training program. When you begin your program, start with level 1 for seated, standing, and moving activities.

FIGURE 8.3

Sample Progressive Balance Program

	Level 1	Level 2	Level 3	Challenge
Seated balance activities*	Seated chair lean	Add arm movements: • Raise one arm at a time to the front and then to the sides • Raise both arms to the front and then to the sides	Combine arm and leg movements	• Sit on a pillow • Sit on a stability ball • Close one eye • Close both eyes • Turn your head to the right and then to the left
		Add leg movements: • Raise one knee at a time • Raise one leg (straightened) at a time		
Standing balance activities*	Upright stance (four variations: wide stance, narrow stance, semitandem, tandem)	In all four variations, add: • Forward and backward sway • Lateral sway (side to side)	Add arm movements to sway: • Raise one arm at a time to the front and then to the sides • Raise both arms to the front and then to the sides	• Close one eye • Close both eyes • Turn your head to the right and then to the left • Hold an item, such as a book
Movement balance activities	Walk forward and backward	• Wide-stance walk • Narrow-stance walk • Walk on heels • Walk on toes	• Tandem walk forward and backward • Walk while carrying an item • Walk with head turns	• Barefoot • One eye closed • Recite a poem • Surface change (mat, sand, etc.) • Obstacles
	Walk side to side	• Sidestep on heels • Sidestep on toes • Turn in a circle	• Sidestep while carrying an item • Sidestep with head turns • Crossover walk: cross one foot over the other foot	

*The descriptions and photos of these activities can be found at the end of the chapter, beginning on page 161.

Once you have successfully completed level 1 for at least two sessions, then move on to level 2, which builds on the basic activities from level 1. When you feel comfortable with the level 2 activities for at least two sessions, consider adding some level 3 options. You can add challenge activities to any level, but add only one challenge at a time to ensure safety.

To maintain your flexibility and move efficiently throughout your life, you should strive to participate in a stretching program at least two to three days per week. Typically, about 10 minutes of stretching is required to target all the major muscle groups. Static stretches should be held 15 to 60 seconds with about four repetitions of each stretch. For dynamic stretches, include 5 to 12 repetitions or continuous movement for 30 to 60 seconds. You can perform stretching exercises on their own or after a cardiorespiratory or resistance training session. In addition, by including balance activities in your exercise session, you will benefit in your daily activities and potentially reduce your risk of falls.

FLEXIBILITY STRETCHES

The exercises to improve flexibility that have been listed throughout this chapter are provided here, organized by type—either static or dynamic. Each stretch includes a description and photos to help you perform it correctly.

Static Stretches

Static stretches, as discussed in detail previously in this chapter, are simple exercises that you can use to improve your flexibility. Remember to always warm up before stretching.

Neck

- *Forward flexion*: Facing forward, move your head forward to tuck your chin into your chest; hold.

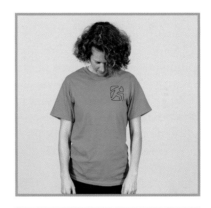

- *Lateral flexion*: Facing forward, allow your head to tilt to the side so your ear moves toward your shoulder; hold. Repeat on the other side.

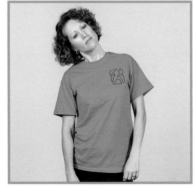

Shoulders

- *Arms across chest*: Facing forward, straighten your right arm and draw it across your chest. Your arm should be as straight as possible, and you should feel gentle tension in your right shoulder. Grasp your right arm with your left hand and apply gentle pressure with your left hand to increase the tension in your right shoulder. Repeat on the other side.

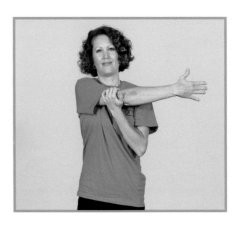

- *Arm hug*: Cross your arms around your body with your elbows pointing forward. Let your upper body round, and squeeze your arms toward each other.

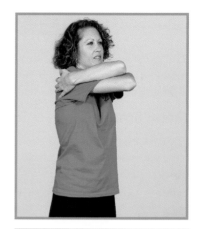

- *Pillar/overhead reach*: Facing forward, stand upright and extend your arms above your head, keeping your shoulders in a neutral position (in line with your hips). Interlock your fingers and use your palms to press upward. You can also involve your trunk muscles (torso) by slightly rotating to one side of your body and back. Hold when you feel tension in your torso on the side opposite the reach.

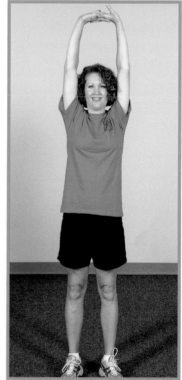

- *Kneeling cat*: Adopt a crawl position on your hands and knees (*a*). Draw in your abdominals and contract your buttocks, and then round your spine throughout its entire length (*b*).

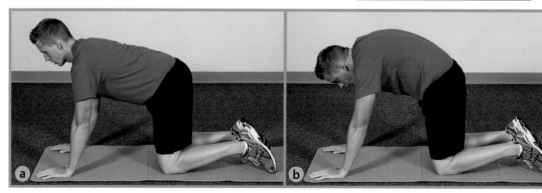

• *Supine rotational stretch*: Lie faceup on the floor and bend your knees so that your feet are flat on the floor. Straighten your arms out from your sides across the floor to stabilize your upper body (*a*). Slowly move both legs with your knees bent to the right side of your body while keeping your upper back against the floor and your abdomen oriented toward the ceiling (*b*). Repeat by moving your legs to the left side.

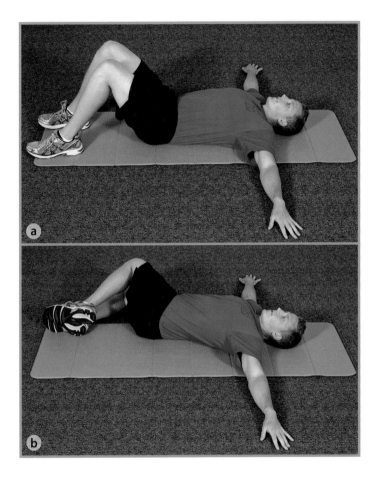

Chest

- *Chest stretch*: In this stretch, your shoulders should be relaxed, not elevated. Straighten your arms toward your back, keeping them at or a little below shoulder height. A good cue for this stretch is "Open arms wide".

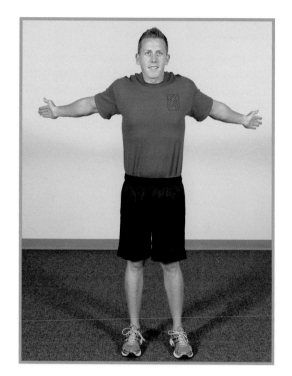

- *Progressive chest stretch*: Place your arms against an open doorway and lean forward until you feel gentle tension across your chest. This exercise also stretches the biceps.

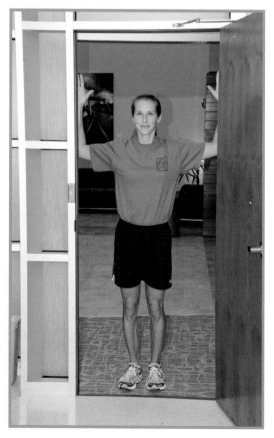

Biceps

- *Biceps wall stretch*: Position your arm from your hand to your inner elbow against a wall and turn your body away from it, exhaling slowly. Repeat on the other side.

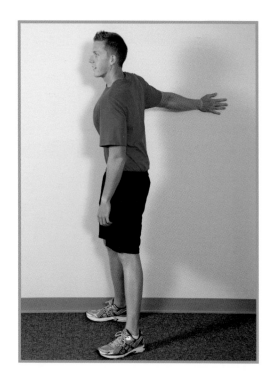

Triceps

- *Elbow behind the head*: Facing forward, bring your right arm up, bend from your elbow, and drop your hand behind your head, trying to reach your left shoulder with your right hand. The left hand can be placed on the right elbow to assist with this stretch. Repeat on the other side.

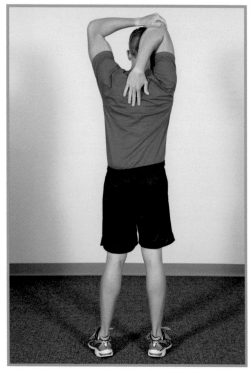

- *Seated hip rotator stretch*: Sit upright on a sturdy, nonmovable chair. Cross your right ankle onto your bent left knee (*a*) and gently press down on your right knee until tension develops in the outer portion of your right thigh (*b*). Repeat on the other side.

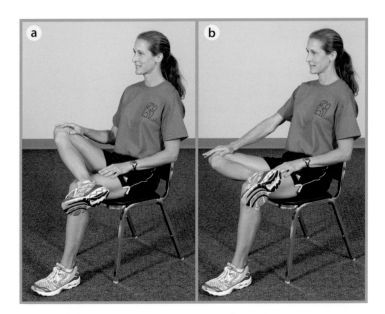

- *Supine hip rotator stretch*: Lie faceup on floor with your knees bent so your feet are flat on the floor and cross your right ankle onto your bent left knee (*a*). Lift your left foot off the floor and wrap your hands around your left leg and draw it into your body (*b*). Focus on opening up your right knee until tension develops in the outer portion of your right thigh. Repeat on the other side.

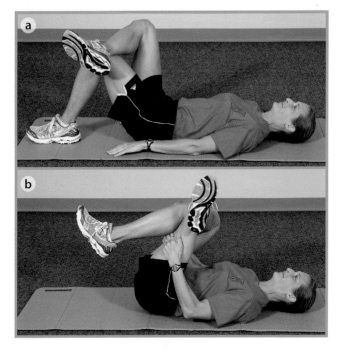

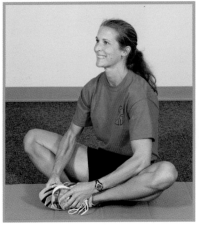

- *Butterfly stretch*: Sit upright on the floor with the soles of your feet together. Draw your knees to the floor and lean forward from your hips and use your elbows to press your legs downward.

- *Kneeling hip flexor stretch*: Kneel on both knees with your upper body lifted. Plant your right foot on the floor until you reach a 90 degree angle with both your front and back legs (*a*). Shift your weight forward while keeping your upper body lifted (*b*). Repeat on the other side.

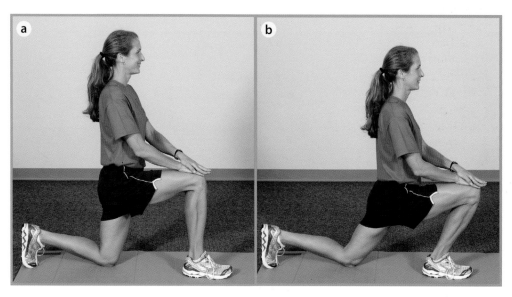

- *Standing hip flexor stretch*: Stand erect and keep your hands on your hips. Step forward with your right foot into a lunge position (*a*). Your right foot will be in front of your body and your left foot will be behind your body; your left heel may be elevated to facilitate this movement. Shift your hips forward and maintain this position, feeling tension develop in your hips, quadriceps, and buttocks (*b*). Repeat on the other side.

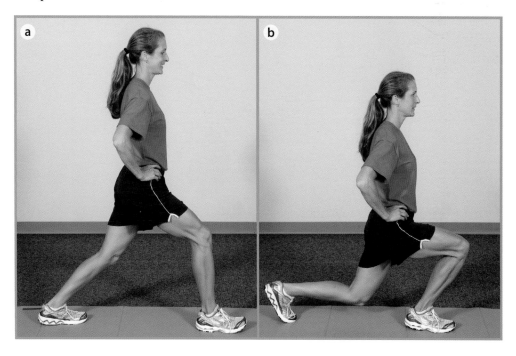

- *Seated hamstring stretch*: Sit upright on the floor with both legs straight and hands resting on your legs (*a*). Slowly walk your hands forward toward your feet, keeping your chest lifted (*b*).

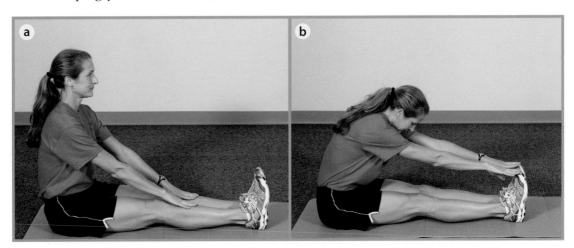

- *Standing hamstring stretch*: Standing upright, bring your right foot slightly ahead of your left foot. Slowly draw your hips back while slightly bending your left knee and straightening your right knee (*a*). Bring the toes of your right foot off the floor and toward your body (*b*). Hold and then return to the starting position. Repeat with the other leg.

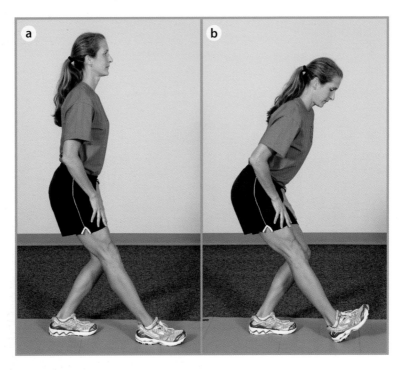

- *Prone quadriceps stretch*: Lie facedown on the floor with your legs straight. Draw your right heel back toward your buttocks using your left hand. Be sure to keep your knees together.

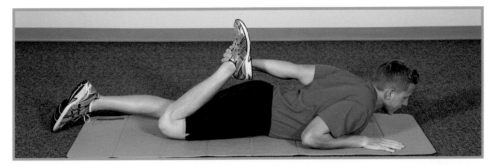

- *Side-lying quadriceps stretch*: Lie on the floor on your right side. Bend your left knee, keeping your knees and hips in a straight line (keep your knees together and do not twist your leg to the side). Draw your left heel back toward your buttocks with your left arm. Repeat on the other side.

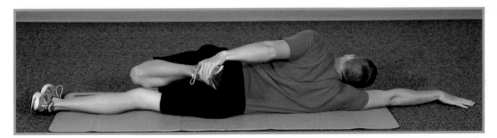

- *Standing quadriceps stretch*: While in a standing position (you can hold on to a chair for support), bend your right knee toward your buttocks. Grasp your right ankle with your left hand. Be sure to keep your knees close together and your ankle behind your buttock; do not twist your leg outward. Gently pull your thigh back slightly. Repeat on the other side.

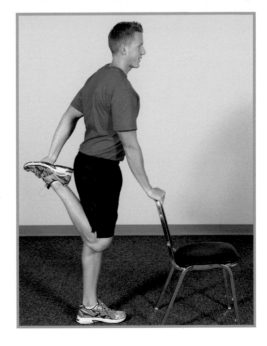

• *Seated calf stretch*: Sit upright with both legs straightened out in front of you (*a*). Draw your toes toward your upper body (*b*).

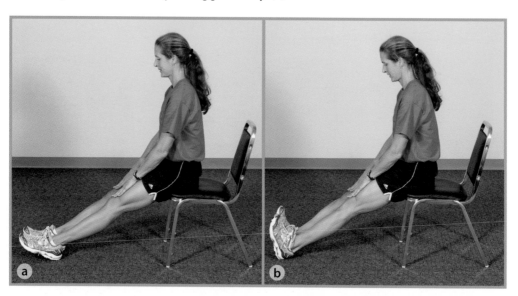

• *Standing calf step stretch*: Stand with your legs extended on the edge of an immovable step and grasp a banister or handrail for support. Move your right foot so your heel back is off the edge of the step (*a*). Slowly drop your right heel until tension develops in your right calf (*b*). Repeat on the other side.

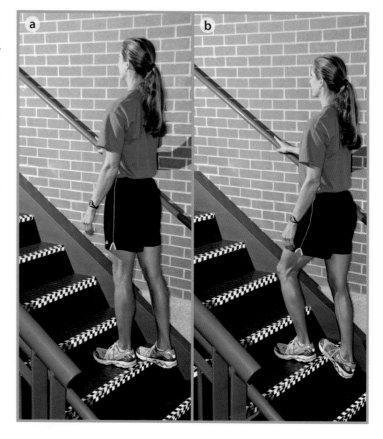

Dynamic Stretches

Dynamic stretches, as discussed in detail previously in this chapter, are more active than static stretches. Remember to always warm up before any stretching activity.

Arms and Shoulders

- *Arm circle*: Stand with your feet shoulder-width apart and your knees slightly bent. Raise both arms to the side at shoulder height with your palms out. Make small circles with your arms extended, gradually increasing the size of the circles.

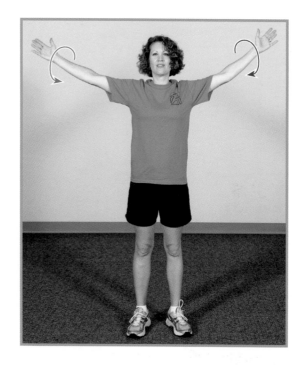

- *Shoulder shrug*: Lift both shoulders toward your ears (*a*) and then lower them away from your ears (*b*).

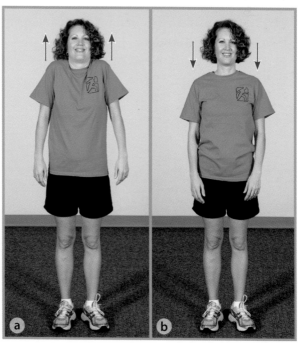

- *Pendulum leg swing (front to back)*: Place your right hand on the back of a chair for balance. Lift your left leg and swing it forward (in front of your body) (*a*) and back (behind your body) (*b*). Begin with small swings and progress to larger swings. Switch to the opposite leg.

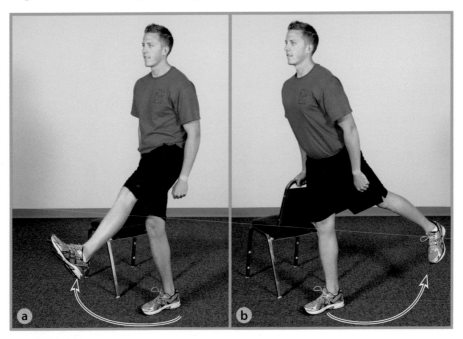

- *Pendulum leg swing (side to side)*: Place both hands on the back of a chair for balance. Swing your left leg out to the left (*a*), and back across your body to the right (*b*). Begin with small swings and progress to larger swings. Switch to the opposite leg.

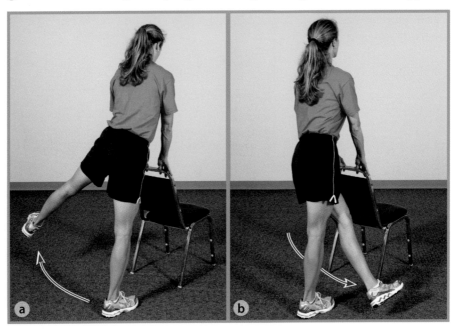

- *Internal hip rotation*: Stand upright with your feet shoulder-width apart. Raise your left foot toward the side of your body and tap the outside of your left heel with your left hand. Allow your knee to rotate inward. Switch and tap the outside of your right heel with your right hand. Alternate tapping each foot. Progress to walking forward while alternating feet.

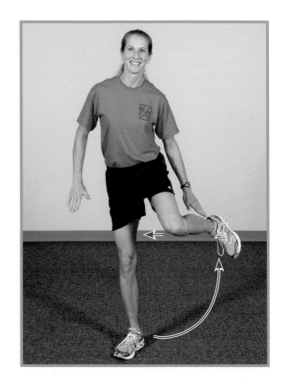

- *External hip rotation*: Stand upright with your feet shoulder-width apart. Raise your left foot in front of your body and tap the inside of your left heel with your right hand. Allow your knee to point away from your body. Switch and tap the inside of your right heel with your left hand. Alternate tapping each foot. Progress to walking forward while alternating feet tapping.

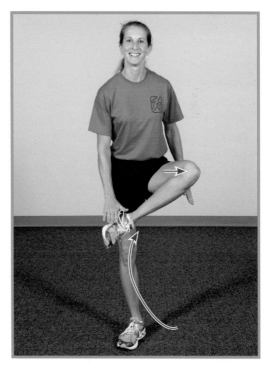

- *Side shuffle*: Stand with your feet shoulder-width apart, your knees slightly bent, and your hands on your hips. Take one step to the left with your left foot (*a*); then bring your right foot in to meet your left foot (*b*). Begin with small steps, progress to larger steps, and then progress to a shuffle. Switch to the opposite direction.

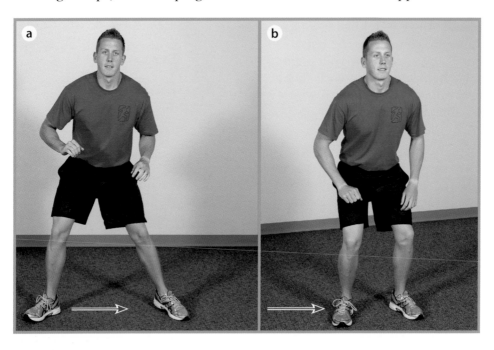

Quadriceps

- *Butt kick*: Begin marching in place. Pull your heel in closer toward your buttock with each step. Progress to moving forward (walking or jogging) while kicking your buttocks.

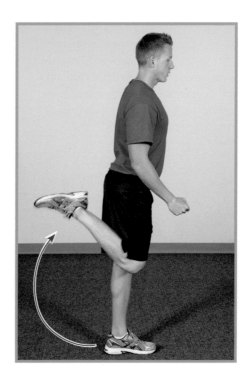

Hamstrings

- *High knees*: Begin marching in place. Raise your knees higher and higher with each step. Progress to moving forward (walking or jogging) with high knees.

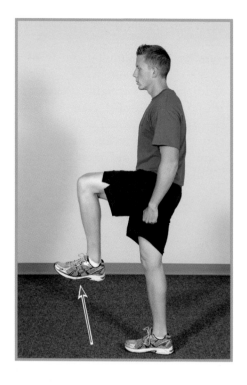

Ankles

- *Dynamic foot range of motion*: Sit upright in a chair with both legs together and straightened in front of you. Point your toes away from your body and pull your toes toward your body (*a*). Rotate your feet clockwise and counterclockwise (*b*).

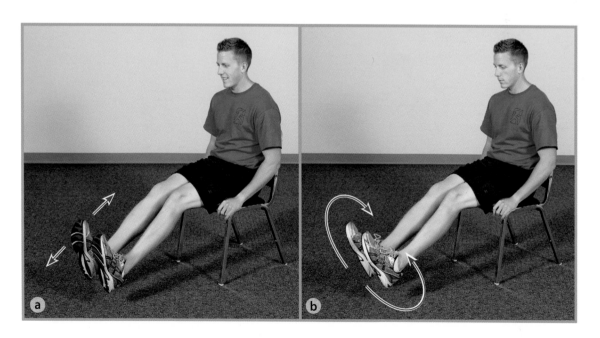

Combined Movements

- *Soldier walk*: Simultaneously rotate your right arm forward and raise your left leg (straight). Reach your right hand toward your left lower leg and toes. Switch to the opposite side. Progress to alternating to the opposite side and then to walking while alternating sides.

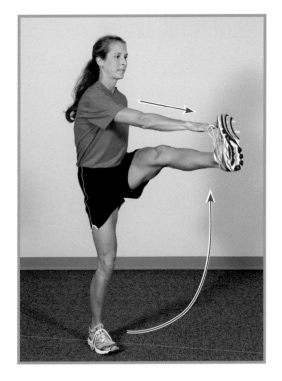

- *Wood chop*: Stand with your feet wider than shoulder width. Reach both arms down toward the outside of your left foot while bending your knees slightly (*a*). Move your arms diagonally across your body and end by reaching above your right shoulder (*b*). Switch to the opposite side.

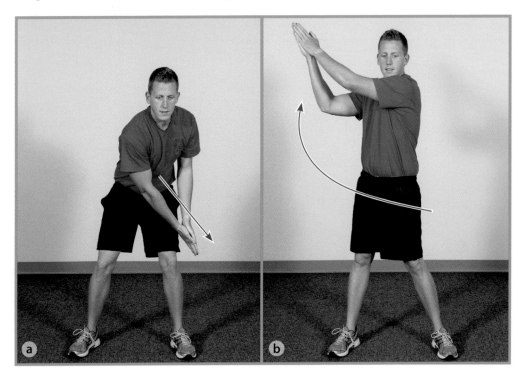

BALANCE AND MOVEMENT ACTIVITIES

Balance and movement activities challenge your stability. Creating situations in which you feel unsteady will improve your balance. The activities in this section provide a number of options, ranging from relatively easy to more challenging.

Balance

- *Seated chair lean*: While seated on the edge of a chair, lean forward (*a*), backward (*b*), or side to side (*c*).

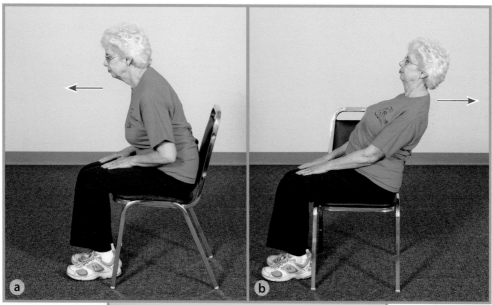

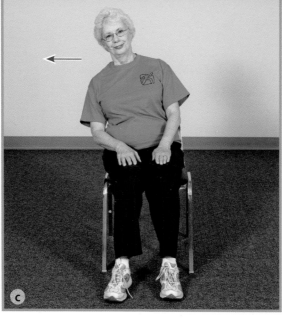

- *Upright stance*: Maintain a standing position with the following variations of foot positions: wide stance, in which your feet are hip-width apart (*a*); narrow stance, in which the insoles of your feet are touching each other (*b*); semitandem, in which your feet are in a split stance, one foot forward and the other foot out and to the back (*c*); and tandem, in which your feet are placed heel to toe (*d*).

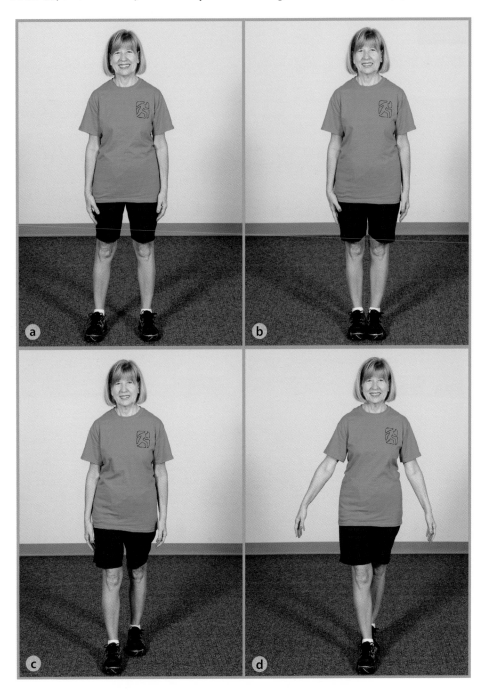

- *Side-to-side shuffle and forward/backward walk*: For a side-to-side shuffle, take 10 side steps to the right and 10 side steps to the left. Your eyes should look straight ahead. For a forward or backward walk, take 10 steps forward and then take 10 steps backward. Your eyes should look straight ahead.

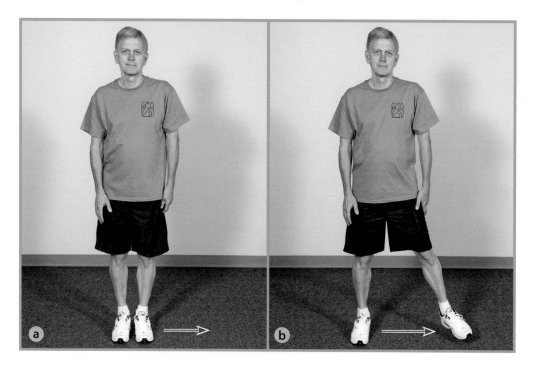

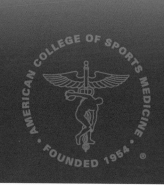

part **III**

Fitness and Health for Every Age

No matter your age, a physically active lifestyle and wise nutritional choices allow for an ongoing evolution of your fitness ID. Change is part of life, and your exercise program and diet evolve over time as well. The upcoming chapters provide age-specific recommendations for both physical activity and nutrition. Each age group (children and adolescents, adults, older adults) has unique areas of focus related to exercise and diet. Watch your fitness evolve as you merge your goals and lifestyle with the dietary recommendations and physical activity guidelines presented in this section.

chapter 9

Children and Adolescents: Up to Age 17

I t is never too early in life to start developing healthy habits. Active youth have a better chance of growing into healthy adults.[21] Risk factors for chronic diseases such as heart disease, high blood pressure, type 2 diabetes, and osteoporosis have their roots early in life.[21] Regular physical activity and good nutrition are two ways to lower the chance of developing risk factors for these diseases.[10] Kids who are active typically display higher levels of aerobic and muscular fitness and have a lower percentage of body fat. Anxiety and depression may also be reduced in children and adolescents who are physically active on a regular basis.[21]

Although the benefits of physical activity are well established, the activity levels of youth are below desired levels and tend to decrease with age. Similarly, a gap exists between recommended diets for youth and what the majority of youth actually consume.[10] Thus, it is vital that adults provide opportunities for children and adolescents to be physically active and that they encourage wise nutritional choices.

Because children and adolescents are not small versions of adults, this chapter provides physical activity recommendations that are appropriate for youth from infancy through adolescence. Providing a variety of enjoyable activities is vital to motivate youth to be active and to continue being active as adults. This chapter also addresses healthy eating for youth, including how adults involved in the lives of children and adolescents can modify the environment to encourage healthier eating choices.

FOCUS ON NUTRITION

As discussed in chapter 4, good nutrition is important in the pursuit of optimal health. The U.S. government's *Dietary Guidelines for Americans* points out that youth decrease their risk of developing heart disease by consuming diets with sufficient (but not excessive) calories—in particular, diets in which calories come from a variety of nutrient-dense foods and beverages (including fruits, vegetables, dietary fiber, whole grains, lean protein, low-fat dairy, and low-sodium items), while keeping the intake of added sugar, refined carbohydrate, and fat (saturated and total) low.[22]

Encouraging children to eat well can be challenging. Childhood is a pivotal time to provide good examples and encourage healthy choices.[20] Letting children observe others enjoying fruits, vegetables, and whole grains is a great way to promote healthy nutritional behaviors. One way to set a good example is to plan ahead and have fruits such as oranges and bananas available for snacks, rather than grabbing a less-nutritious choice at the checkout line. You can also have children assist in preparing meals or snacks or with simple tasks such as tearing lettuce for a salad or adding veggie toppings to a pizza.

Although the "clean plate club" was used in the past to prompt kids to eat, the current recommendation is to encourage them to stop eating when they're full, rather than when their plates are clean. Children who understand the concept of being full are less likely to become overweight.[20] Offer a number of healthy eating options and let your child make food selections. This approach lets the child decide what to eat, while still allowing you to provide needed guidance. Because children often don't eat enough at meals to remain full until the next meal, a good option is to plan for three meals, plus a couple of snacks, each day.[20] Snacks should be nutritious and should not substitute for skipping meals.

Although younger children are influenced to a great extent by parents, guardians, and other adults, older children and adolescents eat more meals and snacks outside of the home and make more personal decisions about what to eat. One factor that has a pervasive impact on food choices is the media.[10] Consider, for example, the number of television advertisements that focus on sugary breakfast cereals, cookies, candy, and fast-food restaurants. Then, count the number of advertisements for fruits and vegetables (if you can find any at all). Of course, there is no comparison! Because adolescents tend to consume more sweetened beverages, french fries, pizza, and other fast-food items, many do not meet healthy eating recommendations for fruits, vegetables, dairy foods, wholes grains, lean meats, and fish.[10] This results in too much fat in the diet and insufficient intake of nutrients such as calcium and iron, as well as vitamins A, D, and C, and folic acid.[10] Unfortunately, many adolescents skip breakfast and actually consume about one third of their calories from snacks, with sweetened beverages being a major contributor.[10]

Where and Why Do Youth Fall Short?

The dietary intake of some nutrients, including calcium, potassium, fiber, magnesium, and vitamin E, appear to be low for many youth.[22] The low intake of fiber may be linked to underconsumption of whole grains, fruits, and vegetables. Also, low magnesium and potassium intake is reflected in insufficient fruit and vegetable

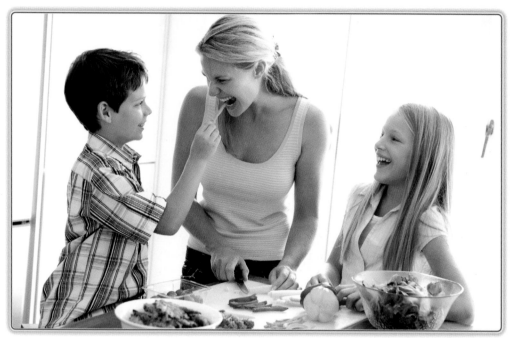

Involve children in making positive nutritional choices.

consumption. Low calcium intake usually results from insufficient intake of milk and milk products. Vitamin E intake can be improved by consuming fortified cereals, as well as various nuts and oils.

Making some simple substitutions in dietary choices can help to address these areas of deficiency and improve the nutrient content of children's diets. Following are some practical ways to address these nutritional concerns:

- Substitute whole fruit for fruit juice.
- Replace starchy vegetables (e.g., white potatoes) with dark green vegetables (e.g., broccoli) and orange vegetables (e.g., carrots, sweet potatoes).
- Increase the consumption of low-fat or skim milk in place of soda.
- Eat breakfast on a daily basis, including cereals fortified with vitamin E.

Replacing less nutritious items with more nutritious ones can improve the diets of youth.

Where and Why Do Youth Need to Cut Back?

Although experts promote the consumption of fruits, vegetables, and whole grains for optimal health, the top sources of calories for U.S. youth are grain desserts (e.g., cakes, cookies, doughnuts, pies, and granola bars), pizza, and sugar-sweetened beverages (soda and fruit drinks).[22] As a result, the amount of added sugar and fat consumed is excessive. The *Dietary Guidelines* suggests that children (as well as adults) need to reduce their consumption of solid fats and added sugars (SoFAS is a new abbreviation used for these dual targets). Nearly 40% of the calories youth consume are SoFAS![22] See *Major Sources of SoFAS* for a look at what kids are consuming.

Youth need to consume a diet that provides needed nutrients for normal growth and development, immunity, and cognitive function. Solid fats and added sugars (SoFAS) are overconsumed by youth and often result in excessive intake of calories with little nutritional value. Reducing the consumption of SoFAS may be one of the most important steps to stemming the growing prevalence of obesity in youth.

How Are Youth Consuming Solid Fats?

Top sources of solid fats for youth are pizza, grain desserts, whole milk, regular cheese, and fatty meats. Sources vary somewhat by age, with younger children consuming more whole milk and teenagers getting their major contributions from fried potatoes.

How Are Youth Consuming Added Sugars?

Added sugars come from soda (the number one source by far), fruit drinks, grain desserts, dairy desserts, and candy. Soda makes up one third of the weight of beverages consumed by youth. On average, youth consume 171 calories each day from sugar-sweetened beverages (soda and fruit drinks combined).

Adapted from U.S. Department of Agriculture and U.S. Department of Health and Human Services, 2010.

Because of the high calorie content but limited nutrient value of the foods youth often consume (e.g., soda and high-fat fried foods), the overall caloric intake of youth is higher than desired. When the number of calories consumed is not matched by physical activity, overweight and obesity result. Foods with a high fat content are considered calorie dense, meaning that, per gram, the calorie content is high and the nutrient content is relatively low. Ideally, foods should be high in nutrients (i.e., nutrient dense) relative to the number of calories they contain. Table 4.4 on page 69 of chapter 4 gives some examples of reduced calorie, lower-fat alternatives to higher-fat foods. In addition to making simple substitutions, adults can make other changes that can address overweight and obesity in youth, such as the following:[22]

- Limit fast-food meals.
- Limit screen time (TV, computer).
- Don't let youth skip breakfast.
- Keep a check on portion size.

Taken together, these are action-oriented steps that can help address the growing problem of overweight and obesity in youth.

What Should the Nutrition Focus Be for Children and Adolescents?

Obviously, improving the diets of children and adolescents will require greater attention to making nutritious choices at home, at school, and in community settings. Promoting good nutrition early in life and providing positive role models for healthy eating are two important ways of improving the eating patterns of youngsters. The purpose of making healthy dietary choices is not just to avoid chronic disease (although the benefits related to heart disease and other chronic conditions are clear); it is also to meet nutrient requirements that lead to the best possible level of function and the ability to engage in physical activity. Food is the fuel for physical activity, and selecting the best fuel provides the nutrients needed for optimal performance during day-to-day activities and strenuous physical activity.

Normal growth requires good nutrition.[20] As with adults, children's weight in relation to height can be assessed easily via the body mass index (BMI) as described on page 26 of chapter 2. However, BMI is a bit more complex for youth because of various growth patterns. As a result, BMI-for-age charts are recommended for youth between the ages of 2 and 20 (see figure 9.1 or go to www.cdc.gov/growthcharts/ and enter *BMI calculator* into the search window for an easy online calculator and individualized interpretation).[6]

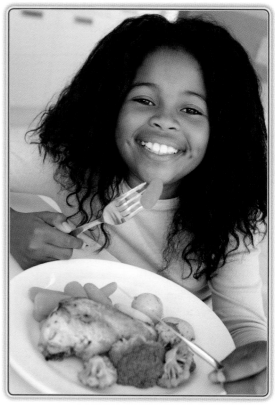

Following the *Dietary Guidelines* provides the best nutrition for kids.

Implementing Dietary Guidelines for Youth

The American Heart Association's dietary strategies for youth (2 years of age and older) are intended to provide the best nutrition possible.[10] Following are tips for optimizing nutrition:

- Use recommended portion sizes when preparing and serving foods.
- Remove the skin from poultry before eating.
- Reduce salt intake, including salt from processed foods.
- Reduce added sugars including sugar-sweetened drinks and juices. The consumption of sweetened beverages and fruit juice should be limited to 4 to 6 ounces (113-170 ml) for children 1 to 6 years of age and 8 to 12 ounces (227 to 340 ml) per day for those 7 to 18 years of age.[10]
- Limit high-calorie sauces such as Alfredo, cream sauce, cheese sauces, and hollandaise.
- Ensure that "whole grain" is the first ingredient on the food label when looking to select products that are actually mainly whole grain.
- Eat legumes (beans) and tofu in place of meat for some entrees.
- Read food labels (especially for breads, breakfast cereals, and prepared foods such as soups) to check for salt and sugar content. When possible, choose high-fiber, low-salt, low-sugar alternatives.

Adapted from Gidding, Dennison, Birch, et al., 2005, p. 2062.

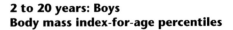
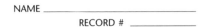

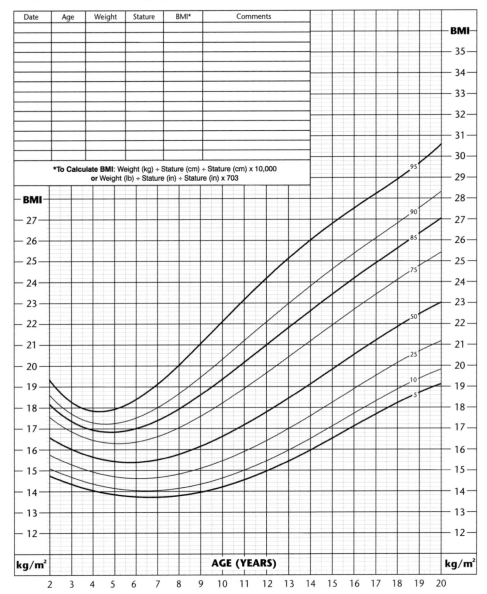

Figure 9.1a Body-mass-index-for-age charts for boys.

Reprinted from Centers for Disease Control and Prevention, 2009.
From ACSM, 2011, *ACSM's complete guide to fitness & health* (Champaign, IL: Human Kinetics).

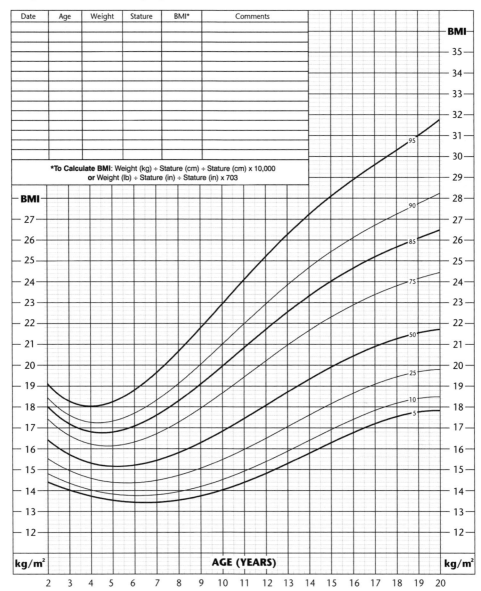

Figure 9.1*b* Body-mass-index-for-age charts for girls.

Reprinted from Centers for Disease Control and Prevention, 2009.
From ACSM, 2011, *ACSM's complete guide to fitness & health* (Champaign, IL: Human Kinetics).

Follow the horizontal line matching the child's BMI until it intersects with the vertical line for the child's age; note the percentile line closest to this point of intersection. Typically, a healthy weight is considered between the 5th percentile and the 85th percentile. Risk for overweight is considered from the 85th percentile to the 95th, and a classification of overweight is given for youth at the 95th percentile and above.[6] BMI does not consider body composition, and thus if a youth is determined to be overweight or at risk of overweight, a follow-up with a health care provider would be appropriate.

Consuming an appropriate number of calories and foods from various categories results in optimal nutrition. See table 9.1 for age-specific daily calorie and serving size recommendations for grains, fruits, vegetables, and milk and dairy items for boys and girls.[10] Note that the calorie recommendations in table 9.1 are for an inactive child; about 200 calories would need to be added for a moderately active child and 200 to 400 calories per day for a very physically active child.[10]

Table 9.1 Daily Estimated Calories[1] and Recommended Servings for Children and Adolescents

	1 Year	2-3 Years	4-8 Years	9-13 Years	14-18 Years
Calories[2]	900 kcal	1000 kcal	1400 kcal for males; 1200 kcal for females	1800 kcal for males; 1600 kcal for females	2200 kcal for males; 1800 kcal for females
Fat	30%-40% kcal	30%-35% kcal	25%-35% kcal	25%-35% kcal	25%-35% kcal
Milk/dairy[3]	2 cups[6]	2 cups	2 cups	3 cups	3 cups
Lean meat/ beans	1.5 oz	2 oz	4 oz for males; 3 oz for females	5 oz	6 oz for males; 5 oz for females
Fruits[4]	1 cup	1 cup	1.5 cups	1.5 cups	2 cups for males; 1.5 cups for females
Vegetables[4]	3/4 cup	1 cup	1.5 cups for males; 1 cup for females	2.5 cups for males; 2 cups for females	3 cups for males; 2.5 cups for females
Grains[5]	2 oz	3 oz	5 oz for males; 4 oz for females	6 oz for males; 5 oz for females	7 oz for males; 6 oz for females

[1]Calorie estimates are based on a sedentary lifestyle. Increased physical activity will require additional calories: by 0-200 kcal/d if moderately physically active; and by 200-400 kcal/d if very physically active.

[2] For youth 2 years and older; adopted from Table 2, Table 3, ad Appendix A-2 of the *Dietary Guidelines for Americans* (2005)[14], http://www.healtheirus.gov/dietaryguidelines. Nutrient and energy contributions from each group are calculated according to the nutrient-dense forms of food in each group (e.g., lean meats and fat-free milk).

[3]Milk listed is fat-free (except for children under the age of 2 years). If 1%, 2%, or whole-fat milk is substituted, this will utilize, for each cup, 19, 39, or 63 kcal of discretionary calories and add 2.6, 5.1, or 9.0 g of total fat, of which 1.3, 2.6, or 4.6 g are saturated fat.

[4]Serving sizes are 1/4 cup for 1 year of age, 1/3 cup for 2 to 3 years of age, and 1/2 cup for ≥4 years of age. A variety of vegetables should be selected from each subgroup over the week.

[5]Half of all grains should be whole grains.

[6]For 1-year-old children, calculations are based on 2% fat milk. If 2 cups of whole milk are substituted, 48 kcal of discretionary calories will be utilized. The American Academy of Pediatrics recommends that low-fat/reduced fat milk not be started before 2 years of age.

Reprinted with permission. *Circulation.* 2005; 112: 2061-2075. © American Heart Association, Inc.

A CLOSER LOOK
Erica

Erica is a 10-year-old female who is 4 feet 6 inches (137 cm) tall and 100 pounds (45.4 kg) (BMI = 24.1). This places her at approximately the 95th percentile on the BMI-for-age chart, thus classifying her as potentially obese. Her parents are concerned about her weight gain over the past couple of years and develop the following plan after meeting with Erica's pediatrician and talking over options with Erica:

- Erica's parents created an activity chart on which Erica tracks her physical activity (e.g., walking to school, taking the dog for a walk around the neighborhood park, riding her bike). Erica's parents are doing the same. The first one to reach 300 minutes of activity picks the next weekend family outing (e.g., window shopping at the mall, a picnic at a local park, a day at the beach). At that point, everyone starts over and again works up to another 300 minutes. Each family member has found ways to increase activity and the low-level competition has created a fun atmosphere of encouraging more activity.

- Erica's family has agreed to limit TV viewing to one program per night. In the past, the television was the focus of the family life and often was accompanied by snacking on high-calorie, low-nutrient items. Now they are shooting baskets, playing Frisbee golf, and doing dance videos (even Dad!) together. Replacing the screen time with fun activities not only provides more physical activity, but also cuts down on the consumption of unneeded calories.

- On the nutritional side, the family commits to decreasing the number of visits to fast-food restaurants. Preparing some bulk meals on the weekend allows them to quickly and easily prepare workday and schoolday meals. This additional preparation is done together as a family and the meals are more nutritious than those that the family had been consuming.

- Breakfast is another new commitment. Erica's parents often just grabbed coffee for breakfast, and Erica typically ate little before rushing off to school. Setting the alarm clock to go off 20 minutes earlier allows everyone in the family time for breakfast together.

- Soda consumption was routine for all the family members and accompanied almost every meal and snack. Soda has been replaced with low-fat milk for Erica at breakfast and dinner. Water flavored with a lemon has been substituted at other meals and snacks.

All of these changes are steps toward helping Erica (and her parents) increase physical activity and create a more nutritious diet.

As with physical activity, eating patterns established early in life can carry forward into adulthood. Setting a positive example and providing opportunities to make good nutrition choices are keys to developing a solid foundation for healthy eating in youth. The following tips can help a family eat well:[20]

- *Make half your grains whole.* Select whole grain foods more often (e.g., whole wheat bread, brown rice, oatmeal, low-fat popcorn).

- *Vary your veggies.* Eat a variety of vegetables, and in particular, seek out dark green and orange vegetables (e.g., spinach, broccoli, carrots, sweet potatoes).
- *Focus on fruits.* Fruits can be part of meals or snacks, whether they are fresh, frozen, canned, or dried.
- *Eat calcium-rich foods.* Low-fat and fat-free milk and other milk products should be consumed several times a day to help build strong bones.
- *Go lean with protein.* Protein can be found in lean or low-fat meats, chicken, turkey, and fish, as well as dry beans and peas.
- *Change your oil.* Good sources of oil are fish, nuts, and liquid oils (e.g., corn, soybean, canola, and olive oil).
- *Don't sugarcoat it.* Check labels and choose foods and beverages that do not have sugar and sweeteners as one of their primary ingredients.

Finally, the U.S. Department of Agriculture nutrition pyramid for kids, shown in figure 9.2, is an excellent resource. The website mypyramid.gov also includes resources for younger age groups including downloadable posters and kid-friendly materials.

FOCUS ON PHYSICAL ACTIVITY

Since the 1970s, the prevalence of obesity in American youth has increased from 5% to 10.4% among those age 2 to 5 years, from 6.5% to 17.0% for those age 6 to 11 years, and from 5% to 18.1% for youth age 12 to 19 years.[6] Although the current prevalence of obesity in American youth is startling, the projected outcome of a lifetime of unhealthy body weight is even more disheartening. Overweight youth tend to continue to be overweight adults and thus have a higher risk of obesity-related diseases.

Budget-related cutbacks in physical education and increased time spent in sedentary activities have led to an escalation in the overweight status of youth and have contributed to a substantial reduction in childhood physical activity.[5] Over half of young boys and three out of four young girls do not engage in daily physical activity![5] The long-term consequences of high levels of body weight and physical inactivity include a greater risk of early death and the presence of chronic health conditions such diabetes and certain forms of cancer.[9, 18]

Benefits of Physical Activity for Children and Adolescents

Engaging in regular physical activity during childhood and adolescence can enhance cardiovascular and musculoskeletal health, can produce beneficial changes in blood lipid (cholesterol) levels, and has been tied to higher levels of physical self-concept and academic performance.[3, 19] Because youth who are overweight are more likely to become overweight adults,[8] physical activity from an early age can play a key role in developing good health and avoiding unhealthy weight gain.[16] The fact that inactivity and low physical activity patterns tend to be harder to modify with age[17] further emphasizes the need to encourage youth to develop and maintain an active lifestyle.

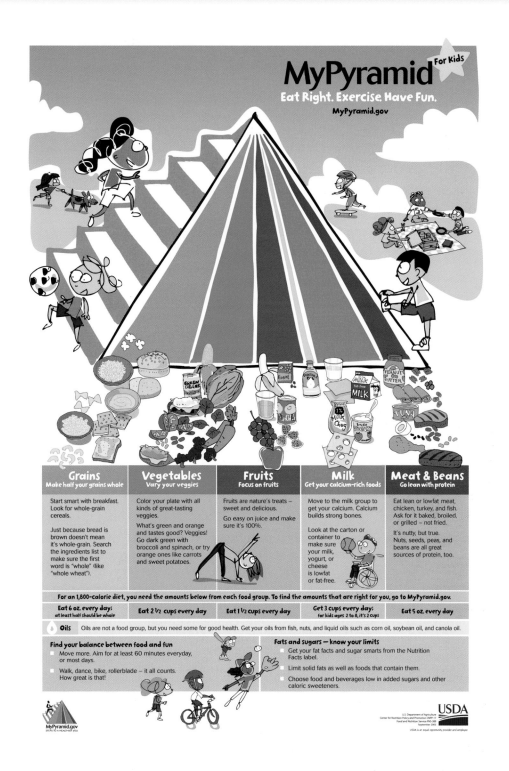

Figure 9.2 MyPyramid for kids.

U.S. Department of Agriculture

Medical Screenings and Physical Activity

Most healthy children and adolescents can begin a physical activity program without a visit to a physician or health care provider. However, if a preexisting condition exists (e.g., asthma, diabetes, or obesity), or if there are any other special circumstances or concerns, then consulting with a physician or health care provider before increasing activity is warranted. Often, simple adjustments can be made to the activity program, such as starting out with a lower amount of activity and progressing more slowly. For youth involved in competitive sports, a sport physical is typically required to ensure that no health conditions exist that could limit the ability to endure the rigors of a particular sport.

The next section presents physical activity guidelines for each developmental phase of the child relative to the frequency, intensity, time, and type (i.e., FITT profiles) of recommended physical activity. The intensity range of physical activity varies from moderate to vigorous. Moderate physical activities (such as briskly walking to school) can be performed and maintained easily, whereas vigorous activities (such as running on the playground) are more intense and feature substantial increases in heart rate, breathing rate, and sweating and often require more rest periods.[21]

Physical Activity for Infants, Toddlers, and Preschoolers

How early is too early to encourage children to be active? This is an issue the National Association for Sport and Physical Education (NASPE) has addressed for children up to 5 years of age in a document titled "Active Start."[13] Now in its second edition, "Active Start" highlights the roles parents, child care providers, and teachers play in motivating children to be active, which include serving as active role models and creating environments that facilitate play and movement exploration.[14] NASPE's overall position is that all children from birth to age 5 should engage daily in physical activity that promotes movement skillfulness and foundations in health-related fitness. The following sections provide guidance for and examples of age-appropriate activities for infants (birth to 1 year), toddlers (1 to 3 years), and preschoolers (3 to 5 years).

Infants (Birth to 1 Year)

From the first days of life, the ability to move and explore allows infants to begin to understand and make sense of their surroundings. During the first year of life, infants start to develop and repeat movement patterns as muscles learn to respond to information from the brain. Consequently, infants need numerous opportunities to participate in a variety of physical activities that promote skill development and movement competency. The acquisition of new movement skills also helps newborn children adapt to new physical surroundings.[1]

FITT Profile for Infants   Parents and caregivers should play with infants several times a day during waking hours, especially when they are alert and happy. Although parents and caregivers should take advantage of opportunities to engage infants in active play, the intensity level of physical activity will be determined by the child. When infants are not interested in engaging in active play, for instance, they typically communicate this by crying or looking away. A variety of positive facial, nonverbal, and verbal expressions should be used to motivate infants to be active.

Infants should be encouraged to participate in a variety of activities that promote the development of basic movement skills such as reaching, grasping, holding, squeezing, crawling, sitting, and standing. Examples of activities include playing games such as pattycake and peek-a-boo; placing objects of different sizes, textures, colors, and shapes within or just beyond their reach; or assisting with movement skills such as sitting, crawling, standing, and stepping. Infants may also enjoy banging objects to music, crawling across a surface decorated with bright-colored objects, bouncing in a baby seat, or lying or sitting in a supported position while reaching out and manipulating a suspended mobile.

Recommended Activity Settings for Infants   Infants should be placed in settings during the day that promote movement and exploration of their surroundings. If the play environment is too small, or if the infant is placed in sedentary or restrictive settings (e.g., a baby seat or play pen) for extended periods, a delay may occur in learning and practicing fundamental behaviors such as rolling over, sitting, crawling, creeping, and standing. Play equipment should be nontoxic, contain no sharp edges or points, and be free of pieces that can be swallowed. Playing, rolling, and crawling activities can be performed on a rug or blanket that is at least 5 feet by 7 feet (1.5 by 2.1 m).[13]

Toddlers (1 to 3 Years)

Once a child can walk, a new vista of physical activity choices emerges. Learning to stand and walk in an upright, hands-free posture allows the toddler to acquire and refine fundamental movements (e.g., walking, running, jumping, leaping, throwing, catching, kicking, bouncing) that form the basis of many sport, fitness, and dance activities. Although the ability to perform these core movement patterns is a partial by-product of physical growth, an environment that is supportive, stimulating, and provides opportunities for the toddler to safely engage in structured and unstructured physical activity is also essential. Regular exposure to age- and developmentally appropriate physical activities helps toddlers become more confident in their attempts to master the physical environment, while developing cardiorespiratory endurance, strength, balance, and flexibility.

FITT Profile for Toddlers   When alert and awake, toddlers should engage in multiple bouts of short-burst, moderate to vigorous bouts of physical activity in both indoor and outdoor settings. Although the length of these bouts will vary depending on the age and developmental stage of the child, at least 30 minutes of structured physical activity and at least 60 minutes (up to several hours) of unstructured physical activity should be accumulated each day.[14] Toddlers should not be sedentary for longer than 60 minutes at a time, except when sleeping.[14]

Structured physical activities for toddlers are planned and directed by an adult (parent or caregiver) and can include activities such as action-oriented follow-along songs, dancing to rhythms of taped music or music videos, moving through an obstacle course that provides opportunities to employ manipulative or movement skills, and simple chase games. Unstructured physical activity is initiated by the toddler as he or she explores the surrounding environment. Examples might include playing on and around playground structures, moving on a variety of riding toys (e.g., tricycles, scooters) while wearing a safety helmet, and digging and building in a sandbox. A toddler's interest in being physically active can be enhanced by using age-appropriate toys and equipment in a variety of movement environments.

Recommended Activity Settings for Toddlers Indoor and outdoor play areas for toddlers should meet or exceed recommended safety standards and be large enough to facilitate large-muscle activities. Play environments should also be child-proofed, accessible, and inviting. Each toddler should have a minimum indoor activity space of 35 square feet (3.3 sq m) of activity room and an outdoor activity space of at least 75 square feet (7 sq m).[13]

Preschoolers (3 to 5 Years)

The preschool years are an optimal time to learn and refine movements in a variety of activity settings so the child develops fundamental motor skills before entering kindergarten. Motor skills are a learned sequence of movements that allow the child to move and function to complete physical tasks in a smooth and coordinated fashion. Promoting the development of needed movement patterns at this stage of life will carry forward into the future. The period from 3 to 5 years of age is also a good time to help children develop good nutritional habits; expend enough calories to ward off excessive weight gain; and increase heart fitness, muscular strength, flexibility, and bone density. The physical activity profile of a preschooler will depend on a number of factors, including age, maturity, ability, and previous exposure to motor learning and development. Consequently, parents and caregivers should keep in mind that children at a given age demonstrate varying degrees of proficiency in performing motor tasks.

FITT Profile for Preschoolers Parents and caregivers of preschoolers should plan structured physical activity sessions that are moderate to vigorous in intensity and last between 6 and 10 minutes. A minimum of 60 minutes of structured physical activity should be accumulated daily.[14] Although preschoolers have the capacity to sustain structured, developmentally appropriate physical activity for longer durations (e.g., 30 to 45 minutes), they should also be encouraged to accumulate multiple shorter bouts of structured activity each day. In addition to engaging in structured activity, preschoolers should participate in inside and outside unstructured physical activity lasting at least 60 minutes to several hours a day at self-selected intensity levels.[14] With the exception of sleeping, periods of sedentary activity lasting more than one hour should be avoided.[14]

Preschoolers can enjoy an array of structured physical activities, including obstacle courses that promote movement and manipulative skills, mimicking animal movements to develop strength and flexibility, and cardiorespiratory activities that improve aerobic fitness. Playing imitative games (such as "Simon Says") using a variety of movement patterns, dancing to music of various tempos and rhythms, and receiving formal instruction in various motor skills are other structured forms of physical activity that are appropriate for preschool children. Unstructured physical activities for 3- to 5-year-olds include climbing on playground structures; playing with bats and balls; running up and down inclined surfaces; riding a variety of wheeled riding toys (while wearing a safety helmet); and chasing bubbles, balls, and hoops. Active play that involves "dressing up," going on treasure hunts, and performing specific movement patterns (e.g., galloping like a horse) while another child or other children mimic the activity, are other less formal activity options for the preschool child.

Recommended Activity Settings for Preschoolers   Activity spaces for preschoolers should be large enough to accommodate child-directed play or physical activities supervised by adults. The play environment should have the capability of being modified or reconfigured to allow for different types of activity. Ideally, each child should have a minimum indoor space of 5 feet by 7 feet (1.5 by 2.1 m) for structured movement activities and a minimum of 75 square feet (7 sq m) of outdoor play space.[13] Larger play areas may be required to accommodate activities such as running, skipping, and kicking.

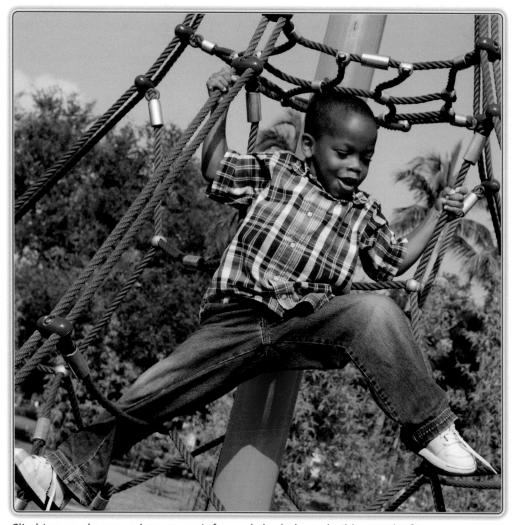

Climbing on playground structures is fun and also helps to build muscular fitness.

Physical Activity for Children and Adolescents

The association between physical activity and good health in school-aged youth is well established.[15, 19, 21] Regular physical activity during childhood and adolescence has beneficial effects on cardiovascular and musculoskeletal health, body composition, and blood lipid levels.[19] In addition, benefits to mental health (e.g., decreased anxiety and depression, improved self-concept) and academic performance have been linked to physical activity and fitness levels in schoolchildren.[19]

Physical Activity Guidelines for Children and Adolescents

Current guidelines indicate that school-aged youth (ages 6 to 17) should accumulate a minimum of 60 minutes, and up to several hours, of age-appropriate physical activity on all, or most, days of the week.[15, 19, 21] Conversely, experts recommend that children and adolescents avoid extended periods (greater than two hours) of inactivity during school hours, as well as outside of school time.

The physical activity profile of children and adolescents should feature activities that stimulate the aerobic system, increase muscular fitness, and produce stronger bones. School-aged youth should also participate in activities that are enjoyable and appropriate for their age, developmental status, and personal preferences. As described in the next session, a variety of physical activities, games, and sports can be used to meet the recommended guidelines.

FITT Profile for Aerobic Fitness   The majority of children's daily 60-minute activity period should include rhythmic, large-muscle, moderate to vigorous aerobic physical activities. Moderate-intensity activity can be considered a level 5 or 6 on a 10-point scale of effort (in which 0 is sitting at rest and 10 is the highest level of effort possible).[21] Vigorous-intensity aerobic activity (level 7 or 8 on the 10-point scale) should also be performed at least three days a week.[21] Because youth frequently engage in short bursts of activity interspersed with brief rest intervals, any time spent in moderate or vigorous aerobic activities can be counted toward meeting the aerobic guidelines. However, a majority of the one-hour target time should be spent being active. For example, during a 20-minute recess, a child might accumulate 12 minutes of physical activity in periods lasting between a few seconds and several minutes, and 8 total minutes of rest. Some activities, such as bicycling, can be classified as either moderate or vigorous, depending on how intensely energy is being expended. Table 9.2 lists aerobic activities for children and adolescents that can be performed at moderate or vigorous intensities.

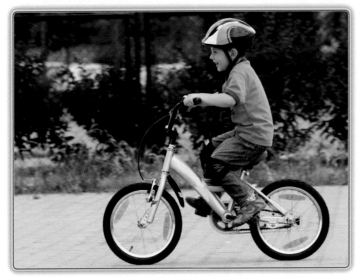

Kids of all ages enjoy bike riding, which is a great way to increase aerobic fitness.

Table 9.2 **Examples of Aerobic Activities for Children and Adolescents**

	Children	Adolescents
Moderate intensity	• Active recreation such as hiking, skateboarding, and rollerblading • Bicycle riding • Brisk walking	• Active recreation such as canoeing, hiking, skateboarding, and in-line skating • Riding a stationary or road bike • Brisk walking • Housework and yardwork, such as sweeping and pushing a lawn mower
Vigorous intensity	• Active games involving running and chasing, such as tag • Bicycle riding • Jumping rope • Martial arts, such as judo and karate • Running • Sports such as soccer, ice or field hockey, basketball, swimming, and tennis • Cross-country skiing	• Active games involving running and chasing, such as flag football • Bicycle riding • Jumping rope • Martial arts, such as judo and karate • Running • Sports such as soccer, ice or field hockey, basketball, swimming, and tennis • Cross-country skiing • Vigorous dancing

Adapted from U.S. Department of Health and Human Services, 2008.

FITT Profile for Muscular Fitness and Bone Strengthening Current recommendations are that a portion of the 60-minute period of daily physical activity of children and adolescents include muscle strengthening activities at least three days a week.[21] The primary targets of strengthening should be the major upper- and lower-body muscle groups (e.g., legs, hips, back, abdomen, arms, chest, shoulders). Table 9.3 lists games and resistance training exercises that promote muscle strengthening. An example of a properly aligned weight machine is shown in figure 9.3.

The American College of Sports Medicine supports the use of resistance training for youth, provided the training program is properly designed and competently supervised.[7] Myths still abound regarding resistance training for youth, including that growth plates can be injured resulting in stunted growth or that strength gains are not possible in younger kids. In reality, resistance training improves muscular strength and endurance in youth and helps strengthen bones while having no negative effect on physical growth. In addition, resistance training potentially decreases the incidence and severity of injury rather than causing injury.[4]

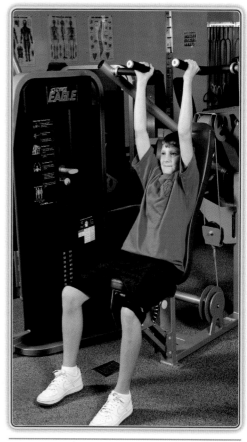

Figure 9.3 Youth can benefit from properly designed and supervised resistance training.

To keep resistance training sessions safe, adults must ensure that children and adolescents are mature enough to follow directions. Sessions should also be supervised by a knowledgeable adult who understands standard safety guidelines. Youth should be instructed to use controlled movements for all resistance training activities. In addition, proper technique is a pivotal requirement and should be emphasized rather than focusing on how much weight can be lifted. A warm-up and cool-down should be part of each resistance training session.

So, how young is too young to start resistance training? Strength training has been used with boys and girls as young as 7 to 8 years of age.[7] Options include using rubber tubing or weight machines specially designed for children. Younger children may also be able to engage in muscle-strengthening activities such as push-ups (either regular or modified) or sit-ups. The goal of resistance training is to improve musculoskeletal strength as part of a well-rounded fitness program that also features the development of endurance, flexibility, and agility.

The guidelines for resistance training outlined in chapter 7 can be modified for children and adolescents by having them do one to three sets of 8 to 15 repetitions of a given exercise.[2] Resistance training can occur two or three days a week with one day between sessions to allow the muscles to respond and recover.[7] The intensity of training should not be maximal (i.e., to the point of muscle failure). Rather, training intensity should be moderate and focused on learning and performing resistance exercise with good technique.[7]

When muscles contract, they pull on bones and stimulate bone growth. Hence, muscle-building activities that generate high-impact forces, such as running, jumping, and basketball, also cause bones to become stronger and denser. Because weight-bearing physical activity during childhood has a positive and potentially lasting influence on bone strength,[12] it is essential for children and adolescents to participate in bone-building activities. As with muscle-strengthening activities, bone fitness activities should be performed at least three days a week as part of the 60-minute period of daily physical activity.[21] Table 9.3 identifies various activities that can be used to increase bone strength in school-aged youth.

Table 9.3 **Examples of Muscle- and Bone-Strengthening Activities for Children and Adolescents**

	Children	Adolescents
Muscle strengthening	• Games such as tug-o-war • Push-ups (knees on floor) • Resistance exercises using body weight or resistance bands • Rope or tree climbing • Sit-ups, curl-ups, or crunches • Swinging on playground equipment or bars	• Games such as tug-o-war • Push-ups or pull-ups • Resistance exercises using resistance bands, free weights, and weight machines • Climbing wall • Sit-ups, curl-ups, or crunches
Bone strengthening	• Games such as hopscotch • Hopping, skipping, jumping • Jumping rope • Running	• Hopping, skipping, jumping • Jumping rope • Running • Sports such as gymnastics, basketball, volleyball, and tennis

Adapted from U.S. Department of Health and Human Services, 2008.

Tracking Changes in Youth Fitness

Children and adolescents present a wide range of interests and fitness levels. Although some enjoy competitive sports and others prefer recreational activities, youth of all ages can meet the guidelines presented in this chapter. Fitness assessments for youth (e.g., FITNESSGRAM assessments outlined in chapter 2) can be used to determine whether sufficient fitness is present to provide the important health benefits discussed in this chapter. BMI can also be tracked from year to year (because it is age related). Chapter 2 provides instruction on how to conduct youth fitness assessments as well as how to interpret the results. For youth, results are considered as falling in a healthy fitness zone (HFZ) or in need of improvement. Figure 9.4 can be used to track a child's progress over time. A goal can be to have all assessments in the healthy fitness zone or above. It should be noted that FITNESSGRAM testing is an integral part of many school physical education programs.

FIGURE 9.4
Fitness Assessment Progress Chart for Youth*

	Current	6-month assessment	1-year assessment
One-mile run	____ HFZ or above ____ Needs improvement	____ HFZ or above ____ Needs improvement	____ HFZ or above ____ Needs Improvement
Curl-up	____ HFZ or above ____ Needs improvement	____ HFZ or above ____ Needs improvement	____ HFZ or above ____ Needs improvement
Push-up	____ HFZ or above ____ Needs improvement	____ HFZ or above ____ Needs improvement	____ HFZ or above ____ Needs improvement
Sit-and-reach	____ HFZ or above ____ Needs improvement	____ HFZ or above ____ Needs improvement	____ HFZ or above ____ Needs improvement
BMI-for-age	____ Percentile	____ Percentile	____ Percentile

*HFZ = Healthy fitness zone
From ACSM, 2011, *ACSM's complete guide to fitness & health* (Champaign, IL: Human Kinetics).

Children and adolescents who do not yet meet the aforementioned guidelines should gradually raise their physical activity levels over time and aim to be active more frequently, for longer time periods, or both.[21] Youth who are already meeting the physical activity recommendations should consider becoming more active, especially in view of recent research suggesting that additional health benefits can be realized when minimum recommended levels of physical activity are exceeded.[11] Lastly, youth who exceed the recommended activity guidelines should continue to maintain their level of performance and vary their physical activity routines to avoid injury.[21]

Although children and adolescents can meet the recommended physical activity guidelines by participating in the activities listed in tables 9.2 and 9.3, they should also look for opportunities to be active throughout the day. Examples of lifestyle physical activity include walking or riding a bicycle with friends, taking a "physical activity break" from studying or playing video games, or helping with active household chores such as vacuuming and washing the family car. Having a posted checklist is a way to visually promote these lifestyle activities. After all the items are checked off, a small reward may be given (e.g., gift card, tickets to a sporting or fitness event, new exercise clothes). Exploring local parks, trails, or greenways allows the entire family to be active together.

An even simpler approach to promoting physical activity in youngsters is to maximize outside time and minimize inside time (it's much harder to be sedentary when outdoors and very easy to be sedentary when inside). Parents, family members, and teachers who participate in regular physical activity can also be real-life models of how to integrate activity and movement into everyday living.

Practical Examples of Meeting the Physical Activity Guidelines for Children and Adolescents

An endless number of routines that combine aerobic activity with muscle-strengthening and bone-building activities can be created to meet current physical activity recommendations for children and adolescents. Even youth not interested in competitive sports can enjoy meeting these recommendations. Adults can present kids with a daily "physical activity menu" that lists several activities from which to choose, providing variety and promoting creativity. Figures 9.5 and 9.6 show one-week activity plans for Latoya, a female 8-year-old elementary school student whose focus is on active play, and Antonio, a 14-year-old male junior high student who is more interested in organized sport-related physical activity. The plans for both youngsters are age appropriate. Notice how physical activity is woven into Latoya's daily routine, and how general activity is incorporated into Antonio's weekly routine along with organized sports play.

Consider Latoya's physical activity profile for the sample week and see how she has incorporated both moderate-intensity aerobic activity and some vigorous-intensity aerobic activity, as well as activities that will help to strengthen her muscles and bones:

- *Vigorous-intensity aerobic activity*: Swim (S, F); jump rope (M, W), play tag and run (M), engage in active play (T, Th), play soccer (M,W), wash the family car (S), play basketball (W)
- *Moderate-intensity aerobic activity*: Play Frisbee golf (T, Th), walk (S, F, Sat)
- *Muscle-strengthening activity*: Swing on monkey bars (T, Th), climb (W), do sit-ups (T, Sat)
- *Bone-building activity*: Play hopscotch (Th), jump rope (M,W), play tag and run (M), play basketball (W), climb (W)

Consider Antonio's physical activity profile for the sample week. He meets and exceeds the guidelines regarding at least one hour of moderate to vigorous physical activity each day and includes vigorous activity on at least three days each week (actually, almost daily!).

- *Vigorous-intensity aerobic activity*: Flag football (M, F), basketball (T, Th, F), skateboarding (W), tennis (Sat)
- *Moderate-intensity aerobic activity*: Lawn mowing (S), baseball (T, Th), yard-work (Sat)
- *Muscle-strengthening activity*: Weightlifting (M, W, Sat)
- *Bone-building activity*: Volleyball (W), basketball (T, Th, F)

FIGURE 9.5

Sample One-Week Activity Program for Latoya
(8-year-old female elementary school student)

Day	Activities
Sunday	• Walk the dog (30 minutes) • Help wash the family car (20 minutes) • Swim in the neighborhood pool (30 minutes)
Monday	• Jump rope (5 minutes) • Play tag and run during recess (15 minutes) • Play soccer during physical education class (40 minutes)
Tuesday	• Do sit-ups at home (5 minutes) • Play Frisbee golf at school (40 minutes) • Swing on monkey bars (5 minutes) • Engage in active play with friends at school (15 minutes)
Wednesday	• Jump rope (5 minutes) • Climb up and down playground equipment during recess (15 minutes) • Participate in intramural soccer after school (30 minutes) • Play basketball at home with her brother (10 minutes)
Thursday	• Play Frisbee golf at school (40 minutes) • Hopscotch (10 minutes) • Swing on the monkey bars (5 minutes) • Engage in active play with friends during recess (20 minutes)
Friday	• Walk with a friend in the neighborhood (30 minutes) • Swim in the neighborhood pool (30 minutes)
Saturday	• Walk in a nearby park with her family (60 minutes) • Do sit-ups and stretching exercises (10 minutes)

FIGURE 9.6

Sample One-Week Activity Program for Antonio
(a 14-year-old male junior high school student)

Day	Activities
Sunday	• Mow the lawn using a push mower (1 hour)
Monday	• Play flag football in physical education class (45 minutes) • Lift weights at home (45 minutes)
Tuesday	• Play basketball at school (30 minutes) • Play baseball after school (1 hour)
Wednesday	• Play volleyball in physical education class (45 minutes) • Skateboard at home (15 minutes) • Lift weights at home (45 minutes)
Thursday	• Play basketball at school (30 minutes) • Play baseball after school (1 hour)
Friday	• Play flag football after school (1 hour) • Play basketball with friends at home (30 minutes)
Saturday	• Do general yardwork (30 minutes) • Lift weights at home (45 minutes) • Play tennis at the local park (1 hour)

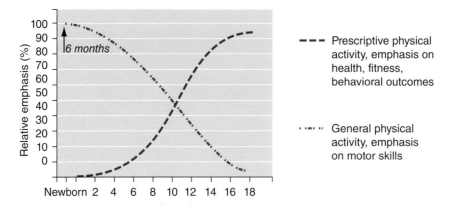

Figure 9.7   Relative contributions of motor skill development and prescriptive physical activity during childhood and adolescence.

Reprinted by permission from Strong, Malina, Blimkie, et al., 2005, p. 736.

This section of the chapter has presented an integrated approach to physical activity from infancy to adolescence. Movement exploration and the acquisition of basic motor skills start early and continue during the first years of life. Once children enter school, their movement repertoire expands and motor skill patterns undergo further refinement. The school years are also a time when youth receive specialized instruction in physical education and gain familiarity with playing various games and sports. With the onset of adolescence, greater emphasis can be placed on using physical activity to improve and maintain cardiovascular and musculoskeletal health. Figure 9.7 illustrates how the relative contributions of motor skill development and physical activity as an agent for improving health and fitness change from birth to age 18.

The benefits of physical activity and exercise for children and adolescents are numerous. With a balanced nutritional plan to complement an activity program, youth can thrive in daily activities as well as in sport and recreational endeavors. Healthy youth also have a better chance of growing into healthy adults. It is never too early, or too late, to develop good habits.

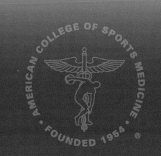

chapter 10

Adults:
Ages 18 to 64

I f you are a healthy adult between the ages of 18 and 64 years, this chapter is for you. (If you are between the ages of 50 and 64 years and have a chronic condition or functional limitation, then chapter 11 provides more appropriate guidance.) Adulthood should be a time of experiencing life to the fullest. With robust health and fitness, you can fully embrace your diverse roles within your family, community, and workplace. Unfortunately, throughout this age span, a shift toward sedentary behavior tends to occur, as noted in figure 10.1. Leisure time inactivity increases—or in other words, active leisure pursuits decrease. In addition, although ideally 100% of adults would engage in both aerobic activity and resistance training, the percentage of adults engaging in these activities decreases with age. Although this is a bit discouraging, let's focus on the positive side – on you! By reading this book, you are taking steps to change your personal health path. By focusing on nutrition and physical activity, you can claim a healthier and more active life.

FOCUS ON NUTRITION

Nutrition is the process of taking food into your body so your body can use that food to provide energy for daily activities and exercise. Too often the word *nutrition* paints pictures of unappealing foods and denial of taste. Eating healthy does not mean surviving on dry toast and carrot sticks. A balanced diet should include a variety of appetizing foods that provide needed nutrients, as described in chapter 4. Food can have nonnutrition-related functions as well. For example, social celebrations, holiday get-togethers, and expressions of support to a family facing an illness or tragedy often include food. Food is part of everyday life. Rather than seeing nutrition as an obstacle, you can focus on positive food choices as part of your new healthy lifestyle.

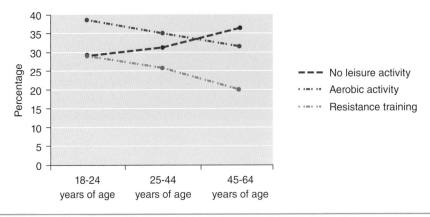

Figure 10.1 Activity patterns of adults in America.
Source: Centers for Disease Control and Prevention Wide-ranging Online Data for Epidemiologic Research.

You may be asking yourself, Does nutrition really have much of an impact? To drive home the importance of nutrition, consider that an estimated 16% of deaths in men and 9% of deaths in women have been attributed to missing the mark with regard to nutrition.[3] Hitting the mark does not have to be a mystery. The U.S. government's *Dietary Guidelines for Americans* provides a summary and synthesis of research related to nutrition and food to provide guidance related to healthy eating.[3]

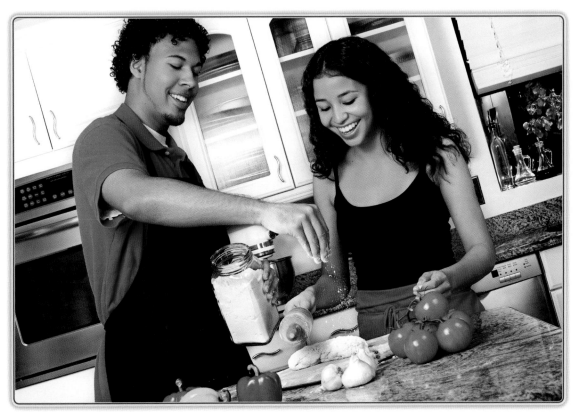

Focus on positive food choices as part of your healthy lifestyle.

Where and Why Do Adults Fall Short?

The *Dietary Guidelines* points out that American adults often are lacking in their consumption of calcium, potassium, fiber, and magnesium, as well as vitamins A, C, and E.[3] Finding foods containing these vitamins and minerals is not difficult. Table 10.1 lists some examples of good sources. Reflect on your own eating habits and consider small changes you can make to ensure that you consume adequate amounts of these nutrients.

Table 10.1 **Examples of Food Sources for Nutrients and Fiber Often Lacking in the Adult Diet**

Nutrient	Food source
Calcium	Milk, yogurt, cheese Cereal or oatmeal, calcium fortified Soy beverages, calcium fortified Pink salmon with bone Collards, spinach, kale, okra, or turnip greens, cooked from frozen
Potassium	Potato, sweet potato, baked Tomato paste, puree, juice, and sauce Milk, yogurt Clams, halibut, yellowfin tuna, rainbow trout, Pacific rockfish, cod Banana, cantaloupe
Magnesium	Nuts (Brazil nuts, almonds, cashews, pine nuts, peanuts, hazelnuts) Pumpkin and squash seed, roasted kernels Halibut, pollock, walleye, haddock, yellowfin tuna, cooked Spinach, lima beans, cooked from frozen Brown rice, beans (great northern, white, black, navy)
Vitamin A	Organ meats (liver, giblets) Baked sweet potato Collards, spinach, kale, turnip greens, cooked from frozen Carrot juice, carrots cooked from fresh, carrots raw Sweet red pepper, Chinese cabbage, mustard greens, cooked
Vitamin C	Red or green sweet peppers, raw or cooked Orange, kiwi, strawberries, pineapple, mango, guava Broccoli, cantaloupe Tomato juice, grapefruit juice, vegetable juice cocktail Brussels sprouts, kale, cauliflower, cooked
Vitamin E	Cereals, fortified Nuts (almonds, hazelnuts, pine nuts, peanuts, Brazil nuts) Sunflower seeds, roasted Oils (sunflower, cottonseed, safflower, canola) Peanut butter
Fiber	Beans (navy, kidney, black, white, pinto, lima, great northern) Bran or oat bran cereal Sweet potato Whole wheat English muffin, spaghetti Apple, pear, banana, raspberries, blackberries, dates, dried figs,

Adapted from U.S. Department of Health and Human Services and U.S. Department of Agriculture, 2005, pp. 56-65.

Falling short in regard to these nutrients as well as others is likely related to an underconsumption of vegetables, fruits, whole grains, milk and milk products, and oils.[5] Take a second look at table 10.1 to identify a couple of items in each row that you could add to your diet. In addition, women of reproductive age should consume foods containing folic acid and iron.[5] Specifically, pregnant women should consume 400 micrograms of folic acid per day to prevent neural tube defects in their babies (for more information on nutrition during pregnancy, see chapter 18). Low iron levels are common among women, which is why experts recommend that women consume iron-rich foods (e.g., meat, poultry, fish, fortified cereals, whole grains). When consuming products such as fortified cereals and grains, you may also want to consume foods rich in vitamin C (e.g., orange juice along with your fortified cereal), which help your body absorb the iron.[5]

Where and Why Do Adults Need to Cut Back?

Although adults may underconsume some nutrients, they often overconsume others. Particularly, adults are consuming too many calories as well as too much salt, added sugars, cholesterol, and fat (in particular, saturated and trans fats).[3] To maintain body weight, the number of calories consumed in foods and beverages must equal the number of calories the body uses for basic functions as well as to provide energy for work, activities of daily living, and exercise. Shifts in this balance as a result of even small amounts of extra calories on a daily basis can be to blame for the gradual increase in body weight often seen throughout adulthood. One of the benefits of a physically active lifestyle is the additional calories used on a daily and weekly basis. For more detailed information on weight management, see chapter 13.

Salt (or more technically, sodium) intake is linked with higher blood pressure (see chapter 15 for more information on how sodium can be related to high blood pressure). Middle-age as well as older adults may be more salt sensitive than others.[3] To decrease the risk of developing high blood pressure, keep a handle on your sodium intake. Naturally occurring sodium and added salt within the cooking process or at the table account for some of your total intake. Most salt consumption, however, is related to what manufacturers add to processed foods. Snack favorites that typically are high in sodium include pretzels, potato or tortilla chips, and salsa. Some items vary in their sodium content among manufacturers. Soup is a good example of a product that can be very high in sodium or reasonable, in the case of some new lower-sodium options. Keep an eye on product labels. Low-sodium products have less than 140 milligrams of sodium, or less than 5% of the Daily Value for sodium.[3]

Other areas of overconsumption include saturated and trans fats, cholesterol, and added sugars. Chapter 4 explains how to shift from higher-fat and higher-calorie foods to lower-fat and lower-calorie options. In addition, chapter 4 provides guidance on detecting evidence of added sugar on food labels. By paying closer attention to food labels, you can optimize your choices.

What Should the Focus Be for Adults?

Adults should focus on an adequate intake of all vitamins and minerals and, in particular, those listed previously as often being underconsumed. The focus should be on natural sources rather than highly processed food items. Compared to natural foods, processed foods tend to supply relatively few vitamins and minerals and have more calories. Eating mostly processed food can lead to being overweight or obese while also being undernourished in regard to micronutrients.[5] The *Dietary Guidelines for Americans* offers the following recommendations for food groups to include:[3, 5]

- *Fruits and vegetables*: Consume more fruits and vegetables (at least 2.5 cups of vegetables is associated with a decreased risk of cardiovascular disease). When selecting vegetables, choose from each of the five subgroups, which include dark green vegetables, orange vegetables, legumes, starchy vegetables, and other vegetables.
- *Whole grain products*: Keep your focus on whole grains. At least half of the grains you consume should be whole grain.
- *Milk products*: Consume 3 cups of milk (fat-free or low-fat) or equivalent dairy products per day.

Simple changes can have an impact over time. Bringing an apple, orange, or container of cut vegetables to work may help you avoid grabbing a less nutritious, high-calorie item from a vending machine. Ideally, food selections should be nutrient dense. This simply means that the food item packs the biggest punch possible with regard to vitamins, minerals, and fiber for the least number of calories.[5] Compare 100 calories of jelly beans to 100 calories from orange slices. First, the orange offers a greater quantity (over a cup's worth) for the same 100 calories (see figure 10.2)! Second, the orange provides calcium, potassium, vitamin C, and folic acid among other vitamins and minerals. In contrast, 100 calories of jelly beans (about 25 pieces) provide some potassium and sodium along with added sugar. The potassium in the orange is over 375 milligrams compared to 10 milligrams in the jelly beans. This simple example clearly demonstrates the benefits of consuming natural, nutrient-dense foods.

With regard to areas of typical overconsumption (fats, sugars, sodium, and calories), keep your focus on nutrient-dense fruits, vegetables, and whole grains. By doing so, you will be in line with the following *Dietary Guidelines*:[3, 5]

- Total fat intake should be 20% to 35% of total calories with limits on saturated fats (less than 10% of calories or even progressing to less than 7%) and trans fats (as low as possible). The main source of fat should be polyunsaturated and monounsaturated fats.

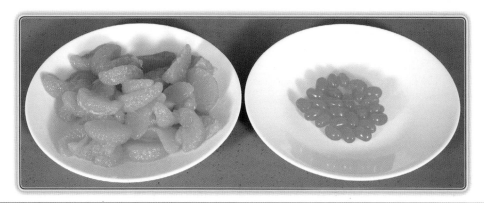

Figure 10.2 To understand nutrient density, compare 100 calories of jelly beans to 100 calories of orange slices.

- Carbohydrate intake should be mainly from fiber-rich fruits, vegetables, and whole grains rather than added sugars or sweeteners.
- Sodium consumption should be less than 2,300 milligrams per day (this amounts to about a teaspoon); less than 1,500 milligrams per day may be even better.
- Body weight should be within a healthy range; overweight and obesity are related to too many calories, too little physical activity, and often both. See chapter 13 for information on how nutrition and physical activity together can help you maintain or regain a healthy body weight.

With these guidelines in mind, you may realize that your current diet is right on track, or you may see that changes are needed. If facing the latter, consider a series of substitutions rather than a sudden overwhelming overhaul. Food should be enjoyed, and with some attention, it can also be good for your health.

FOCUS ON PHYSICAL ACTIVITY

Incorporating an exercise program into your busy day may seem impossible. Adulthood is full of responsibilities at home as well as at work. Time spent on exercise may feel frivolous or even selfish. Actually, a regular exercise program is one of the most important investments you can make for your future and that of your family. If you have been reading from the beginning of this book, you are aware of the impressive list of benefits from exercise—physical as well as mental. Your personal health is valuable, but it requires attention on a regular basis.

Each day you have the opportunity to make investments in your future health. As with a financially solid retirement plan, you need to start early and continue for the greatest benefit. You don't need to spend hours per day to be healthy, but it does require a time commitment. Ashley (see *A Closer Look*) found out how quickly fitness is lost (and, unfortunately, how quickly weight is gained) when she neglected physical activity and nutrition. Take some time to reflect on the reasons you can benefit from including exercise in your weekly plan. This reflection is a process you will want to repeat in the future because your areas of focus will likely change over time. Chapter 3 has additional guidance about formulating your personal expectations and goals as well as hints for fitting exercise into your busy schedule.

The benefits of exercise for adults of all races and ethnicities, both males and females, have been clearly documented.[4] As discussed in more detail in chapter 1, physical activity reduces the risk of premature death from heart disease as well as some cancers.[4] If you improve your fitness with regular aerobic exercise, you can reap the rewards of lower blood pressure, better cholesterol levels, and a decreased risk of both heart disease and stroke.[4] Regular exercisers can also lower the risk of developing type 2 diabetes, colon cancer, and breast cancer. In addition, adults who engage in a regular activity regimen have a healthier body weight and body composition as well as other benefits such as increased bone strength, improved sleep quality, and lower risk of depression.[4] These benefits are impressive—and are yours for the taking!

Considering the numerous health benefits of regular exercise, it is surprising how many people are not active. Although the reasons vary widely, for some, fear of being injured or having a heart attack during physical activity overrides any benefits they might gain from being active. Risks of adverse events during physical activity are real, but for most people they are outweighed by the benefits.[4]

A CLOSER LOOK

Ashley

Ashley is a 28-year-old young professional who has been working for her current employer for five years. Her job includes a significant amount of computer work and time sitting at her desk. In addition, she meets with customers, often over lunch. The combination of a relatively sedentary job and high-calorie lunches has resulted in Ashley's gaining 25 pounds (11.4 kg) since her days as a college student. An invitation to her 10-year high school class reunion prompted Ashley to do some personal reflection. She realizes she is not happy with her body weight and would like to lose at least 15 pounds (6.8 kg) before her reunion three months from now; plus, she is frustrated with feeling tired all the time. Compounding her inactivity during the day, she does little activity once back at her apartment in the evening, except to grab some dinner and watch TV.

Ashley is in need of a balanced exercise program including aerobic exercise, resistance training, and flexibility exercises. To lose weight, she will need to adjust her calorie intake (food consumption) as well as her calorie expenditure (physical activity). Following the concepts outlined in chapter 13 will allow Ashley to lose weight gradually and to maintain her weight loss over time. Aerobic exercise combined with resistance training will help her meet her weight loss goal as well as help her deal with her stress. Ashley has found some no-cost ways to be active including taking advantage of the fitness facility at her place of work, walking in her neighborhood after work, and exercising with workout DVDs from the local library (which include aerobic dance, balance ball workouts, and power yoga). By making a series of small changes in her diet in combination with increased physical activity, she improves the likelihood of losing the 15 pounds and of keeping the weight off.

Ashley's example shows the importance of taking time to reflect on what is important. For Ashley, the issues were both her physical appearance and feeling tired all the time. By reflecting on your own concerns, you can start planning to address them. Also, including exercise doesn't have to come with a big price tag. Ashley found simple ways to include activity that didn't have a monetary cost.

To help minimize risks, begin at a low to moderate intensity and build your fitness slowly over time.[1] Check through your personal risk factors for heart disease using the screenings in chapter 2. If needed, consult with your physician or health care provider to determine whether you need to modify any general exercise guidelines because of your personal health history and situation.

Physical Activity Guidelines for Adults

Adults need to move beyond the usual light or even sedentary daily activities to include physical activity focused on aerobic fitness, muscular fitness, and flexibility. The American College of Sports Medicine strongly supports the inclusion of these three components to provide a complete and balanced physical activity program.

Aerobic Fitness

Aerobic fitness refers to how your body is able to take in and use oxygen during physical activities. Assessment of aerobic fitness can require complex laboratory assessments, but chapter 2 outlined two simple ways to estimate your fitness (for more details on the one-mile walk test and the 1.5-mile run test, see chapter 2). The final score from whichever test you complete is an estimate of your $\dot{V}O_2$max, or the maximal amount of oxygen your body can use during activity. The higher the value is, the better your aerobic fitness is. You can compare your score to those of others of your sex and age in table 2.2 on page 30 of chapter 2.

As you may have noted when looking up your score, $\dot{V}O_2$max tends to decrease with age. Loss of fitness occurs as a result of the physical changes associated with aging, but it also is influenced by activity level. Sedentary, or inactive, lifestyles speed up the age-related decline in fitness. In contrast, maintaining a physically active lifestyle with focused attention on aerobic activities can help you retain your fitness. Although a balanced exercise program isn't the elusive fountain of youth, maintaining (or beginning) an exercise program will provide a better quality of life.

The U.S. government's *Physical Activity Guidelines for Americans,* as well as the ACSM, recommends that adults engage in regular aerobic physical activity.[1, 4] The following provide substantial health benefits:[1, 4]

- Moderate-intensity aerobic activity at least 30 minutes per day five days per week (or a weekly total of at least 150 minutes), or
- Vigorous-intensity aerobic activity at least 20 to 25 minutes per day three days per week (or a weekly total of 75 minutes), or
- A combination of moderate-intensity and vigorous-intensity aerobic activity at least 20 to 30 minutes per day three to five days per week

Moderate intensity refers to activities that noticeably increase your heart rate and breathing. An example is brisk walking. Vigorous-intensity activities substantially increase heart rate and breathing. Examples are jogging and running. For more details on aerobic fitness, see chapter 6.

For additional health benefits such as lowering the risk of colon and breast cancer, the *Physical Activity Guidelines* suggests a greater amount of physical activity, which can be achieved by one of the following targets:[4]

- 300 minutes of moderate-intensity activity per week, or
- 150 minutes of vigorous-intensity activity, or
- A combination of moderate- and vigorous-intensity activity (e.g., approximately 40 to 60 minutes per day three to five days per week)

Exceeding the preceding levels may provide even more benefits (e.g., a lower risk of premature death), although scientists have not yet determined what the upper limit is, above which no additional health benefits accrue.[4]

Muscular Fitness

Muscular fitness includes muscular strength (how much you can lift in one maximal effort) as well as muscular endurance (maintaining a muscle contraction or contracting a muscle repeatedly without tiring). Muscular fitness is a vital component of an exercise program.[4] Loss of muscle is a common result of aging and is technically referred to as sarcopenia. As muscle function is lost, the ability to generate force declines.[2] This loss of muscle translates into difficulty lifting, pushing, pulling, and

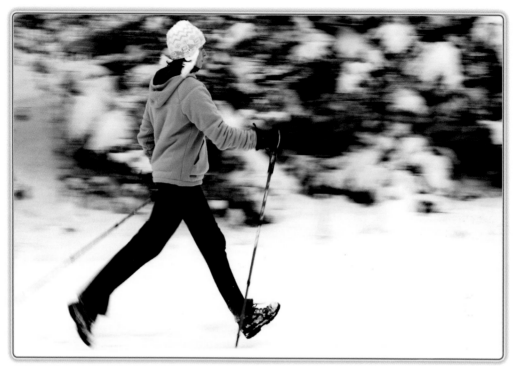

Take advantage of seasonal opportunities to exercise.

other activities of daily living. In addition, muscular fitness is vital for full participation in most recreational and sporting activities.

The *Physical Activity Guidelines for Americans* and ACSM both suggest resistance training a couple of days per week to maintain muscular fitness or improve your current fitness level. You should resistance train each of the major muscle groups two or three times per week, ensuring that you have at least 48 hours of recovery time between these sessions (i.e., don't resistance train the same body part two days in a row). Each session should include two to four sets of 8 to 12 repetitions and a rest between sets of two to three minutes.[1] For more details on resistance training, see chapter 7, which includes activity suggestions.

Flexibility

Flexibility is a fitness attribute that can influence your ability to perform activities in your day-to-day life. The ability to reach, bend, and turn provides freedom of motion. Many recreational activities and sports also benefit from a full range of motion (e.g., golf, tennis, and swimming). Therefore, stretching is recommended for all adults.

Stretching should target all of the major joints in the body and should be done when the muscles are warm to be most effective.[1] ACSM recommends that adults stretch at least two to three days per week. When using static stretching, hold the stretch for 15 to 60 seconds and repeat this at least four times. For dynamic stretching, be sure to use controlled movements and bring the targeted body part through its range of motion. More complete details on flexibility and stretching are found in chapter 8.

Programs to Meet and Exceed the Physical Activity Guidelines for Adults

Chapters 6, 7, and 8 provide detailed information on activities to promote aerobic fitness, muscular fitness, and flexibility. Now it is time to put these components together into a weekly program.

As you begin an exercise program, be realistic. Reflect on the type of program that will work with your schedule. Remember, you can split your activity into several shorter bouts over the course of the day (each should be at least 10 minutes long). Including 10 minutes of brisk walking in the morning, at noontime, and in the evening is a way to meet the target for moderate-intensity aerobic activity. For others, one 30-minute period may work better. No one pattern is right or wrong. The *best* exercise program is one you enjoy and continue to follow for years to come. Note how Joaquin (see *A Closer Look*) found activities that work with his schedule and how he enjoys and is also encouraged by his wife's participation with him.

Easing into your exercise program is recommended to decrease your risk of injury and avoid muscle soreness, which can lead to discouragement. Figures 10.3, 10.4, and 10.5 offer sample activity programs for beginning exercisers, intermediate-level exercisers, and more established exercisers, respectively. Note that each program includes aerobic activity, resistance training, and stretching. Each of these components is needed for a balanced exercise program. You may find that you are able to easily progress through the levels of the program, or you may need to take an extra couple of weeks at each level. ACSM, in conjunction with the *Physical Activity Guidelines*, recommends the following:

- *Aerobic activity*: Typically three to five days per week depending on the intensity of the activity
- *Resistance training*: Typically two or three days per week
- *Stretching for flexibility*: A minimum of two to three days per week

Sample Beginner Exercise Program for Adults*

Week	Aerobic	Resistance	Stretching**	Comments
1-2	Three days per week; 10–20 minutes per day; light intensity (level 3 or 4)	Two days per week; one set, 8–12 reps of six exercises***	Two days per week; 10 minutes of stretching activities	An easy beginning aerobic activity is walking. Select a comfortable pace. If you haven't been very active, target 10 minutes at a time for your aerobic activity. Include some stretching activities (see chapter 8) after your walk. For resistance training, see chapter 7, page 131, for details on what activities to include.
3-4	Three days per week; 20–30 minutes per day; light to moderate intensity (level 4 or 5)	Two days per week; one or two sets, 8–12 reps of six exercises***	Two days per week; 10 minutes of stretching activities	The focus for the next couple of weeks will be getting comfortable with at least 20 minutes of aerobic exercise at least three days per week. Continue with your resistance training program.
5-7	Three or four days per week; 30–40 minutes per day; moderate intensity (level 5)	Two days per week; two sets, 8–12 reps of six exercises***	Two days per week; 10 minutes of stretching activities	For the next three weeks, get comfortable with up to 40 minutes of aerobic exercise at least three days per week (for each week, add 5–10 minutes per session). Continue with your resistance training program, completing two sets per exercise and adding more weight if the 12 repetitions for a given exercise now feel easy.
8-10	Three or four days per week; 35–50 minutes per day; moderate intensity (level 5 or 6)	Two days per week; two sets, 8–12 reps of six exercises***	Two days per week; 10 minutes of stretching activities	Over the past couple of months you have been developing a good aerobic fitness base. For some variety, you can consider other activities such as biking or swimming (for more ideas, see chapter 6). If you like walking, you can also keep doing that. For your resistance training program, consider adding some variety and trying some other exercises (see chapter 7 for details).

*All activity sessions should be preceded and followed by a 5- to 10-minute warm-up and cool-down.

**Include stretching activities after aerobic exercise to improve flexibility. For specific stretches to target the major muscle groups, see chapter 8.

***Resistance training is more fully outlined in chapter 7. Beginners should select one exercise for each of the following body areas: hips and legs, chest, back, shoulders, low back, and abdominals.

FIGURE 10.4

Sample Intermediate-Level Exercise Program for Adults*

Week	Aerobic	Resistance	Stretching**	Comments
1-2	Three or four days per week; 35–50 minutes per day; moderate intensity (level 5 or 6)	Two days per week; one or two sets, 8–12 reps of 8 to 10 different exercises***	Two or three days per week; 10 minutes of stretching activities	You should be doing aerobic activity for a total of 150–200 minutes per week (moderate-intensity activity). For resistance training, include exercises for biceps and triceps (in addition to the body areas previously targeted) and add exercises for the quadriceps and hamstrings in the second week, so you will have included a total of 10 exercises (see chapter 7 for details).
3-5	Three to five days per week; 30–60 minutes per day; moderate intensity (level 5 to 6)	Two days per week; one or two sets, 8–12 reps of 10 different exercises***	Two or three days per week, 10 minutes of stretching activities	The focus for the next three weeks is to increase the time you spend in aerobic exercise or to increase the intensity, but don't do both at the same time. If you feel more comfortable with moderate-intensity activity, 200 minutes per week is appropriate. If you feel ready to increase intensity (e.g., jogging rather than walking), you can cut back on the time to 20–30 minutes per day and still realize the same benefits (note that the target for vigorous-intensity activity is 75–100 minutes per week). You may want to consider a mix of moderate- and vigorous-intensity activity as well (see chapter 6 for more details). Continue with your resistance training program.
6-10	Three to five days per week; 30–60 minutes per day; moderate intensity (level 6)	Two days per week; two sets, 8–12 reps of 10 exercises***	Two or three days per week, 10 minutes of stretching activities	For your aerobic activity, you can either increase the time spent per day or increase the number of days per week. Ultimately, you want your weekly total to be 200–300 minutes of moderate-intensity activity or 100–150 minutes of vigorous-intensity activity (recall that two minutes of moderate activity equals one minute of vigorous activity) or a combination of moderate and vigorous activity. For your resistance training, consider trying some difference exercises this week while still targeting the same muscle groups (see chapter 7 for details).

*All activity sessions should be preceded and followed by a 5- to 10-minute warm-up and cool-down.

** Include stretching activities after aerobic exercise to improve flexibility. Target all the muscle groups, holding each for 15–60 seconds. For specific stretches to target the major muscle groups, see chapter 8.

***Resistance training is more fully outlined in chapter 7. Select one exercise for each of the following body areas: hips and legs, chest, back, shoulders, low back, and abdominals. As you progress, you will expand the number of body areas you target by adding quadriceps and hamstrings as well as biceps and triceps. This provides 10 body areas to target. Examples of exercises you can include for each body area are found in table 7.2 on page 133 of chapter 7.

FIGURE 10.5

Sample Established Exercise Program for Adults*

Week	Aerobic	Resistance	Stretching**	Comments
1-2	• Five days per week for moderate exercise, or • Three days per week for vigorous exercise, or • Three to five days per week for a mix of moderate and vigorous exercise	Two days per week; two sets, 8–12 reps of 10 different exercises***	Two or three days per week, minimum; 10 minutes of stretching activities	Congratulations on your ongoing commitment to exercise. To find specific aerobic activities, see chapter 6. Ultimately, you want your weekly total to be 200–300 minutes of moderate-intensity activity or 100–150 minutes of vigorous-intensity activity (recall that two minutes of moderate activity equals one minute of vigorous activity) or a combination of moderate and vigorous activity. See chapter 7, page 131, for details on resistance training activities to include.
3-4	Two or three days per week of moderate activity and one or two days of vigorous activity	Two days per week; two sets, 8–12 reps of 10 different exercises***	Three days per week, minimum; 10 minutes of stretching activities	For the next couple of weeks, try mixing up your activities. Try a new aerobic activity or change the intensity of an activity you already do on a regular basis. Continue with your resistance training program.
5-6	• Five days per week for moderate exercise, or • Three days per week for vigorous exercise, or • Three to five days per week for moderate and vigorous exercise	Two days per week; two sets 8–12 reps of 10 exercises***	Three days per week, minimum; 10 minutes of stretching activities	Continue with your aerobic training program. For your resistance training, consider trying some different exercises (see chapter 7 for details). If you typically use machines, try a couple of new exercises using dumbbells to provide your muscles with a new challenge. Be sure to maintain good form when trying new activities.
7-8	• Five days per week for moderate exercise, or • Three days per week for vigorous exercise, or • Three to five days per week for moderate and vigorous exercise	Two days per week; three sets, 8–10 reps of 10 exercises***	Three days per week, minimum; 10 minutes of stretching activities	Continue with your aerobic training program. For your resistance training, consider doing three sets rather than two (see chapter 7 for details). You may need to cut back on your reps to add the additional set.

* All activity sessions should be preceded and followed by a 5- to 10-minute warm-up and cool-down.

** Include stretching activities after aerobic exercise to improve flexibility. For specific stretches to target the major muscle groups, see chapter 8.

***Resistance training is more fully outlined in chapter 7. Select one exercise for each of the following body areas: hips and legs, chest, back, shoulders, low back, abdominals, quadriceps, hamstrings, biceps, and triceps. Examples of exercises you can include for each body area are found in table 7.2 on page 133 of chapter 7.

Each activity in figures 10.3 through 10.5 presents a range of days to match your goals as well as your strengths and weaknesses. The simple fitness assessments in chapter 2 can provide some insight into areas in which you may need to spend some additional time. Repeating the fitness assessments periodically (e.g., every three to six months) can be helpful for charting your progress. This is covered in the next section on tracking your progress.

Tracking Your Progress

No matter where you start (beginner, intermediate, established), advancing your fitness can provide additional health and fitness benefits. You can progress in aerobic conditioning by manipulating the FITT components in the sample activity programs in figures 10.3 through 10.5. Increasing the number of days per week (frequency) or the number of minutes you spend in each exercise session (time) are two simple ways to progress. How hard you exercise (intensity) is another factor. Keep in mind that both moderate- and vigorous-intensity activities are ways to improve your health. If you find moderate-intensity activity more attractive, you will have to spend more time exercising than if you did vigorous-intensity activity. Similarly, you can improve your muscular fitness by manipulating the number of

FIGURE 10.6

Fitness Assessment Progress Chart for Adults

	Assessment 1 (baseline)	Assessment 2*	Assessment 3**
Body composition assessments			
Body mass index			
Waist circumference			
Cardiorespiratory fitness assessments			
Rockport One-Mile Fitness Walking Test ($\dot{V}O_2$max estimate) *or* 1.5-mile run test ($\dot{V}O_2$max estimate)			
Muscular fitness assessments			
1-repetition maximum (for strength)			
Curl-up test (for endurance)			
Push-up test (for endurance)			
Flexibility assessment			
Sit-and-reach test			

*From baseline: Two months for a beginner, three months for an intermediate exerciser, and four months for an established exerciser
**From baseline: Four months for a beginner, six months for an intermediate exerciser, and eight months for an established exerciser
From ACSM, 2011, *ACSM's complete guide to fitness & health* (Champaign, IL: Human Kinetics).

resistance training sessions you do per week, the amount of weight or resistance you use, and even the type of resistance activities you do.

As you adjust these FITT components, you can gauge your body's response in a number of ways. If you are a beginner or intermediate exerciser, you can use the fitness assessments in chapter 2 every two to four months. If you are an established exerciser, assessing every four to six months would likely provide sufficient feedback because changes will likely not be as dramatic. The degree of improvement will naturally become less the more fit you become (because you will be getting closer to your maximal capacity). At this point, increasing the time between assessments to six months will still help you gauge your status without becoming an undue burden. Figure 10.6 is a chart for recording your scores or rankings.

Between fitness assessments, you can note your progress in less objective ways, including the following for aerobic conditioning:

- Your resting heart rate is lower.
- When doing the same activity, your heart rate and perception of effort are lower.
- Your heart rate returns to resting levels faster following your workout.
- You are able to complete the same number of minutes of activity, but at a higher intensity.
- You are able to continue longer at the same intensity.
- You are increasing the total time you spend exercising each week.

By tracking your workouts, you can watch for these positive signs of improving fitness.

For resistance training, you may observe the following as evidence of improvements:

- You are able to lift the same weight 12 times rather than just 8 before becoming fatigued.
- You are able increase the weight lifted or the resistance you overcome.
- You are able to complete more body weight exercises (e.g., push-ups, curl-ups).
- You increase the number of sets completed targeting a particular muscle group.

For flexibility, you may observe that you are able to reach farther or hold a position with less tension than you could earlier in your stretching program.

Figure 10.7 is targeted for beginners and intermediate-level exercisers and highlights some simple ways to chart your progress in aerobic conditioning in addition to the standardized fitness assessments.

As you progress from week to week, ask yourself these questions:

- Is the same workout easier than it was last week?
- Is my heart rate lower for the same level of intensity?
- Can I go for an extra 10 minutes per session?
- Could I increase the intensity slightly and still complete the same length of workout?
- Is my resting heart rate lower?

If you answer yes to most of these questions, you are right on track. If you answer no to a number of the questions, you may need to slow the pace of your progress to ensure that your body has sufficient time to adapt. Because each person is unique, a cookie-cutter approach to exercise does not work. To improve, you need to provide your body with a new challenge, but you also need to allow your body enough time to respond and improve. This is why increases in time or intensity are done slowly over a number of weeks. When assessing the success of your exercise program, don't forget the E of FITTE—enjoyment! Continue to look for activities that you enjoy doing so you can maintain your activity.

Figure 10.8 provides some markers of progress in resistance training for beginners and intermediate exercisers. Note that the formal fitness assessments described in chapter 2 should be done at least a couple of months apart to give your body time to respond to the training.

To help you track the status of your flexibility, figure 10.9 has some simple weekly markers. The standardized fitness assessments outlined in chapter 2 are not needed on a weekly basis. Including them every two to four months allows you to gauge your progress without becoming overly focused on the scores.

For established exercisers, improvements in fitness will likely be in much smaller increments. As you age, maintaining your fitness level can also be a potential goal. Figure 10.10 is a summary chart that may be helpful for established exercisers. Writing down your workouts can be helpful so you can look back on them. An activity chart provides a weekly accounting of how many sessions you have targeting aerobic fitness, muscular fitness, and flexibility (see figure 3.2 on page 55 of chapter 3 for an example).

FIGURE 10.7
Aerobic Fitness Progress Chart for Beginners and Intermediate-Level Exercisers

	Resting heart rate (record once per week)	Total time spent in aerobic exercise (minutes per week)	Time spent in moderate and vigorous activity (minutes per week)	
			Moderate	Vigorous
Week 1				
Week 2				
Week 3				
Week 4				
Week 5				
Week 6				
Week 7				
Week 8				
Week 9				
Week 10				

From ACSM, 2011, *ACSM's complete guide to fitness & health* (Champaign, IL: Human Kinetics).

FIGURE 10.8

Muscular Fitness Progress Chart for Beginners and Intermediate-Level Exercisers

	Number of resistance training sessions per week	Number of reps per set	Number of sets per muscle group	Number of different exercises within the session
Week 1				
Week 2				
Week 3				
Week 4				
Week 5				
Week 6				
Week 7				
Week 8				
Week 9				
Week 10				

From ACSM, 2011, *ACSM's complete guide to fitness & health* (Champaign, IL: Human Kinetics).

FIGURE 10.9

Flexibility Progress Chart for Beginners and Intermediate-Level Exercisers

	Time spent stretching per session	Number of stretching sessions per week
Week 1		
Week 2		
Week 3		
Week 4		
Week 5		
Week 6		
Week 7		
Week 8		
Week 9		
Week 10		

From ACSM, 2011, *ACSM's complete guide to fitness & health* (Champaign, IL: Human Kinetics).

FIGURE 10.10

Fitness Progress Chart for Established Exercisers

	Resting heart rate (record once per week)	Total time spent in aerobic exercise (minutes of moderate and vigorous activity per week)	Number of resistance training sessions per week	Number of resistance training exercises per session	Number of reps per set	Number of sessions per week of stretching activities
Week 1		Moderate: ____ minutes Vigorous: ____ minutes				
Week 2		Moderate: ____ minutes Vigorous: ____ minutes				
Week 3		Moderate: ____ minutes Vigorous: ____ minutes				
Week 4		Moderate: ____ minutes Vigorous: ____ minutes				
Week 5		Moderate: ____ minutes Vigorous: ____ minutes				
Week 6		Moderate: ____ minutes Vigorous: ____ minutes				
Week 7		Moderate: ____ minutes Vigorous: ____ minutes				
Week 8		Moderate: ____ minutes Vigorous: ____ minutes				
Week 9		Moderate: ____ minutes Vigorous: ____ minutes				
Week 10		Moderate: ____ minutes Vigorous: ____ minutes				

From ACSM, 2011, *ACSM's complete guide to fitness & health* (Champaign, IL: Human Kinetics).

Regardless of your current fitness level, recording your exercise and reflecting on your progress allows you to check off short-term goals (e.g., increasing the number of minutes per week, increasing the intensity, including different resistance training exercises) as you continue to move to your long-term goals (e.g., reaching the "Good" category for aerobic fitness, losing weight, improving your flexibility).

Adulthood can be a hectic and busy time. Too often, personal health and fitness take a back seat just when you can least afford it. Taking charge of your diet and physical activity will provide many benefits (e.g., lower risk of heart disease and type 2 diabetes) as well as a better quality of life. Within your diet, keep a focus on fruits, vegetables, whole grains, and low-fat dairy products while avoiding the overconsumption of fat (especially saturated and trans fats), sodium, and sugar. Physical activity along with a solid nutritional plan will help you maintain your desired body weight as well as promote your overall fitness. Aerobic activities, resistance training, and stretching together provide a comprehensive program to maximize the benefits to your health.

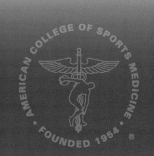

chapter 11

Older Adults:
Ages 65 and Older

Does old age simply happen? Or can you play an active role in deciding your fate as you grow older? Many studies now suggest that maintaining a high level of physical activity may help postpone some of the negative consequences of growing older. Avoiding a sedentary lifestyle may be one of the most effective means of promoting independence and maintaining a high quality of life in old age. For the purposes of this chapter, the term *older adults* refers to anyone age 65 or older. The guidelines presented in this chapter would also be appropriate for adults age 50 to 64 with chronic conditions or functional limitations that affect their ability to be active.[13]

Advances in medicine over the past century have resulted in declines in infectious diseases and increases in the average lifespan.[36] As a result, chronic diseases such as heart disease, type 2 diabetes, obesity, and certain cancers have now become the top causes of death.[31, 32, 36, 44, 47] Because these conditions take time to develop, older adults have a higher relative risk. The good news is you can take action to lessen your risk or avoid many of the chronic conditions that affect older adults by addressing biological risk factors such as hypertension, obesity, and high cholesterol. In addition, you can avoid some lifestyle factors that increase risk, including an unhealthy diet, physical inactivity, smoking, and alcohol abuse.

FOCUS ON NUTRITION

Eating well is an important component of developing a healthy, active lifestyle. The National Institute on Aging (NIA) emphasizes that following a healthy eating plan is an essential component of successful aging. The NIA recommends that all older adults follow a dietary regimen based on the U.S. government's *Dietary Guidelines for Americans*,[43] as discussed in chapter 4. The major components of a healthy diet for older adults are as follows:

- Increasing the consumption of vegetables, fruits, whole grains, and fat-free or low-fat milk and milk products
- Including healthy forms of protein in the diet such as lean meats, poultry, fish, beans, eggs, and nuts
- Limiting the consumption of saturated fats, trans fats, cholesterol, salt, and added sugars
- Balancing calories from foods and beverages with calories burned through physical activities to maintain a healthy weight

Where and Why Do Older Adults Fall Short?

The *Dietary Guidelines* are based on compelling research[44] but need to be put into practice on a regular basis to be of any benefit. As highlighted for adults in chapter 10, suboptimal consumption of calcium, potassium, fiber, magnesium, and vitamins A, C, and E often continues into older adulthood.[45] With age, the metabolic rate does decrease resulting in fewer calories required to maintain body weight.

Tips for Healthy Eating for Older Adults

The NIA has developed a number of tips for healthy eating, which are summarized as follows:
- Eat a variety of fruits and vegetables. Eating fruits and vegetables of different colors gives your body a wide range of valuable nutrients, including fiber, folic acid, potassium, and vitamins A and C.
- Eat a diet rich in foods that contain fiber such as dry beans, fruits, vegetables, and whole grain foods.
- Season your foods with lemon juice, herbs, or spices, instead of butter and salt.
- Look for foods that are low in cholesterol and fat, especially saturated fats (mostly in foods that come from animals) and trans fats (found in many cakes, cookies, crackers, icings, margarines, and microwave popcorn). Saturated fats and trans fats can have a negative effect on blood cholesterol levels.
- Choose and prepare foods with little salt.
- Choose poultry and lean cuts of meat. Trim away extra fat and remove the skin from chicken and turkey before cooking. Broil, roast, bake, steam, microwave, or boil foods instead of frying them.
- Reaching and maintaining a healthy weight are important for your overall health and well-being. The secret is to balance your "energy in" and "energy out" over the long run. "Energy in" is the calories from foods and beverages you consume each day, and "energy out" is the calories you burn for basic body functions and during physical activity.
- Watch your portion sizes. Controlling portion size helps limit calorie intake, especially when eating foods that are high in calories.

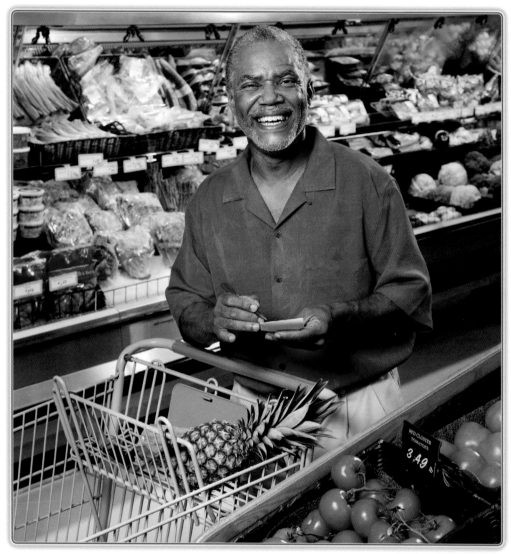

Healthy eating is an essential part of successful aging.

As calorie consumption drops, ensuring that you are consuming nutrients in sufficient qualities can become more difficult.

Adults over the age of 50 should pay special attention to consuming sufficient vitamin B_{12}.[45] Your health care provider should check your B_{12} status. Because many older adults have difficulty absorbing naturally occurring B_{12} from food, they should consume products fortified with B_{12} because this crystalline form is more easily absorbed.[45] The RDA for B_{12} is 2.4 micrograms per day. Ready-to-eat cereals are an example of a food typically fortified with B_{12}.

Similarly, older adults may benefit from consuming extra vitamin D from fortified foods (e.g., milk products) and supplements.[43] Vitamin D status depends on the amount taken in as well as the amount formed by the action of sunlight on the skin. Because older adults may have difficulty forming vitamin D in their skin, they should try to consume about 20 micrograms of vitamin D each day.[43]

Where and Why Do Older Adults Need to Cut Back?

Older adults are not unique in regard to excessive consumption of calories in relation to the number of calories they use each day. Because metabolic rate naturally decreases with age, one way to remain in caloric balance is to expend more calories in exercise and physical activity.

Older adults are encouraged to aim for the lower sodium intake (no more than 1,500 mg each day) and to meet the potassium recommendation (4,700 mg each day) with food.[45] Adults over the age of 50 have a 90% risk of high blood pressure. Because of the impact sodium can have on blood pressure (for more information, see chapter 15), sodium intake should be kept in check. Increasing potassium intake may help lessen the negative impact sodium can have on blood pressure.[45] As a caution, older adults who are taking medications that could interfere with the normal excretion of potassium, or who have kidney disease, should consult with a doctor regarding appropriate potassium intake to avoid excessive levels in the blood.[45]

What Should the Focus Be for Older Adults?

Older adults benefit from nutrient-dense foods, especially given their lower calorie requirements. Nutrient-dense foods include vegetables (including cooked dry beans and peas), fruits, whole grains, and fat-free or low-fat milk and milk products.[45] These foods provide the most nutrients for the least amount of calories—thus, they are "dense" when it comes to nutritional value per calorie. Following the *Dietary Guidelines* (as outlined in chapter 4) is recommended.

FOCUS ON PHYSICAL ACTIVITY

Although the interrelationships among heart disease risk factors may seem complex and are unique to each person, the World Health Organization has identified regular physical activity as probably the single most effective way to decrease your risk.[27] Researchers have found that people who are highly active have a much lower risk of heart disease (as well as death from all other causes) compared to people of a similar age who are only moderately or less active.[11] A physically active lifestyle can make a difference!

How much physical activity do you need to stay healthy? How hard do you have to exercise to maximize health benefits? What type of exercise is best? These questions are often asked by older adults who are about to embark on an exercise program. Although precise answers to these questions depend on a wide variety of factors including current levels of health and fitness, prior exercise experience, and personal preference, a number of guidelines exist with regard to how much and what type of exercise older adults need.

Recommendations from ACSM and the American Heart Association (AHA) for the frequency, intensity, and duration of exercise for older adults are summarized in the following section. They address aerobic fitness, muscular fitness, flexibility, and balance. If you have been inactive, ease into a new activity program gradually. Don't worry about reaching the target levels immediately. Before beginning, refer to the health screening tools in chapter 2 to ensure that you are ready to start being physically active. Consulting with your health care provider is always an appropriate step if you have any specific questions or concerns.

Benefits of Physical Activity for Older Adults

Although there used to be some skepticism about the health benefits of exercise and physical activity, over the past 20 to 30 years a substantial number of research studies have confirmed many benefits for older adults who participate in regular physical activity. The U.S. government's *Physical Activity Guidelines for Americans* conclude that, compared to less active people, more active people have lower rates of all-cause mortality, coronary heart disease, high blood pressure, stroke, type 2 diabetes, metabolic syndrome, colon cancer, breast cancer, and depression.[40]

The benefits of activity for older adults are significant.[13, 27] Although no amount of physical activity can stop the biological aging process, there is evidence that regular physical activity can minimize the physiological effects of an otherwise sedentary lifestyle and increase healthy life expectancy by limiting the development and progression of chronic disease and disabling conditions.[16] Importantly, not only does physical activity benefit your physical health, but also strong evidence suggests that it can improve psychological health and well-being. Regular physical activity can favorably influence a broad range of body systems and thus may be a lifestyle factor that discriminates between those who experience successful aging and those who do not.

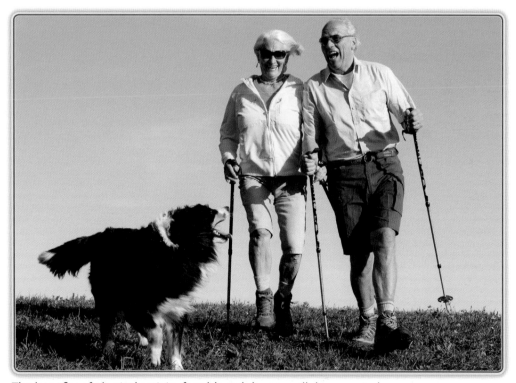

The benefits of physical activity for older adults are well documented.

Regular exercise can be an important element in the management of many diseases. Physicians often recommend exercise as part of the treatment of numerous medical conditions faced by older adults including coronary heart disease,[15, 31, 39] hypertension,[12, 30, 39] peripheral vascular disease,[25] type 2 diabetes,[34] obesity,[46] elevated cholesterol,[9, 39] osteoporosis,[16] osteoarthritis,[2, 3] claudication,[38] and chronic obstructive pulmonary disease.[5] Furthermore, in a joint statement, ACSM and AHA[27] concluded that physical activity is valuable in the treatment and management of depression and anxiety disorders,[11] dementia,[14] pain,[4] congestive heart failure,[32] syncope,[10] stroke,[17] back pain,[19] and constipation.[24] In addition, there is some evidence that physical activity prevents or delays cognitive impairment[1, 23, 47] and disability,[20, 29, 35] and improves sleep.[21, 36] What an overwhelming list of benefits! Physical activity and exercise can play a major role in your life.

The World Health Organization (WHO) suggests that the benefits of physical activity for older adults are in three general areas—physiological, psychological, and social (see *Threefold Focus on Benefits of Physical Activity for Older Adults*). The WHO guidelines conclude that regular physical activity provides substantial health-related benefits. In addition, it is cheap, safe, and readily available.

Threefold Focus on Benefits of Physical Activity for Older Adults

Following are lists of the physiological, psychological, and social benefits of physical activity for older adults based on the WHO guidelines.[47]

Physiological Benefits

Immediate physiological benefits of physical activity in older adults are as follows:

- *Glucose levels*: Physical activity helps regulate blood sugar (glucose) levels.
- *Catecholamine activity*: Some "activity-related" hormones are stimulated by physical activity.
- *Improved sleep*: Physical activity has been shown to enhance sleep quality and quantity in people of all ages.

Long-term physiological benefits of physical activity in older adults are as follows:

- *Aerobic, or cardiorespiratory, endurance*: Substantial improvements in almost all aspects of cardiorespiratory functioning have been observed following appropriate physical training.
- *Resistance training, or muscle strengthening*: People of all ages can benefit from muscle-strengthening exercises. Resistance training can have a significant impact on the maintenance of independence in old age.
- *Flexibility*: Exercise that stimulates movement throughout the range of motion assists in the preservation and restoration of flexibility.
- *Balance and coordination*: Regular activity helps prevent or postpone age-associated declines in balance and coordination that are a major risk factor for falls.
- *Velocity of movement*: Typically, movement and reaction time slows with age. People who are regularly active can often postpone these age-related declines.

Psychological Benefits

Immediate psychological benefits of physical activity in older adults are as follows:

- *Relaxation*: Appropriate physical activity enhances relaxation.
- *Reduced stress and anxiety*: There is evidence that regular physical activity can reduce stress and anxiety.
- *Enhanced mood state*: Numerous people report elevations in mood state following appropriate physical activity.

Long-term psychological benefits of physical activity in older adults are as follows:

- *Improved general well-being*: Improvements in almost all aspects of psychological functioning have been observed after periods of extended physical activity.
- *Improved mental health*: Regular exercise can make an important contribution to the treatment of several mental illnesses, including depression and anxiety.
- *Cognitive improvement*: Regular physical activity may help postpone age-related declines in how the brain and nerves process information and thus improve reaction time.
- *Improved motor control and performance*: Regular physical activity helps prevent or postpone age-associated declines in the control of muscle contraction for either precise or more general movements.
- *Skill acquisition*: New skills can be learned and existing skills refined by all people regardless of age.

Social Benefits

Immediate social benefits of physical activity in older adults are as follows:

- *Empowerment*: Rather than voluntarily adopting a sedentary lifestyle, participation in appropriate physical activity can help empower older adults and assist them in playing a more active role in society.
- *Enhanced social and cultural integration*: Physical activity programs, particularly when carried out in small groups or in social environments, enhance social and intercultural interactions for many older adults.

Long-term social benefits of physical activity in older adults are as follows:

- *Enhanced integration*: Regularly active people are more likely to stay engaged in society and more likely to contribute actively to the social milieu.
- *Formation of new friendships*: Participation in physical activity, particularly in small groups and in other social environments, stimulates new friendships and acquaintances.
- *Widened social and cultural networks*: Physical activity frequently provides opportunities to widen social networks.
- *Role maintenance and new role acquisition*: A physically active lifestyle helps foster the stimulating environments necessary for maintaining an active role in society, as well as for acquiring positive new roles.
- *Enhanced intergenerational activity*: Physical activity can be shared across generations and thus provides opportunities for old and young to interact together.

Physical Activity Guidelines for Older Adults

The *Physical Activity Guidelines* clearly state that "regular physical activity is essential for healthy aging"[40]—not just *helpful* or *suggested*, but *essential*. For adults over the age of 65 with no chronic conditions, the guidance provided applies and includes aerobic fitness, muscular fitness, and flexibility. In addition, balance training is recommended for older adults at risk of falling. Older adults with chronic conditions should achieve as much physical activity as possible, within the limitations of their abilities, in consultation with their health care providers.[40]

Aerobic Fitness

Aerobic exercises are those that require the body to move in a rhythmic fashion for a period of time. Examples include walking, jogging, biking, and playing tennis, of which walking is the most common aerobic activity for older adults. For older adults, any type of exercise that does not impose excessive impact stress on the body is recommended. Aquatic exercise and stationary cycling may be advantageous if you have limited tolerance for weight-bearing activity. For more information on aerobic activities, see chapter 6.

On a scale of 0 to 10 for level of physical exertion, consider moderate intensity to be a level 5 or 6. This would be considered a medium level of effort in which you feel your breathing rate and heart rate increase. Vigorous intensity would be a level 7 or 8 and would produce greater increases in breathing and heart rate. For moderate-intensity activities (such as walking), accumulate at least 30 minutes or up to 60 minutes per day (for greater benefit). You can do this in multiple bouts of at least 10 minutes each or continuously. The goal is to be active a total of 150 to 300 minutes per week. If you enjoy more intense activity, then shoot for at least 20 to 30 minutes per day or more to total 75 to 150 minutes per week. Vigorous activity may include jogging or running for healthy older adults or walking more briskly for those who are more deconditioned.

A CLOSER LOOK
Alex

Alex is a 70-year-old man who retired last year from his job in lawn care maintenance. He had worked for most of his adult life in the outdoors and thus was quite active (e.g., mowing, trimming grass, lifting bags of seed and soil, working on landscaping). In addition, he had always enjoyed water sports (sailing, scuba diving) and most evenings could be found walking the ocean beach near his home. Now retired, Alex still wants to maintain his fitness. Without the physical stresses of his lawn care job to promote muscular fitness, he has begun a formal resistance training program for the first time in his life since his days as an athlete in high school. He maintains his aerobic fitness with evening walks along the beach, followed by some stretching activities (for flexibility). He also takes advantage of a local path to ride his bike for 45 minutes at least three days per week. For balance training, he joins a group of seniors who meet twice a week at a beachfront pavilion for tai chi. Alex enjoys his activity program and has found that he is maintaining his fitness (even showing some improvement in his flexibility) with his new plan of action.

If you are engaging in moderate-intensity activities, experts recommend that you exercise a minimum of five days per week; if your exercise is vigorous, a minimum of three days per week is recommended. If you like to mix the level of intensity on various days, consider three to five days per week as your target. If you find that you are unable to meet the minimum recommendation of 150 minutes per week because of a chronic health condition, try to be as active as your abilities and condition allow. Remember, any activity is better than no activity. Whatever your current fitness level is, you can benefit from doing a bit more.

Muscular Fitness

Resistance training is described in detail in chapter 7. Regardless of your age, strengthening your muscles will benefit you in your day-to-day activities. A number of types of resistance exercises are outlined in chapter 7, including lifting weights (using dumbbells or machines), using resistance bands, and doing calisthenics (e.g., push-ups, pull-ups, sit-ups). With these types of resistance training you should perform 8 to 10 exercises involving the major muscle groups with 10 to 15 repetitions each. You can also consider other activities such as stair climbing, heavy gardening, and carrying heavy loads as muscle strengthening.

Including resistance training at least two days per week is recommended. Be sure to wait at least 48 hours between exercise sessions for a given muscle group to give your body time to adapt. Using the 0 to 10 scale described previously, resistance training should be between moderate (level 5 or 6) and vigorous (level 7 or 8). You need to use the muscles at a level higher than you typically do during routine daily activities to see improvements.

Flexibility

Flexibility tends to decrease with age, but you can work to maintain the flexibility you need for daily activities with a regular stretching program. You should plan to include some time stretching at least two days per week. Remember to do a general warm-up first (e.g. walking, light calisthenics). By increasing the temperature in your muscles, you will increase the ability of your muscles to stretch.

Stretching should be done to the point where you can feel tightness in the muscle but not to the point of discomfort or pain. On the 0 to 10 scale, moderate intensity (level 5 or 6) is the target for your stretching activities. Static stretches that target all the major muscle groups and involve placing the joint and muscle into a stretched position for about 15 to 60 seconds are recommended. Avoid bouncing or jerking stretches because these could increase the potential for injury. For help with setting up a stretching program, refer to chapter 8, in particular focusing on the static stretches.

Balance

Balance training is recommended for people who fall frequently or have mobility problems. Although there are currently no specific recommendations regarding balance training for older adults, most balance and fall prevention programs include the following:

- Progressively more difficult postures that gradually reduce your base of support (e.g., two-legged stand, semi-tandem stand, tandem stand, one-legged stand)

- Dynamic movements that challenge your center of gravity (e.g., tandem walk, circle turns)
- Stressing postural muscle groups (e.g., standing on just your heels or toes)
- Reducing sensory input (e.g., standing with your eyes closed)

For details on balance training, see chapter 8, which includes pictures of exercises you can try. In general, balance training two or three days per week is recommended for older adults.

Special Considerations for Beginners

If you have been sedentary for many years, start out slowly when beginning a new exercise program, especially if you are frail or have chronic conditions that affect your ability to perform physical tasks. Increases in exercise intensity and duration should be gradual and tailored to your tolerance and preference. Taking it easy and being patient are good strategies for deconditioned seniors. For some older adults, muscle-strengthening activities and balance training may need to precede aerobic training activities. If chronic conditions prevent activity at the recommended minimum level, you should perform physical activities as tolerated so as to avoid being sedentary.

Concerns for safety have been identified as a barrier to exercise by many older adults.[8] Of course, there is always a risk of injury when doing physical activity. The good news is that a prudently advanced program can provide many benefits that ultimately outweigh the risks. Increasing your physical activity level gradually over time will lessen the chance of injury. Keeping your exercise intensity at a level appropriate for your current fitness level will optimize safety. If you do have any questions or concerns, consult with your health care provider or a certified fitness professional.

Some risks are associated with regular physical activity, but the risks of being sedentary are much greater! Low-intensity physical activity reduces the risks of injury and muscle soreness and may be perceived as less threatening than moderate- or high-intensity activity. Although lower risk is associated with lower-intensity exercise, the consensus is that moderate physical activity has a better risk-to-benefit ratio, and as such should be the goal for most older adults.

Although speaking with a health care provider is always a good idea, the involvement of a primary care provider before beginning a program of physical activity is not always necessary. The decision to do so depends on your health condition and the level of intensity and mode of physical activity you plan to pursue. Having a strategy to manage your risk and prevent activity-related injuries is recommended.[17] A website has recently been developed to help older adults identify the physical activity program most suited to their personal needs, preferences, and health condition: the Exercise Assessment and Screening for You (EASY) screening tool.[33]

EASY helps you or your health care provider identify types of exercise or physical activity regimens that can be tailored to meet your existing health condition, illness, or disability. The EASY tool includes six screening questions that emphasize the importance of engaging in regular exercise, attending to health changes, recognizing a full range of signs and symptoms that might indicate potentially harmful events, and becoming familiar with simple safety tips for initiating and progressively increasing physical activity patterns.[43] EASY is an inclusive approach that tailors physical activity to the needs of virtually all older adults. EASY is found at www.easyforyou.info.

Fitness Assessments Specific to Older Adults

Chapter 2 outlined some simple assessments that you can use to measure your fitness level and track your progress. You may want to substitute those with some of the following assessments, which have been established specifically for people between the ages of 60 and 94. Regular and accurate performance feedback can assist you in developing realistic expectations of your own progress.[26]

Normal ranges for men are found in table 11.1, and normal ranges for women are found in table 11.2. If your score is over the range listed, consider yourself above average; if your score falls short of the range listed, consider yourself below average.

Chair Stand

The chair stand assessment, as shown in figure 11.1, is used to determine lower-body muscular fitness. This test involves counting the number of times in 30 seconds you can stand from a seated position while keeping your arms folded across your chest.

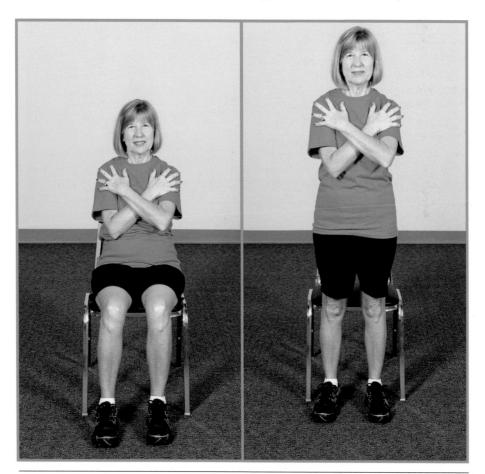

Figure 11.1   Chair stand.

Arm Curl

The arm curl assessment, as shown in figure 11.2, is used to determine upper-body muscular fitness. This test involves counting the number of dumbbell curls you can complete in 30 seconds. Men should use an 8-pound (3.6 kg) dumbbell, and women should use a 5-pound (2.3 kg) dumbbell.

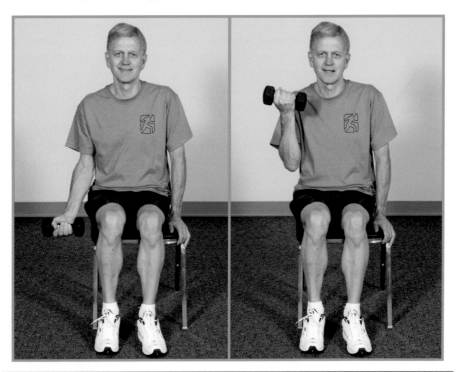

Figure 11.2 Arm curl.

6-Minute Walk

The 6-minute walk test is used to measure aerobic fitness. This test requires you to determine the distance you can walk in 6 minutes around a 50-yard (45.7 m) rectangular area (see figure 11.3 for the setup).

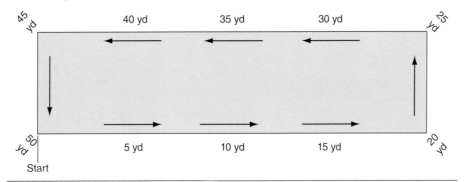

Figure 11.3 Setup for 6-minute walk test.

Adapted by permission from Rikli and Jones, 2001, p. 65.

8-Foot Up and Go

The 8-foot up and go test is used to assess agility and balance. This test involves timing how many seconds it takes you to get up from a seated position, walk 8 feet (2.4 m), turn, and return to a seated position (see figure 11.4).

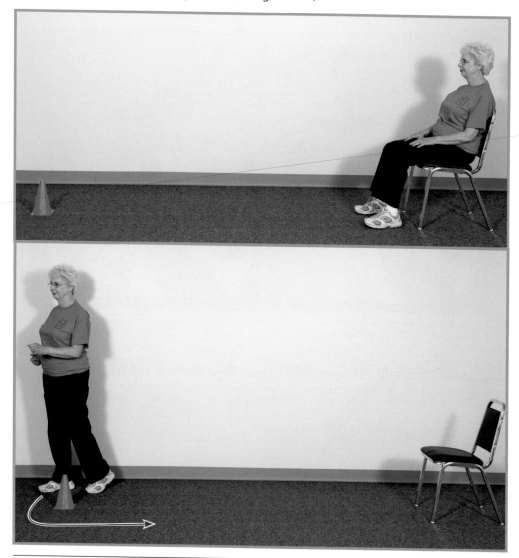

Figure 11.4   8-foot up and go.

Modified Sit-and-Reach

The sit-and-reach test was included in chapter 2 to assess flexibility, but you may prefer to use a modified version, as shown in figure 11.5. In this version, you sit in chair (rather than having to get down on the floor) with your foot extended and measure the distance between your fingers and toes.

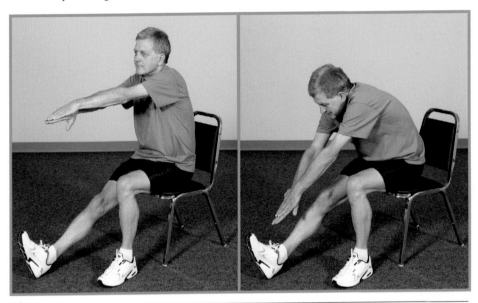

Figure 11.5 Modified sit-and-reach.

Table 11.1 Normal Ranges for Fitness Test Scores for Men

	60–64 years of age	65–69 years of age	70–74 years of age	75–79 years of age	80–84 years of age	85–89 years of age	90–94 years of age
Chair stand test (number of stands)	14–19	12–18	12–17	11–17	10–15	8–14	7–12
Arm curl test (number of repetitions)	16–22	15–21	14–21	13–19	13–19	11–17	10–14
6-minute walk test (number of yards)	610–735	560–700	545–680	470–640	445–605	380–570	305–500
8-foot up and go test (number of seconds)	3.8–5.6	4.3–5.9	4.4–6.2	4.6–7.2	5.2–7.6	5.5–8.9	6.2–10.0
Chair sit-and-reach (number of inches)	−2.5 to +4.0	−3.0 to +3.0	−3.0 to +3.0	−4.0 to +2.0	−5.5 to +1.5	−5.5 to +0.5	−6.5 to −0.5

Adapted by permission from Rikli and Jones, 2001, p. 87.

Table 11.2 Normal Ranges for Fitness Test Scores for Women

	60–64 years of age	65–69 years of age	70–74 years of age	75–79 years of age	80–84 years of age	85–89 years of age	90–94 years of age
Chair stand test (number of stands)	12–17	11–16	10–15	10–15	9–14	8–13	4–11
Arm curl test (number of repetitions)	13–19	12–18	12–17	11–17	10–16	10–15	8–13
6-minute walk test (number of yards)	545–660	500–635	480–615	435–585	385–540	340–510	275–440
8-foot up and go test (number of seconds)	4.4–6.0	4.8–6.4	4.9–7.1	5.2–7.4	5.7–8.7	6.2–9.6	7.3–11.5
Chair sit-and-reach (number of inches)	−0.5 to +0.5	−0.5 to +4.5	−1.0 to +4.0	−1.5 to +3.5	−2.0 to +3.0	−2.5 to +2.5	−4.5 to +1.0

Adapted by permission from Rikli and Jones, 2001, p. 87.

Programs to Meet and Exceed the Physical Activity Guidelines for Older Adults

A commitment to your exercise program is vital to fully realize the benefits outlined in this chapter. Social support from family and friends has been associated with long-term exercise adherence in older adults.[28] Examples of social support strategies include peer support (e.g., tell a friend and bring a friend, the exercise buddy system) and professional health educator support (telephone counseling, mail follow-up). Reaching out to others may not only help you, but also benefit others.

For many seniors, aging is associated with a loss of perceived control.[22] You can turn this attitude around and feel confident in your ability to succeed by participating in physical activity.[43] Seizing chances to practice various activities and gain mastery will enhance your self-efficacy. Tailoring your exercise program to your needs and interests can help motivate you to initiate and maintain a routine of regular physical activity.[37] You have choices—choosing a physically active lifestyle is a step in the right direction!

Older adults need to include physical activity focused on aerobic fitness, muscular fitness, flexibility, and balance. ACSM strongly supports the inclusion of these four components, as outlined in the *Physical Activity Guidelines,* to provide a complete and balanced physical activity program.

- *Aerobic activity*: Typically three to five days per week depending on the intensity of the activity
- *Resistance training*: At least two days per week
- *Stretching for flexibility*: A minimum of two days per week
- *Balance training*: Typically two or three days per week

Notice that each activity component includes a recommended range of days to give you the freedom to create a program based on your goals and also on areas on which you may need to focus. Figures 11.6, 11.7, and 11.8 provide activity programs for beginners, intermediate, and established exercisers, respectively. The simple fitness assessments in chapter 2, as well as additional fitness assessments in this chapter, will give you some insight into what areas you may need to spend some additional time. Repeating fitness assessments periodically (e.g., every three to six months) is helpful in charting your progress. This will be covered in the next section on tracking your progress.

Tracking Your Progress

Maintaining progress, or finding new activities or exercise formats, helps to advance your fitness no matter where you start (beginner, intermediate, established). You can progress in the various areas by manipulating the FITT components in the sample activity programs in figures 11.6 through 11.8. For aerobic activity, increasing the number of days per week (frequency) or the number of minutes you spend in each exercise session (time) are two simple ways to progress. How hard you exercise (intensity) is another factor. Both moderate- and vigorous-intensity activities are ways to improve your health. A wide range of activities may fall into these categories, so gauge your level of exertion using the 10-point scale previously described. Brisk walking might feel moderate (level 5 or 6) to a healthy 65-year-old but could be considered vigorous (level 7 or 8) to an 80-year-old. You need to exercise at a level that feels good to you. Similarly, you can improve your muscular fitness by manipulating the number of resistance training sessions you do per week, the amount of weight or resistance you use, and even the type of resistance activities you do.

FIGURE 11.6

Sample Beginner Exercise Program for Older Adults*

Week	Aerobic	Resistance	Stretching**	Balance	Comments
1-3	Three days per week; 10–20 minutes per day; light intensity (level 3 or 4)	Two days per week; one set, 10–15 reps of six different exercises***	Two days per week; 10 minutes of stretching activities	Two days per week; 10 minutes of balance activities	An easy beginning aerobic activity is walking. Select a comfortable pace. If you haven't been very active, target 10 minutes at a time for your aerobic activity. Include some stretching activities (see chapter 8) after your walk. For resistance training, see chapter 7, page 131, for details on what activities to include. For balance training, see chapter 8 page 159 for details on what activities to include.
4-6	Three days per week; 20–30 minutes per day; light to moderate intensity (level 4 or 5)	Two days per week; one or two sets, 10–15 reps of six different exercises***	Three days per week; 10 minutes of stretching activities	Two or three days per week; 10 minutes of balance activities	The focus for the next three weeks will be getting comfortable with at least 20 minutes of aerobic exercise at least three days per week. Gradually increase your intensity to a moderate level by the sixth week. Continue with your resistance training program and add an additional set by week 5. Add an additional session of balance training by the sixth week.
7-9	Three or four days per week; 30–40 minutes per day; moderate intensity (level 5)	Two days per week; two sets, 10–15 reps of six different exercises***	Three days per week; 10 minutes of stretching activities	Three days per week; 10 minutes of balance activities	For the next three weeks, try to increase your total time spent in moderate aerobic activity (either 40 minutes per day three days per week or 30 minutes per day four days per week). Continue with your resistance training program, completing two sets per exercise and adding more weight if you are able to do 15 repetitions relatively easily.
10-12	Three or four days per week; 35–50 minutes per day; moderate intensity (level 5 or 6)	Two days per week; two sets, 10–15 reps of six different exercises***	Three days per week; 10 minutes of stretching activities	Three days per week; 10 minutes of balance activities	Over the past couple of months you have been developing a good aerobic and muscular fitness base. For some variety, you can consider other activities such as stationary biking or swimming (for more ideas, see chapter 6). If you like walking, you can also keep doing that. For your resistance training program, consider adding some variety and trying some other exercises (see chapter 7 for details).

*All activity sessions should be preceded and followed by a 5 to 10 minute warm-up and cool-down.

**Include stretching activities after your aerobic exercise to improve flexibility. For specific stretches to target the major muscle groups, see chapter 8.

***Resistance training is more fully outlined in chapter 7. Beginners will select one exercise for each of the following body areas: hips and legs, chest, back, shoulders, low back, and abdominals.

FIGURE 11.7

Sample Intermediate-Level Exercise Program for Older Adults*

Week	Aerobic	Resistance	Stretching**	Balance	Comments
1-3	Three or four days per week; 35–50 minutes per day; moderate intensity (level 5 or 6)	Two days per week; two sets, 10–15 reps of six to ten different exercises***	Two or three days per week; 10 minutes of stretching activities	Three days per week; 10 minutes of balance activities	You should be doing aerobic activity for a total of 150–200 minutes per week (for moderate-intensity activity). For resistance training, add exercises for biceps and triceps during the second week and add exercises for the quadriceps and hamstrings in the 3rd week, so you will include 10 different exercises by the third week (see chapter 7 for details).
4-6	Three to five days per week; 30–60 minutes per day; moderate intensity (level 5 or 6)	Two days per week; one or two sets, 10–15 reps of 10 different exercises***	Two or three days per week; 10 minutes of stretching activities	Three days per week; 10 minutes of balance activities	The focus for the next three weeks is to increase the time you spend in aerobic exercise to at least 200 minutes per week by increasing the time spent per day or the number of days per week. Continue with your resistance training program. Consider different balance exercises or move to a higher challenge exercise.
7-10	Three to five days per week; 30–60 minutes per day; moderate intensity (level 5 or 6)	Two days per week; two sets per exercise, 10–15 reps of 10 different exercises***	Minimum of two or three days per week; 10 minutes of stretching activities	Three days per week; 10 minutes of balance activities	For this month, you can either increase the time spent per day or increase the number of days per week for aerobic activities. Ultimately, you want your weekly total to include 200–300 minutes of moderate-intensity activity. As another option, you could increase the intensity of the activity (to a level 7 or 8) while decreasing the time spent to 100–150 minutes of vigorous-intensity activity (recall that two minutes of moderate activity equals one minute of vigorous activity). If this second option is appealing, for a couple of weeks try to combine moderate and vigorous activity (every other exercise session) to allow your body to adapt. For resistance training, consider some different exercises on alternate weeks while still targeting the same muscle groups (see chapter 7 for details).

*All activity sessions should be preceded and followed by a 5- to 10-minute warm-up and cool-down.

** Include stretching activities after your aerobic exercise to improve flexibility. Target all the muscle groups, holding each position for 15–60 seconds each. For specific stretches to target the major muscle groups, see chapter 8.

***Resistance training is more fully outlined in chapter 7. Select one exercise for each of the following body areas: hips and legs, chest, back, shoulders, low back, and abdominals. As you progress, you will expand the number of body areas you target by adding quadriceps and hamstrings as well as biceps and triceps. This provides 10 body areas to target. Examples of exercises you can include for each body area are found in table 7.2 on page 133 of chapter 7.

FIGURE 11.8

Sample Established Exercise Program for Older Adults*

Week	Aerobic	Resistance	Stretching**	Balance	Comments
1-3	• Five days per week for moderate exercise, or • Three days per week for vigorous exercise, or • Three to five days per week for a mix of moderate and vigorous exercise	Two days per week; two sets, 10–15 reps of 10 different exercises***	Two or three days per week; 10 minutes of stretching activities	Three days per week; 10–15 minutes of balance activities	Congratulations on your ongoing commitment to exercise. To find specific aerobic activities, see chapter 6. For resistance training, see chapter 7, and for stretching and balance training, refer to chapter 8.
4-6	Two or three days of moderate activity and one or two days of vigorous activity	Two days per week; two sets, 10–15 reps of 10 different exercises***	Two or three days per week; 10 minutes of stretching activities	Three days per week; 10–15 minutes of balance activities	For the next couple of weeks, try mixing up your activities. Try a new aerobic activity or change the intensity of an activity you already do on a regular basis. Continue with your resistance training program and balance training.
7-9	• Five days per week for moderate exercise, or • Three days per week for vigorous exercise, or • Three to five days per week for a mix of moderate and vigorous exercise	Two days per week; two sets per exercise, 10–15 reps of 10 different exercises***	Two or three days per week; 10 minutes of stretching activities	Three days per week; 10–15 minutes of balance activities	Continue with your aerobic training program. For resistance training, consider trying some different exercises (see chapter 7 for details). If you typically use machines, try a couple of new exercises using dumbbells to provide your muscles with a new challenge. Be sure to maintain good form when trying new activities.
10-12	• Five days per week for moderate exercise, or • Three days per week for vigorous exercise, or • Three to five days per week for a mix of moderate and vigorous exercise	Two days per week; two or three sets per exercise, 10–15 reps of 10 exercises***	Two or three days per week; 10 minutes of stretching activities	Three days per week; 10–15 minutes of balance activities	Continue with your aerobic training program. Consider doing three sets instead of two during one of your resistance training sessions (see chapter 7 for details). You may need to cut back on your reps to add the additional set.

*All activity sessions should be preceded and followed by a 5- to 10-minute warm-up and cool-down.

**Include stretching activities after your aerobic exercise to improve flexibility. For specific stretches to target the major muscle groups, see chapter 8.

***Resistance training is more fully outlined in chapter 7. Select one exercise for each of the following body areas: hips and legs, chest, back, shoulders, low back, abdominals, quadriceps, hamstrings, biceps, and triceps. Examples of exercises you can include for each body area are found in table 7.2 on page 133 of chapter 7.

As you adjust these FITT components, you can gauge your body's response in a number of ways. If you are a beginner or intermediate exerciser, you can use the fitness assessments outlined in this chapter (or those in chapter 2) every two to four months. If you are an established exerciser, assessing every four to six months would likely provide sufficient feedback. Figure 11.9 is a sample form you can use to chart your progress.

Between fitness assessments, you can note your progress in less objective ways, including the following for aerobic conditioning:

- When doing the same activity, your heart rate and perception of effort are lower.
- Your heart rate returns to resting levels faster after your workout.

FIGURE 11.9

Fitness Assessment Progress Chart for Older Adults

	Assessment 1 (baseline)	Assessment 2*	Assessment 3**
Body composition assessments			
Body mass index			
Waist circumference			
Cardiorespiratory fitness assessments (alternative assessments in chapter 2 are the 1-mile walk or the 1.5-mile run)			
6-minute walking test			
Muscular fitness assessments (alternative assessments in chapter 2 are the 1-repetition maximum, curl-up, and push-up tests)			
Chair stand test			
Arm curl test			
Flexibility assessment			
Sit-and-reach			
Balance and agility assessment			
8-foot up and go			

*From baseline: Two months for a beginner, three months for an intermediate exerciser, and four months for an established exerciser
**From baseline: Four months for a beginner, six months for an intermediate exerciser, and eight months for an established exerciser
From ACSM, 2011, *ACSM's complete guide to fitness & health* (Champaign, IL: Human Kinetics).

- You are able to complete the same number of minutes of activity, but at a higher relative intensity.
- You are able to continue longer at the same intensity of activity.
- You are increasing the total time exercising per week.

By tracking your workouts, you can watch for these positive signs of improving fitness.

For resistance training, you may observe the following as evidence of improvements:

- You are able to lift the same weight 15 times rather than just 10 before becoming fatigued.
- You are able increase the weight lifted or the resistance you can overcome.
- You are able to complete more body weight exercises (e.g., push-ups, curl-ups).
- You increase the number of sets completed targeting a particular muscle group.

For flexibility, you may observe that you are able to reach farther or hold a position with less tension than you could earlier in your stretching program. For balance, you may find you can now hold positions longer or you have been able to move on to more advanced exercises (e.g., moving to standing positions, closing eyes).

Figure 11.10 is targeted for beginners and intermediate-level exercisers and highlights some simple ways to chart your progress in aerobic conditioning. On a weekly basis, reflect on the total time spent along with your level of effort.

FIGURE 11.10

Aerobic Fitness Progress Chart for Beginners and Intermediate-Level Exercisers

	Total time spent in aerobic exercise (minutes per week)	Typical perception of effort (on a 10-point scale)
Week 1		
Week 2		
Week 3		
Week 4		
Week 5		
Week 6		
Week 7		
Week 8		
Week 9		
Week 10		

From ACSM, 2011, *ACSM's complete guide to fitness & health* (Champaign, IL: Human Kinetics).

As you progress from week to week, ask yourself these questions:

- Is the same workout easier than it was last week?
- Is my heart rate lower for the same level of intensity?
- Can I go for an extra 5 to 10 minutes per session?
- Could I increase the intensity slightly and still complete the same length of workout?

If you answer yes to most of these questions, you are progressing nicely! If you answer no to a number of the questions, you may not be giving your body sufficient time to adapt. The sample programs are just that—you should feel free to take as many weeks as needed at a particular stage before moving on to the next level. No two people are alike, so don't believe that you need to fit into anyone else's exercise plan but your own. Of course, to progress, you need to provide your body with a new challenge, but you also need to allow your body enough time to respond and adapt. This is why increases in time or intensity are done slowly over a number of weeks. When assessing the success of your exercise program, don't forget the E of FITTE, which stands for enjoyment! Continue to look for activities that you enjoy doing so you can maintain your activity.

Figure 11.11 provides some markers of progress in resistance training for beginners and intermediate exercisers. By tracking your weekly progress, you can ensure

FIGURE 11.11

Muscular Fitness Progress Chart for Beginners and Intermediate-Level Exercisers

	Number of resistance training sessions per week	Number of reps per set	Number of sets per muscle group	Number of different exercises within the session
Week 1				
Week 2				
Week 3				
Week 4				
Week 5				
Week 6				
Week 7				
Week 8				
Week 9				
Week 10				

From ACSM, 2011, *ACSM's complete guide to fitness & health* (Champaign, IL: Human Kinetics).

some improvement when you do your formal fitness assessments. These formal assessments should be done at least a couple of months apart to give your body time to respond to the training.

FIGURE 11.12

Flexibility and Balance Progress Chart for Beginners and Intermediate-Level Exercisers

	Time spent stretching per session	Number of stretching sessions per week	Total time spent in balance training per week
Week 1			
Week 2			
Week 3			
Week 4			
Week 5			
Week 6			
Week 7			
Week 8			
Week 9			
Week 10			

From ACSM, 2011, *ACSM's complete guide to fitness & health* (Champaign, IL: Human Kinetics).

To track the status of your flexibility and balance, consider figure 11.12. In addition to time spent, also consider the difficulty of the exercises you are including (see chapter 8 for a progression of activities).

Fitness levels are more stable for established exercisers. If you are an established exerciser, maintaining your fitness levels may be an appropriate goal. Figure 11.13 is a summary chart for established exercisers. Writing down your workouts can be helpful so you can look back on them. An activity chart provides a weekly accounting of how many sessions you have performed that target aerobic fitness, muscular fitness, and flexibility (see figure 3.2 on page 55 of chapter 3 for an example). Every four to six months you can complete the fitness assessments (see figure 11.9 on page 242).

Regardless of your current fitness level, recording your weekly exercise allows you to reflect on your status. It can be easy to become unbalanced (e.g., walking for aerobic fitness but neglecting resistance training to help with muscular fitness), so taking a moment to reflect on a weekly basis can help you stay on track.

FIGURE 11.13

Fitness Progress Chart for Established Exercisers

	Total time spent in aerobic exercise (minutes of moderate and vigorous activity per week)	Number of resistance training sessions per week	Number of resistance training exercises per session	Number of sessions per week of stretching activities	Number of sessions per week of balance exercises
Week 1	Moderate: ____ minutes Vigorous: ____ minutes				
Week 2	Moderate: ____ minutes Vigorous: ____ minutes				
Week 3	Moderate: ____ minutes Vigorous: ____ minutes				
Week 4	Moderate: ____ minutes Vigorous: ____ minutes				
Week 5	Moderate: ____ minutes Vigorous: ____ minutes				
Week 6	Moderate: ____ minutes Vigorous: ____ minutes				
Week 7	Moderate: ____ minutes Vigorous: ____ minutes				
Week 8	Moderate: ____ minutes Vigorous: ____ minutes				
Week 9	Moderate: ____ minutes Vigorous: ____ minutes				
Week 10	Moderate: ____ minutes Vigorous: ____ minutes				

From ACSM, 2011, *ACSM's complete guide to fitness & health* (Champaign, IL: Human Kinetics).

Although no amount of physical activity can stop the aging process, there is strong evidence that regular physical activity can minimize the physiological effects of aging, increase active life expectancy, and promote independence and quality of life in older age. A combination of aerobic and resistance training activities appears to be more effective than either form of training alone in counteracting the detrimental effects of a sedentary lifestyle on the health and functioning of the cardiovascular system and skeletal muscles. Although clear fitness and performance benefits are associated with higher-intensity exercise training programs in healthy older adults, it is now evident that programs do not need to be of high intensity to reduce the risks of developing chronic cardiovascular and metabolic disease. Healthy eating is another lifestyle choice that contributes to successful aging. Older adults benefit from nutrient-dense foods, including vegetables, fruits, whole grains, and fat-free or low-fat dairy products.

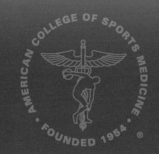
Fitness and Health for Every Body

Some circumstances can affect your fitness ID, including specific health or medical conditions. The upcoming chapters highlight how everyone has the opportunity to make changes to optimize health through physical activity and diet. Benefits of regular physical activity and a healthy diet are well documented for those with heart disease, high blood pressure, high cholesterol, arthritis, and osteoporosis. In addition, body weight and diabetes can be managed well with exercise and diet. Personalizing your fitness program will allow you to reap health and fitness benefits within the limitations that your current health status may present.

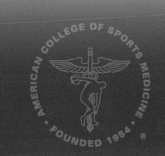

chapter **12**

Cardiovascular and Heart Health

Despite impressive technological advances in medicine during the 20th century, cardiovascular disease (CVD) remains the leading cause of death in the United States and most developed countries. CVD includes stroke and angina pectoris (chest pain) as well as impairment of the heart's ability to pump effectively (congestive heart failure), resulting in inadequate blood flow to body tissues. The good news is that the incidence of CVD is finally decreasing in the United States. Researchers have reported that mortality rates from coronary heart disease fell by more than 40% between 1980 and 2000.[13] Approximately half the decline in cardiovascular deaths was attributed to reductions in major risk factors (obesity and diabetes were notable exceptions) and approximately half to new treatments, medications, and interventions. In contrast, revascularization procedures (coronary bypass surgery and balloon angioplasty) accounted for only 7% of the overall drop in deaths from heart disease. Over the past decade, death from CVD in the United States has been reduced by more than 25%.[24] Nevertheless, heart disease is still too prevalent.

According to the American Heart Association (AHA), coronary heart disease caused approximately one of every six deaths in the United States in 2006.[33] Nearly 2,300 Americans die of CVD each day, an average of one death every 37 seconds. Moreover, people dying of CVD are tragically young. More than 151,000 Americans younger than 65 years died in 2006 from this chronic disease. In 2010, an estimated 785,000 Americans will have a new cardiac event, and approximately 470,000 will have a recurrent attack. An additional 195,000 "silent" (i.e., no painful symptoms) first heart attacks occur each year.

Unfortunately, the recent decline in heart disease incidence may be coming to a screeching halt. Research studies of adolescents and young adults dying from accidental death have found a surprisingly high incidence of mild-to-moderate coronary blockages, a sobering reminder of the gradual evolution of heart disease. Perhaps even more alarming are investigations from the Cleveland Clinic, using a technology called intravascular ultrasound to examine heart arteries, showing unequivocal evidence of coronary heart disease in 85% of adults older than 50 years!

CAUSES OF HEART DISEASE

Investigations begun more than 30 years ago have now refuted the traditional view of heart attacks: that, over time, cholesterol simply builds up on artery walls, eventually occluding (blocking) the flow of blood through the vessel. Numerous studies have now shown that heart attacks often occur at mild-to-moderate coronary blockages (generally less than 70% obstruction).[22] Plaque forming on the inside of the coronary vessels can rupture allowing clot formation to occur, potentially blocking the vessel. This process is believed to be the most important mechanism underlying the rapid progression of less severe blockages to total obstruction.[12] Collectively, these findings suggest a new paradigm for preventing and managing heart disease, and explain the inability of coronary angioplasty or bypass surgery to reduce subsequent coronary events (see *Revascularization Treatments for Cardiovascular Disease*).

Today, cardiovascular disease prevention can be divided into three types: primordial (prevention of risk factors), primary (treatment of risk factors), and secondary (prevention of recurrent cardiovascular events). Much of the success in reducing deaths from CVD over the last 30 years has been through the latter two approaches (i.e., primary and secondary prevention). Now, it is time to focus more effort on primordial prevention (i.e., preventing the development of risk factors) to meet the AHA's 2020 goal of a further 20% reduction in death from CVD and stroke.[24] Men and women with no major cardiovascular risk factors at age 50 have only a 5% and 8% lifetime risk of ever developing CVD, respectively.[25]

Revascularization Treatments for Cardiovascular Disease

Revascularization interventions may be warranted in some situations to help restore blood flow to the heart, which is nourished by the blood vessels on its surface. One way is by angioplasty, in which a thin, very flexible catheter (tube) is inserted into a blocked artery with a balloon that is positioned in the narrowed vessel. As the balloon is inflated, the deposits on the inside of the artery wall are compressed. Often a stent (mesh tube) is placed in the area to prevent the vessel from narrowing again once the balloon is retracted.

Another method to surgically bring blood supply to the heart is to provide another path around the blocked portion of an artery, typically using a vein from the leg or an artery from the chest wall (the internal mammary artery). This vessel is surgically grafted to the blocked heart artery, basically providing a new pathway in which blood can flow, bypassing the narrowed part of the artery. This is referred to as coronary artery bypass graft (CABG).

The American Heart Association has identified several risk factors through extensive clinical studies.[6] Some of these cannot be changed, including increasing age, being male, and heredity (including race—risk is higher in African Americans, Mexican Americans, American Indians, native Hawaiians, and some Asian Americans than in Caucasians). Major risk factors you can modify, treat, or control via lifestyle or with medications include the following:

- *Tobacco smoke.* The risk of heart disease is two to four times higher in smokers than nonsmokers.
- *High blood cholesterol.* Ideally, total cholesterol should be less than 200 mg/dL and LDL cholesterol should be less than 160 mg/dL if you are at low risk for heart disease, but LDL levels should be even lower if you are at higher risk (less than 130 mg/dL or even less than 100 mg/dL if you have existing heart disease).
- *High blood pressure.* High blood pressure is a risk factor because it increases the workload of the heart.
- *Physical inactivity.* Physical activity can have a positive effect on heart health. This is a major focus of this chapter!
- *Obesity and overweight.* Excessive body fat, especially around the waist, increases the risk of heart disease and stroke by increasing the work of the heart.
- *Diabetes.* Approximately 65% of people with diabetes die of some form of heart or blood vessel disease (in particular, risks are greater when blood glucose levels are not controlled).

Other factors related to heart disease risk include stress (your individual response may be a contributing factor), diet and nutrition (as discussed in this chapter), and alcohol. Excessive alcohol intake increases risk, but those who drink moderately may actually have a lower risk than nondrinkers. Women should limit alcohol intake to one drink per day, and men, to two drinks per day. It is not recommended that you start, however, if you are a nondrinker.

HEALTHY APPROACHES TO MANAGING HEART DISEASE

Physical activity and diet are two important lifestyle factors that promote heart health. Lifestyle factors are aspects over which you have control. Nutrition and exercise can contribute to optimizing the health of your heart as well as your overall fitness.

Focusing on Nutrition

Dietary choices play an important role in heart health. The average American diet is high in fat and refined carbohydrates and low in fruits and vegetables, which contributes to elevated cholesterol, high blood pressure, diabetes, and obesity. A nutritious and heart-healthy diet consists of four main components: whole grains, lean protein, healthy fats, and ample fruits and vegetables.[21]

Whole grains can be found in bread, pasta, brown rice, and cereal that are in their more natural state and have not been refined. Whole grains are higher in fiber than refined grains and have been shown to help reduce cholesterol. The AHA recommends at least three 1-ounce (28 g) servings a day of whole grains.[5] This could be a bowl of oatmeal for breakfast, sandwich on whole grain bread for lunch, and brown rice with dinner. Unfortunately, a large percentage of the carbohydrates Americans consume comes from sugar-sweetened beverages and processed foods.

Lean protein can come from either animal or plant-based products such as fish, poultry, legumes, and dairy products. It is important to get enough protein each day, but too much protein in the diet can be harmful because all excess calories are stored as fat. The AHA recommends eating at least four servings per week of nuts, legumes, and seeds.[5]

Several types of dietary fat exist, as discussed in chapter 4. Saturated fats contribute to hardening of the arteries by increasing cholesterol levels, whereas unsaturated fats are actually beneficial for heart health. The AHA recommends that no more than 7% of calories consumed daily come from saturated fats.[5] Another kind of fat called trans fat should be completely avoided because it tends to increase LDL (bad) cholesterol and decrease HDL (good) cholesterol (see chapter 16 for more information on cholesterol).[29] If the words *hydrogenated* or *partially hydrogenated* appear on the ingredient list, the food contains trans fats.

The AHA recommends at least two 3.5-ounce (99 g) servings of fish such as salmon per week; fish is an excellent source of omega-3 fatty acids.[5] In addition to oily fish, flaxseed oil, and canola oil are good sources of these fatty acids. Those who do not consume enough omega-3 fatty acids from foods can take it as a supplement, but foods in their natural form may be even more effective.

Fruits and vegetables are also very important in a heart-healthy diet. They are high in fiber, which helps to reduce LDL cholesterol, and also contain antioxidants that help to balance free radicals in the body. Because fruits are sweet, they are an excellent replacement for high-fat, sugary desserts. The AHA recommends at least 4.5 cups, or 8 servings, of fruits and vegetables per day.[5]

A CLOSER LOOK
Kendra

Kendra is a 57-year-old female who is moderately overweight and has a history of high cholesterol and high blood pressure. She had her first heart attack at age 43, which was treated with balloon angioplasty. Five years later, she had a second heart attack, which was believed to be associated with a coronary spasm during a highly emotional event.

To monitor her heart disease, Kendra undergoes an annual exercise stress test to assess her prognosis and has her blood cholesterol and triglycerides checked every six months. She takes two medications for blood pressure, one for cholesterol, and a blood thinner. She also takes a daily fish oil supplement for heart health. She exercises three to five days per week, focusing on walking, strength training, and yoga. She carefully monitors her resting and exercise blood pressure and heart rate. She also takes an active role in the local WomenHeart support group (www.womenheart.org). In addition to her family, this program provides her with invaluable social support.

Diets high in sodium are linked to high blood pressure, which increases the risk for heart disease and stroke. Foods that are processed, canned, and frozen tend to be high in sodium. The AHA recommends consuming less than 1,500 milligrams of sodium per day. The Dietary Approaches to Stop Hypertension (DASH)[32] plan is specifically beneficial for those with or at risk for hypertension (see chapter 15 for more information on hypertension and the DASH plan). DASH recommendations include avoiding foods that are high in fat, cholesterol, and sodium and instead focusing on fruits, vegetables, whole grains, low-fat dairy products, lean meats, fish, poultry, nuts, seeds, and legumes.

Finally, alcohol should be consumed in moderation. This is defined as no more than two drinks a day for men, and one a day for women, ideally with meals.[29]

Focusing on Physical Activity

Doctors have known for a long time that regular physical activity plays an important role in promoting cardiovascular health. New studies indicate that having a high aerobic fitness level (or capacity) reduces the risk of heart disease, and the reduction is greater than that obtained merely by being physically active.[35] In addition, the muscular system plays an important role in helping people perform occupational and leisure-time activities; as a result, the importance of being able to recruit muscles to do what one wants, when one wants, cannot be overemphasized. Collectively, this capacity is referred to as muscular fitness. Many adults suffer from a variety of musculoskeletal conditions that can be linked to a lack of flexibility—another important, but frequently neglected, component of fitness.

Precautions for Conditions Before Exercise

Using the screening and risk stratification steps outlined in chapter 2 will lead anyone with known CVD or with signs or symptoms to work with a health care provider to develop an individualized exercise program based on personal risk factors and current health status. A medical examination is warranted before initiating an exercise program in these circumstances.

Physical Activity Prescriptions

A complete exercise program includes aerobic activities, resistance training, and flexibility exercises. Although aerobic activities may provide the greatest cardiovascular-specific benefits, resistance training and flexibility exercises are also important parts of a balanced exercise program.

Aerobic Prescription   Regular aerobic exercise decreases the heart rate and blood pressure at rest and at a given submaximal workload. Consequently, the demands on the heart are reduced and signs or symptoms of myocardial ischemia (insufficient blood and oxygen delivery to the heart) may be alleviated. Regular exercise also improves muscle function and increases your ability to take in and use oxygen. As discussed in chapter 2, this is commonly referred to as the maximal oxygen consumption ($\dot{V}O_2$max), or aerobic capacity. As your body's ability to transport and deliver oxygen improves, you will have more energy and less fatigue. This benefit is especially important for deconditioned people and those with heart disease whose aerobic fitness is typically less than that of healthy adults of similar age. Moreover, the greatest relative improvements in cardiorespiratory fitness often occur among the most unfit.

How does an increase in maximal oxygen consumption help you more easily perform occupational and leisure time activities? Scientists have discovered that a given activity (e.g., raking leaves, playing doubles tennis) requires the person to consume a certain amount or volume of oxygen. Those who are not aerobically fit may have to work at the high end of their aerobic capacity to accomplish moderate-intensity activities such as these. On the other hand, aerobically fit people generally consume about the same amount of oxygen while performing these activities, but because they have a higher aerobic capacity, they perform these tasks at a lower percentage of their maximum, thus with less fatigue.

Aerobic exercise training programs can result in modest decreases in body weight and fat stores, blood pressure (particularly in those with elevated resting blood pressure), total blood cholesterol, triglycerides, and LDL cholesterol, and increases in the protective HDL cholesterol. There is also evidence that exercise has favorable effects on insulin resistance (use of blood glucose) and blood clotting. However, although blood pressure, cholesterol, obesity, and diabetes may be favorably affected by regular physical activity, exercise alone should not be expected to alter global risk status. The most effective regimens for coronary risk reduction also include nutritional modification, weight reduction, smoking cessation, stress reduction, and medication usage, if appropriate.

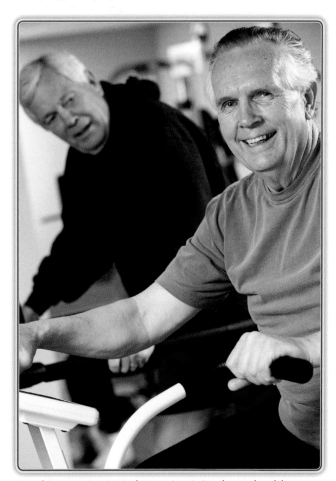

Aerobic exercise is vital to maintaining heart health.

Regular exercisers often report increased self confidence, especially in performing physical tasks; an improved sense of well-being; and reduced feelings of depression, stress, anxiety, and social isolation. The combined results from research studies indicate that exercise-based cardiac rehabilitation in older coronary patients results in mortality rates that are generally 21% to 34% lower than those among people who did not participate.[30] Although the many benefits of aerobic exercise are undeniable, there is no convincing evidence that exercise alone increases the diameter of the coronary arteries or the number of tiny interconnecting blood vessels (called collaterals) that help bring blood to the heart muscle. Moreover, conventional exercise training seems to have little or no effect on improving the pumping effectiveness, or ejection fraction, of a damaged heart or reducing heart rhythm irregularities.[16]

A measure of aerobic fitness, called metabolic equivalents (METs), appears to be one of the most powerful predictors of cardiovascular health and longevity. One MET equals the amount of oxygen your body uses when resting (approximately 3.5 milliliters of oxygen per kilogram body weight each minute). Walking at a pace of 2 or 3 miles per hour (3.2 or 4.8 km/h) uses about 2 and 3 METs, respectively. Tennis requires 6 to 7 METs. Jogging requires 8 to 10 or more METs, depending on the speed. See page 107 of chapter 6 for more information on METs.

Average healthy young to middle-age adults have an aerobic capacity of 8 to 12 METs.[2] In other words, at maximal exercise, they can consume 8 to 12 times the amount of oxygen used at rest. Heart failure patients and those who are elderly or morbidly obese could be as low as 2 to 4 METs. On the other hand, elite endurance athletes, such as Lance Armstrong, are usually in the range of 20 to 25 METs.

Researchers have reported that men and women with and without heart disease who have an aerobic capacity less than or equal to 4 METs have the highest mortality rate.[9] Accordingly, this least-fit, high-risk group may especially benefit from structured exercise, increased lifestyle activity, or both, to improve survival rates.[17] Lifestyle activity includes activities such as household chores and taking the stairs at work. On the other hand, those with an aerobic capacity of 8 METs or higher have the most favorable health outcomes.[20] A recent analysis of studies of healthy men and women concluded that each 1-MET increase in aerobic fitness confers a 15% reduction in cardiovascular events.[20] Thus, inactive people who increase their MET capacity from 5 to 7 could theoretically reduce their risk of dying from heart disease by 30%.

Resistance Training Prescription   Sarcopenia is the loss of skeletal muscle mass that generally accompanies aging, along with associated decreases in muscular fitness. Moderate- to high-intensity resistance training performed two or three days per week for three to six months improves muscular strength and muscular endurance in men and women of all ages by 25% to 100% or more, depending on the training program and the initial level of physical conditioning.[34]

Determining MET Capacity

A progressive treadmill test to peak or symptom-limited effort is the best way to accurately assess your MET capacity. METs may be directly determined by measuring the volume and analyzing the oxygen content of the expired air (via a mouthpiece or face mask) during the last minute of the test. Alternatively, the MET requirement of a given workload can be estimated from the treadmill speed, percentage grade, and exercise duration.[2] Many patients with suspected or known heart disease undergo these tests routinely. Others may have a treadmill exercise test as part of their comprehensive annual physical examination.

MET levels for various aerobic activities other than just treadmill walking or jogging have also been estimated. Because MET values take into account the type of activity and the intensity, you can also use them to summarize your aerobic workout. Chapter 6, page 107, provides steps to determine the number of calories you are using for a particular activity based on the estimated MET values.

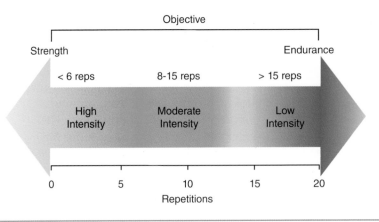

Figure 12.1 Classification of resistance training intensity.

Many middle-aged and older people develop chronic diseases that can be effectively treated by resistance training. Resistance training can favorably modify selected medical conditions and coronary risk factors (e.g., hypertension, glucose tolerance, insulin sensitivity, diabetes mellitus, basal metabolic rate), as well as psychosocial well-being. Regular resistance training has also been shown to reduce the heart rate and systolic blood pressure responses when any given load is lifted.[27] Thus, resistance training can decrease cardiac demands during daily activities such as carrying groceries and lifting moderate-to-heavy objects. Consequently, resistance training is now strongly recommended for both primary and secondary CVD prevention.

Although the traditional resistance training prescription involves performing each exercise three times (e.g., three sets of 10 to 15 repetitions per set), it appears that one set provides similar improvements in muscular strength and endurance.[34] Accordingly, single-set programs performed at least twice a week are recommended rather than multiset programs, especially among novice exercisers, because they are highly effective, less time consuming, and less likely to cause musculoskeletal injury or soreness. Such regimens should include 8 to 10 different exercises, involving those that target the upper and lower extremities, at a load that permits 8 to 15 repetitions per set (see figure 12.1).

Flexibility Prescription   Flexibility is defined as the ability to move muscles and joints through their full range of motion, and can be enhanced by stretching.[1] As discussed in chapter 8, considerable evidence suggests that stretching exercises increase tendon flexibility, improve joint range of motion and function, and enhance muscular performance. Stretching exercises may also enhance functional independence and reduce the susceptibility to falls.

For flexibility to improve, connective tissues and muscles must be elongated through regular, proper stretching, using the overload principle. The amount of stretch is proportional to the applied force, and is modulated by the temperature surrounding a joint. Before stretching, devote at least five minutes to warming up because stretching cold muscles can lead to injury. Your warm-up could be a simple, low-intensity activity, such as walking while moving your arms in wide circles. Your stretching program can be done in conjunction with your aerobic or resistance training at least two days per week, and it should involve all major muscle groups.

Gerald

Gerald is a 51-year-old man who has a family history of high blood pressure. His cholesterol is mildly elevated, and his body mass index (BMI) is 26 kg/m², placing him in the slightly overweight category. Because Gerald was experiencing episodes of intermittent chest pain (angina), his physician ordered an exercise stress test including an ECG. The test showed evidence of insufficient blood flow to the heart muscle, and he was diagnosed with exertion-related angina, caused by coronary artery disease. Subsequently, two stents were inserted after a cardiac catheterization procedure.

After his procedure, Gerald underwent another exercise stress test to determine whether he could safely begin exercising. The test was negative (i.e., the stents were successful at widening the vessel and restoring blood flow) and showed an average level of fitness for a man of his age, corresponding to 9.5 METs. His doctor prescribed medications for blood pressure, cholesterol lowering, and blood thinning. He also referred him to cardiac rehabilitation to begin a supervised cardiovascular risk reduction and exercise program.

Gerald changed to a primarily plant-based diet and started the exercise program, in which he completed 45 to 60 minutes of aerobic exercise three to five days a week, and also participated in a resistance training program three days a week for 45 minutes. With these lifestyle changes, and with regular cholesterol and triglyceride monitoring, he was able to stop taking cholesterol medications after two months, decrease blood pressure medications after 12 months, and reduce his BMI to 21 kg/m².

Gerald underwent another exercise stress test just over a year after his angioplasty procedure to evaluate his cardiac status. The test showed no suggestion of lack of blood flow to the heart muscle. Moreover, he literally doubled his exercise capacity, achieving 19 METs!

Influence of Medications

Sometimes lifestyle changes—the front line in cardiovascular risk reduction—are just not enough. You may need adjunctive drug therapy to better control certain risk factors. Although a detailed description of cardioprotective drugs is outside the scope of this chapter, four major classes of cardiovascular drugs often prescribed will be briefly summarized: aspirin, statins, beta-blockers, and angiotensin-converting enzyme (ACE) inhibitors.

Aspirin Therapy

Aspirin's anticoagulant ability prevents blood platelets from sticking together, thereby lessening the chance of clots forming and occluding narrowed coronary arteries. Regular aspirin use may reduce the likelihood of a heart attack among hospitalized patients with chest pain. When taken during or immediately after a heart attack, aspirin can also minimize heart damage.[14]

Recently, the U.S. Preventive Services Task Force concluded that aspirin decreases the risk of heart attack in men ages 45 to 79 and stroke in women ages 55 to 79 who are at increased risk for, but have not yet experienced, these cardiovascular events.[33]

Both the U.S. Food and Drug Administration and the AHA strongly recommend aspirin for patients who have suffered a heart attack or stroke, who have undergone coronary artery bypass surgery or balloon angioplasty, or who have stable angina pectoris. Indeed, aspirin has been shown to reduce the incidence of recurrent heart attacks by about 25% in patients with known CVD.

What is the optimal dose of aspirin for preventing cardiovascular events? Because the risk of major bleeding from aspirin at 81 milligrams per day is the same as it is with 162 milligrams per day, the most appropriate dose for the primary and secondary prevention of stroke and heart attack is probably 162 milligrams daily.[8] This involves taking two low-dose aspirins, or half of an adult aspirin. Consult with your physician to determine if aspirin therapy is recommended for you.

Statin Drugs

Statins are powerful medications used to treat high blood cholesterol levels. These drugs block cholesterol production in the liver. Because the body needs a certain amount of cholesterol to function, it compensates by drawing on cholesterol found in the bloodstream. This reduces the amount of cholesterol that could damage arteries. Depending on the drug and dosage, statins typically decrease total cholesterol and LDL cholesterol by up to 50%. These drugs generally increase HDL cholesterol by 5% to 15% and reduce triglycerides by 7% to 30%.

Statins do have a downside. In rare cases, statins can cause elevations in some liver enzymes and ultimately result in liver damage. Thus, patients who use statin medications should have their liver enzymes evaluated once or twice yearly. In addition, statins are associated with muscle inflammation, a condition called rhabdomyolysis. The usual complaint is muscle soreness or pain. When this occurs, several weeks off the drugs may be required for the inflammation to totally subside. Thereafter, a different statin can be started at a very low dose and gradually increased to a more therapeutic level.

A CLOSER LOOK
Patty

Patty is a 72-year-old Caucasian woman who is a registered nurse. She has a history of high blood pressure and high cholesterol. Two years ago, while driving home, she became nauseated and short of breath and had severe chest pain. Her husband called 911, and she was rushed to the hospital. Doctors determined that she was having a heart attack and told her that she would need emergency bypass surgery. After reviewing the risks and benefits of the surgery, she decided to undergo triple vessel coronary artery bypass graft surgery.

After surgery she underwent a progressive treadmill stress test to volitional fatigue so that her doctor could clear her to start exercising. Patty enrolled in a cardiac rehabilitation program and began her recovery process. After her surgery she had felt depressed and anxious. She found cardiac rehabilitation to be a tremendously beneficial in improving her fitness level and her emotional well-being. She continues to participate on a regular basis in cardiac rehabilitation because she values the supervision and camaraderie, which help her to stay focused on her exercise and risk reduction goals.

Beta-Blockers

Formally called beta-adrenergic blocking agents, beta-blockers are used to reduce heart rate, treat high blood pressure, relieve angina, ward off dangerous heart rhythm disturbances, and prevent recurrent heart attacks. Referred to by either their generic names, which commonly end in *ol,* or their brand names, these drugs inhibit the activity of the sympathetic nervous system, which is responsible for increasing heart rate and blood pressure. Among heart attack patients, beta-blocker therapy has been shown to reduce the risk of death by 20% and recurrent heart attacks by 25%. A recent analysis concluded that the benefit of beta-blockers is strongly related to the magnitude of reduction in resting heart rate.[7] Each 10-beat-per-minute reduction in resting heart rate is estimated to reduce the relative risk of cardiac death by about 30%.

ACE Inhibitors

ACE inhibitors belong to a class of cardiac drugs called antihypertensives and are normally administered to help lower blood pressure. However, ACE inhibitors are also used to treat heart failure or after major heart attacks that have resulted in considerable heart damage. ACE inhibitors may be referred to by their generic names, which commonly end in *il,* or by their brand names. How do these drugs work? An enzyme in the bloodstream called angiotensin constricts blood vessels and causes the body to retain salt. Therefore, inhibiting angiotensin activity decreases blood pressure. Numerous studies have now shown that ACE inhibitor therapy in selected patients can reduce cardiovascular events by 20% to 25%. Moreover, patients treated with ACE inhibitors often developed heart failure and diabetes less frequently. Another closely related group of drugs called angiotensin receptor blockers (ARBs) can be used as an alternative to ACE inhibitors.

COMMON CONCERNS

Whether you have diagnosed heart disease, or you have two or three risk factors for the development of heart disease (e.g., high blood pressure, obesity, diabetes, cigarette smoking, elevated cholesterol, sedentary lifestyle), your physician has probably recommended that you begin and maintain a regular aerobic exercise program. In either case, as you embark on your journey to improved cardiovascular health, you will likely have a few questions and concerns. Though not an exhaustive list, the following patient profiles illustrate frequently asked questions from patients with multiple risk factors for heart disease or from those with established heart disease.

Profile 1: Carol

Carol is a 57-year-old high school math teacher with the following profile:

- Sedentary lifestyle
- Overweight—height: 64 inches (163 cm); weight: 170 pounds (77 kg); body mass index: 29.0 kg/m^2
- Mild arthritis in knees
- Newly diagnosed with type 2 diabetes mellitus

- Heart attack and subsequent angioplasty (stent placement) three weeks ago
- Given a prescription to attend cardiac rehabilitation by her cardiologist

During her orientation to cardiac rehabilitation, Carol and her husband asked these questions:

▶ *What is body mass index, and what are the normal values?*

Body mass index, or BMI, is a measurement of the distribution of a person's body mass relative to height. Determining BMI is discussed on pages 25-27 in chapter 2. Recall that BMI values greater than 30 kg/m^2 are associated with increased rates of hypertension, elevated blood cholesterol, diabetes, and the development of heart disease.

▶ *I have never liked being physically active, but I know that I need to be. How do I motivate myself in the long term?*

A motive is something that causes a person to act or is a stimulus to action. Understanding the various levels of motivation can be an important first step. As detailed in chapter 5, self-management skills can be used to facilitate motivation (see page 86).

▶ *We are planning a weekend out of town for our 30th wedding anniversary in one month; is sexual activity likely to place excessive demands on my heart?*

Studies show that sexual activity has a favorable effect on health long term; in fact, the Duke First Longitudinal Study of Aging,[28] a 25-year study, found that the frequency of sexual intercourse predicted longevity in the 270 men, ages to 60 to 94, who were studied. Compared with moderate- to vigorous-intensity exercise, sexual activity generally requires less energy expenditure. When with a spouse, sexual activity evokes heart rate and blood pressure responses similar to those evoked by many moderate-intensity daily activities. A simple test for sexual activity readiness is whether you can perform regular aerobic activity (walking at a 2.5 to 3.0 mph, or 4 to 4.8 km/h, pace) without symptoms such as chest pain.

▶ *What exercise precautions should I take regarding my diabetes?*

The American Diabetes Association recommends self-monitoring of blood glucose to gauge whether current medications and dietary and exercise habits are providing optimal blood glucose control.[4] Details on managing diabetes are found in chapter 14.

▶ *What are the signs and symptoms I should watch for that may signify cardiac insufficiency?*

Angina (or angina pectoris) is pain or discomfort as a result of myocardial ischemia, or lack of adequate blood flow to the heart. Pain, pressure, or tightness in the chest, jaw, throat, or upper back that comes on with stress or physical exertion and is relieved with rest or nitroglycerin may signify angina pectoris. Angina can also present itself as increased shortness of breath with minimal activity, or easy fatigability. Those with these signs or symptoms should be evaluated by a physician before continuing a structured exercise program.

Profile 2: Bob

Bob is a 45-year-old attorney with the following profile:

- Elevated low-density lipoprotein (LDL) level (i.e., bad cholesterol)
- High blood pressure for five years
- Overweight—height: 70 inches (178 cm); weight: 220 pounds (100 kg); body mass index: 31.6 kg/m²
- Sedentary lifestyle (however, he enjoys weekly golf using a motorized cart)
- Bob's doctor recommended that he begin a regular exercise program that includes resistance training; however, because of his busy and unpredictable schedule, Bob has difficulty finding opportunities to exercise.

Bob is motivated to make lifestyle changes, but before beginning a regular exercise program, he had the following questions:

▶ *One of my 50-year-old law partners had a heart attack while playing a pickup game of basketball. Can exercise actually trigger cardiac events?*

Although a bout of vigorous exercise (particularly if the activity is infrequent or unaccustomed) can transiently increase the risk of sudden cardiac death or acute myocardial infarction, especially in people with known or occult (hidden) heart disease, the absolute risk of cardiovascular complications is still very low.[31] Moreover, regular aerobic exercise reduces the likelihood of developing heart disease by up to 50%. Thus, the benefits of regular, moderate-intensity exercise far outweigh the associated risks. When beginning an exercise program, one should progress gradually and heed warning signs or symptoms.

▶ *Should I have an exercise stress test before starting my exercise program to screen for exertion-related cardiac abnormalities?*

Those who are classified as being at moderate risk (i.e., with two or more major risk factors for the development of heart disease) who plan to participate in vigorous physical activity, and those who are considered high risk (i.e., with a diagnosis or signs or symptoms of cardiovascular, pulmonary, or metabolic disease) who plan to exercise at moderate or vigorous intensities should have an exercise stress test evaluation before beginning a regular aerobic exercise program.[2] Exercise testing in those considered low risk (i.e., with fewer than two risk factors for the development of heart disease) may be helpful in developing safe and effective exercise programs.

▶ *Can playing golf in the heat pose a problem for me?*

Physical activity in elevated environmental temperatures (greater than 80°F, or 26.7 °C), particularly when associated with high humidity, results in a phenomenon called cardiovascular drift. As a result of cooling mechanisms in the body, heart rates increase beyond levels found under more moderate conditions.[26] Thus, the relative demands on the heart are higher when exercising in elevated temperatures than they are under "normal" environmental conditions. This can place a person at an increased risk for tachycardia (rapid heart rates) or heart rhythm disturbances. To control the exercise environment, people should restrict outdoor activities to the coolest and least humid portions of the day. Alternatively, they should take care to maintain prescribed heart rates during activity. This can be achieved by reducing normal workloads in hot and humid conditions. Proper hydration can also positively influence the effects of cardiovascular drift.

> ▶ *I would like to lose 40 pounds (18 kg) over the next 12 months. Which will be more important in facilitating my weight loss: exercise or diet?*

Research has shown that even modest weight reductions (5% to 10% of total body weight) can result in favorable modifications in coronary risk factors such as hypertension, cholesterol abnormalities, and the development of diabetes. Guidelines from the American College of Sports Medicine[3] suggest that both exercise and diet are important in long-term weight loss success. Therefore, a combination of a reduction in daily caloric intake (i.e., a decrease of 500–1,000 calories per day) and an increase in daily caloric expenditure through physical activity (200–300 minutes per week) is necessary for achieving and maintaining desired weight loss. Of the two interventions (diet and exercise), caloric restriction is generally more important in facilitating weight loss. On the other hand, regular exercise appears essential for preventing weight regain in formerly overweight or obese people. Health care professionals such as exercise physiologists and registered dietitians can assist with the development of a weight loss plan.

Profile 3: Harry

Harry is a 75-year-old retiree with the following profile:

- Hypertension for 30 years; well-controlled for the last 10 years
- Reduced high-density lipoprotein (HDL) level (i.e., good cholesterol)
- Normal weight—height: 69 inches (175 cm); weight: 157 pounds (71 kg); body mass index: 23.2 kg/m²
- Physically active for the last 60 years including 20 years of aerobic exercise sessions four times a week
- Three-vessel coronary artery bypass surgery four months ago (after an exercise stress test that showed probable coronary artery blockages)
- Currently enrolled in cardiac rehabilitation and walking or biking 30 to 45 minutes, four days per week; resistance training twice a week

Harry, a long-time exercise advocate, took the following list of questions to an appointment with his cardiologist:

> ▶ *I enjoy shoveling snow, but the physiologists who monitor me in cardiac rehab recommended that I find a neighborhood kid or a service to do this in the future. Why?*

Cold air, which constricts potentially already blocked coronary arteries, combined with the physical exertion of lifting heavy loads of snow, can create the "perfect storm." Snow shoveling can result in a higher heart rate and blood pressure than when performing a maximal exercise stress test to exhaustion! Combined with the cold temperatures, this increases the risk for cardiac events, such as a heart attack or heart rhythm disturbances.[15] This risk is significant in those with known or occult heart disease. For these reasons, it is best to delegate this activity to a healthy, younger person or service. If hiring a snow removal service is cost-prohibitive, the following recommendations may make snow removal safer:

- Use an automated snow thrower, if possible, because it markedly decreases the demands on the heart.
- Take frequent breaks.
- Never shovel immediately after eating a large meal.
- Be sure to dress appropriately for the cold weather (wear a hat and gloves, dress in layers, and cover your mouth with a scarf if possible).
- Listen to your body; if you feel chest pain, dizziness, nausea, or an unusual shortness of breath, stop and call emergency services.

▶ *My wife and kids are concerned about which activities are appropriate for me; how do I go about identifying safe exercises?*

In general, a given exercise or activity is appropriate if it meets the following criteria. You should evaluate these criteria periodically during every exercise session.

- *Absence of symptoms.* Watch for any untoward signs or symptoms such as chest pain or pressure. If symptoms are present with activity, follow up with a physician before continuing with an exercise program.
- *Appropriate heart rate.* A health care professional can prescribe a target heart rate range (based on your exercise stress test) that results in a safe and generally effective individualized cardiovascular training zone.
- *Appropriate intensity.* Using a talk test or rating exercise as "fairly light to somewhat hard" will result in an exercise level that is appropriate and has a reduced likelihood of resulting in complications (see chapter 6 for details on monitoring intensity).

▶ *My memory is not what it was before my bypass surgery. Is this normal?*

Memory loss after bypass surgery is a relatively common complaint. Many scientific studies demonstrate that postsurgical memory loss is generally transient and not severe enough to permanently affect cognitive functioning.[10, 18] Family and friends of bypass surgery patients may notice lapses in memory for the first few months after surgery; however, most patients can expect a full recovery.

▶ *My HDL is considered low at 35 mg/dL. Can regular exercise improve this value?*

Aerobic exercise and, to a lesser extent, resistance training have been shown to have a modest effect on raising HDL levels. The increases in HDL cholesterol are generally noted after two or three months of regular exercise. In addition, exercise-induced weight loss can also boost HDL values. Finally, if lifestyle modifications do not favorably modify HDL levels, the addition of nicotinic acid (niacin) supplementation, under a physician's care, may be beneficial.[19]

Cardiovascular disease remains the leading cause of death in the United States. Although some risk factors cannot be controlled (e.g., age, genetics, race), you can make lifestyle changes to lower your risk, including increasing physical activity and making wise nutritional choices. Physical activity and diet have the potential to impact cardiovascular disease prevention on all three fronts—prevention of risk factor development, treatment of risk factors, and prevention of initial and recurrent cardiovascular events. Over the years, exercise critics have rhetorically asked, "Fitness for what?" Now, sobering new studies provide exercise enthusiasts with a compelling response: "Fitness for life."

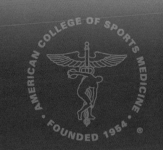

chapter 13

Weight Management

Weight management is a struggle for many people, but controlling body weight has many health benefits. The U.S. Centers for Disease Control and Prevention (CDC) has classified American society as "obesiogenic" due to the environmental factors that promote the excessive intake of unhealthy, high-calorie foods coupled with physical inactivity. This combination has resulted in a culture primed to make its citizens fat. This transformation toward overfatness has not occurred overnight. The number of overweight and obese Americans has gradually increased over the past 20 years. Approximately two-thirds of Americans are now either overweight or obese.[2]

The terms *overweight* and *obesity* are both used to describe situations in which body weight is higher than that recommended for optimal health, because being overweight or obese increases your risk of developing many diseases or health problems. Stated plainly, you are overweight if you weigh more than expected for someone of your stature (height), and you are obese if you weigh a lot more than expected. To be more specific, body mass index (BMI) is used to classify people into four subclasses: underweight, normal, overweight, and obese (see table 13.1). See page 26 of chapter 2 to determine your BMI.

BMI is commonly used because it is very easy to measure and it also correlates strongly with the percentage of body fat. Excess levels of body fat contribute to a number of health concerns including heart disease, hypertension, diabetes, and some cancers.[1] Typically, body fat levels are higher as BMI increases.[1] Table 13.1 indicates that a BMI between 18.5 and 24.9 kg/m² is considered a normal, healthy body weight; this is because BMI within this range is associated with the lowest risk of developing a chronic disease or dying. People classified as overweight have an increased risk of disease and death, and those who are obese have the highest risk of developing a number of diseases.

Table 13.1 Body Mass Index Classification

BMI (kg/m^2)	Classification
Below 18.5	Underweight
18.5–24.9	Normal
25.0–29.9	Overweight
30 or higher	Obese

Determining your BMI is a useful starting point for determining whether you would benefit from losing weight. One thing to keep in mind is that BMI does not distinguish between simply having a higher weight than expected and being overfat.[1] For example, because muscle is much denser than fat, a very muscular male athlete with low body fat could have a BMI that classifies him as overweight or obese. His weight would be higher than expected for his height, but he would not be overfat, and thus not at a higher risk for disease based on body composition. If your BMI is 25 kg/m^2 or greater, use your judgment to determine whether you should make weight loss your goal. If you are an athletic person with large muscles and defined musculature, then BMI may not be the best tool for determining your level of body fatness.[2] In such situations, skinfold measures or bioelectrical impedance (see chapter 2) may be of value, although these techniques require the assistance of a fitness professional.

Body fat distribution is also a predictor of health risk associated with obesity.[1] Accumulation of fat around the abdominal area, often referred to as an apple-shaped physique, carries more risk than fat around the hips and thighs (pear-shaped physique). Taking a measurement of your waist circumference (see pages 27-28 in chapter 2 for guidance on how to do this) is one way to look more closely at abdominal obesity. Waist measures of 35 inches (89 cm) or less for women or 39 inches (99 cm) or less for men classify people as being at low risk for developing chronic disease. Use of both BMI and waist circumference can be helpful in tracking your success at managing your weight.[1]

CAUSES OF OBESITY

The shape and size of your body is due to a combination of both genetic and environmental factors working in unison. In general, your genes create starting points and boundaries that shape how fat or muscular you are likely to become. Although these genetic limits are beyond your control, this does not mean that your body size is beyond your control. Environmental factors such as behaviors and lifestyle choices, including food selections and your level of physical activity, ultimately determine how close to your genetic potential you become.

Genetic Factors

Inherited factors may account for up to 70% of body weight differences in individuals. This is why a child of nonobese parents has only a 10% chance of becoming overweight or obese, but a child with one obese parent has a 40% chance, and a child with two obese parents has an 80% chance of becoming overweight or obese. Research on identical twins provides insight into the importance of genetics in determining body weight. Identical twins raised apart tend to have similar patterns of body fat distribution in spite of different environmental influences.[9]

In addition to body fat, people also tend to inherit specific body types, such as being tall and thin or short and stout. This is important to remember because some people may not be able to achieve a desired body shape no matter how hard they train or how diligent they are about food choices. For example, a very tall and thin person may never be able to put on enough muscle mass to look like a bodybuilder, nor may a very muscular, stocky person ever achieve extreme thinness. Another factor out of your control is where body fat is deposited. Some people naturally gain body fat around the abdominal area, as mentioned previously, whereas others may accumulate fat in their hips and thighs.

Other areas of genetic research include the concept of a thrifty gene and the set point theory. The thrifty gene proposes that humans slow their metabolism and store more body fat in times of food scarcity. This may have been an important survival mechanism many years ago in times of famine, but is not so desirable today when restricting food consumption voluntarily to lower body weight. Whether there is actually a specific gene associated with this phenomenon is a question scientists continue to examine. Regardless, your body's attempt to protect you when you restrict calories can make it difficult to lose weight.

The set point theory proposes that the brain, hormones, and enzymes work in unison to regulate body weight at a genetically determined level. Any attempt to voluntarily change your body weight from the set point initiates a series of body responses that ultimately result in a return to your genetically predetermined weight. These body responses may include becoming more efficient at storing fat or controlling metabolism, hunger, or feelings of fullness with other hormones. As tempting as it may be, you should not use the set point theory as an excuse to conclude that weight control is impossible. You may not attain aesthetic perfection, but you can achieve and maintain a body weight and composition that are best for your health and well-being.[6]

Environmental Factors

It is well established that your environment partly determines your body weight. Although genetic factors limit what you can accomplish, healthy behaviors and choices, such as choosing the correct foods and portion sizes, getting sufficient quantity and quality of physical exercise, and learning behavioral modification techniques certainly can help you reach your genetic potential. Overeating and underexercising are often learned behaviors that can become lifelong habits. Children who are not taught to eat a healthy diet and who are not encouraged to engage in voluntary physical activity begin their lives at a clear disadvantage when it comes to maintaining a healthy body weight. It is very difficult to break old habits when the new behaviors, although healthier, are perceived as comparatively unpleasant. Telling a child who typically eats ice cream while watching television after school that he instead should eat an apple and then play outside may generate a less than enthusiastic response. Over time, new habits can be established by building on small positive changes.

MANAGING YOUR WEIGHT

Establishing or maintaining a healthy body weight requires an understanding of how the body uses food to provide energy. In addition, when weight loss is desired, a plan of action is needed for long-term success.

Energy Balance

Understanding the concept of energy balance (EB) is critical if you want to understand how body weight is regulated in human beings. EB in its simplest form simply compares the amount of energy consumed as food with the amount of energy expended through the combination of resting metabolism, activities of daily living, and voluntary physical exercise. The three possible states of EB are positive, negative, and neutral. Positive EB occurs when you consume more energy (calories) than you expend, resulting in weight gain. Negative EB occurs when you expend more calories than you consume, resulting in weight loss. Neutral EB occurs when the amount of calories you consume equals the amount that you expend,[5] as shown in figure 13.1.

It is important to understand that EB is most meaningful when it is measured over a reasonably long period of time. Being out of EB for one day will have no discernable impact on body weight, but being out of EB over several weeks or months can cause significant weight gain or loss. As an illustration, assume that you eat an extra small handful of your favorite candy per day, and you do this every day for about a month. After only five weeks of this minor 100-calorie daily indulgence, you will have stored an extra pound (0.45 kg) of fat somewhere on your body. Do this for a whole year and you will have gained 10 pounds (4.5 kg) of extra fat. Whereas the small daily positive EB is not discernible to the naked eye, being in positive EB for long periods is definitely noticeable. Unfortunately, most people notice that they are in positive EB only after they have gained weight.

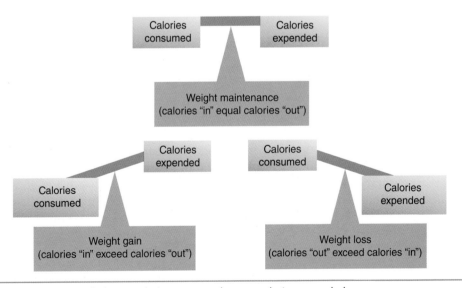

Figure 13.1   Energy balance: calories consumed versus calories expended.

Albert

Albert desires to lose about 10 pounds (4.5 kg). There are approximately 3,500 calories contained in a pound of body fat. This means that for each pound of body fat, he must shift his body into a negative EB of 3,500 calories (for 10 pounds this would be 35,000 calories). For example, for Albert to lose 1 pound (0.45 kg) in the upcoming week, he would need to be in an energy deficit of about 500 calories per day (3,500 calories divided by 7 days). (Note that this is a general estimate; many physiological factors influence the precise rate of weight loss.) Albert can achieve this caloric deficit by reducing his calorie intake, increasing his energy expenditure, or, ideally, combining the two. Here are some examples of how he could achieve this short-term goal: walk 3 extra miles (4.8 km) and drink one fewer nondiet soda per day than normal, or walk only 1 extra mile (1.6 km) and drink two fewer sodas. The most effective approach over the long term is to combine moderate calorie restriction with moderate daily exercise.

Although the concept of EB is relatively straightforward, actually implementing a weight loss program is not quite as simple. Seeking the advice of qualified dietetic and exercise professionals, such as a registered dietitian or an ACSM-certified fitness professional (see chapter 5 for information on finding a certified professional), is a wise approach if you are unsure of how to most effectively balance dietary intake with regular physical activity.

Many external factors control your food intake and physical activity patterns. For example, cultural rituals; childhood experiences; educational and socioeconomic status; nutrition knowledge; convenience; and food flavor, texture, and appearance all influence food intake.[6] Motivation, perceived lack of time, and lack of knowledge may contribute to the choice not to exercise. Qualified dietetic and exercise practitioners have the knowledge and skills to help you control the factors that determine whether you are in positive, negative, or neutral EB.

Estimating Calorie Needs

Probably the first question that comes to mind when contemplating your own body weight is *How many calories do I need?* There are sophisticated laboratory techniques to estimate this, but these tests are not practical for most people. Chapter 4 includes one simple method of estimating needed calories based on body weight and activity level (see table 4.1 on page 61). An alternative method devised by the U.S. Department of Agriculture (USDA) estimates energy needs based on sex, age, and activity level (see table 13.2).

It is important to understand that these methods are only estimates and should not be accepted as absolute values. The estimates are designed to meet the average requirements, but there are definitely interindividual differences that cannot be ignored. You should use these estimates as a starting point, but be prepared to adjust your food consumption if you are not progressing as expected. If you consume the suggested amount of calories and your body weight changes unexpectedly, then you will need to adjust your calorie intake up or down depending on your desired outcome.

Table 13.2 Estimated Calorie Needs Based on Sex, Age, and Activity Level*

| | MALES | | | | FEMALES | | |
| | Activity level** | | | | Activity level** | | |
Age	Sedentary	Moderately active	Active	Age	Sedentary	Moderately active	Active
2	1000	1000	1000	2	1000	1000	1000
3	1000	1400	1400	3	1000	1200	1400
4	1200	1400	1600	4	1200	1400	1400
5	1200	1400	1600	5	1200	1400	1600
6	1400	1600	1800	6	1200	1400	1600
7	1400	1600	1800	7	1200	1600	1800
8	1400	1600	2000	8	1400	1600	1800
9	1600	1800	2000	9	1400	1600	1800
10	1600	1800	2200	10	1600	1800	2000
11	1800	2000	2200	11	1600	1800	2000
12	1800	2200	2400	12	1600	2000	2200
13	2000	2200	2600	13	1600	2000	2200
14	2000	2400	2800	14	1800	2000	2400
15	2200	2600	3000	15	1800	2000	2400
16	2400	2800	3200	16	1800	2000	2400
17	2400	2800	3200	17	1800	2000	2400
18	2400	2800	3200	18	1800	2000	2400
19-20	2600	2800	3000	19-20	2000	2200	2400
21-25	2400	2800	3000	21-25	2000	2200	2400
26-30	2400	2600	3000	26-30	1800	2000	2400
31-35	2400	2600	3000	31-35	1800	2000	2200
36-40	2400	2600	2800	36-40	1800	2000	2200
41-45	2200	2600	2800	41-45	1800	2000	2200
46-50	2200	2400	2800	46-50	1800	2000	2200
51-55	2200	2400	2800	51-55	1600	1800	2200
56-60	2200	2400	2600	56-60	1600	1800	2200
61-65	2000	2400	2600	61-65	1600	1800	2000
66-70	2000	2200	2600	66-70	1600	1800	2000
71-75	2000	2200	2600	71-75	1600	1800	2000
76 and up	2000	2200	2400	76 and up	1600	1800	2000

*Calorie levels are based on the Estimated Energy Requirements (EER) and activity levels from the Institute of Medicine Dietary Reference Intakes Macronutrients Report, 2002.

**Sedentary = less than 30 minutes a day of moderate physical activity in addition to daily activities; moderately active = at least 30 minutes up to 60 minutes a day of moderate physical activity in addition to daily activities; active = 60 or more minutes a day of moderate physical activity in addition to daily activities.

Reprinted from U.S. Department of Agriculture, 2005.

On the USDA Web site (www.mypyramid.gov) you can interactively estimate your energy needs and even devise a personalized meal plan that takes your unique nutrient needs into account. Please be aware that this site is designed for healthy people who are free of disease or medical conditions that could affect nutrient requirements. It does not replace the advice of a registered dietitian who is trained to address the unique needs of people with various medical conditions. Rather, the MyPyramid website is a tool to help you manage your body weight. The site has many other features, including a daily calculation of EB and an estimate of energy expenditure via physical exercise.

Other ways to estimate energy expenditure during exercise include using the MET values to determine caloric expenditure (see chapter 6, page 107) or using exercise equipment that displays the number of calories burned during a session. If you plan to use such readings to help manage your body weight, be sure to enter your age, weight, and sex into the machine's console to achieve the most accurate estimate of calories burned; otherwise, the estimate you receive will be based on the average person and may not be accurate for you. Also, try to use the machines as they were designed to be used. For example, hanging on to the side bars while walking on a treadmill produces erroneous calorie expenditure results because not all of your body weight is being supported throughout the exercise as is assumed in the calorie calculations.

Determining Calorie Expenditure

The amount of calories you burn on a daily basis is commonly referred to as total energy expenditure (TEE). Three major components contribute to TEE: the calories expended at rest; the calories expended during voluntary exercise; and the calories expended during the digestion, absorption, and storage of food after eating. The largest component, which accounts for about 60% to 70% of TEE, is the calories used while the body is resting comfortably, also known as resting metabolic rate (RMR) or basal metabolic rate (BMR).

The term *resting metabolism* is actually a misnomer because the body is never truly at rest. Inside your body is a constant array of activity that must be fueled at all times. For example, your heart beats about 70 times per minute, your neurons fire at light speed 24 hours per day, and your white cells are constantly fighting invaders and replacing old or damaged tissue. All of these activities that keep you alive and allow you to look basically the same from one day to the next are exceedingly costly from an energy standpoint. So, your resting metabolism is essentially what makes you "you," and the more of "you" there is, the greater your RMR is. Thus, it is not surprising that RMR is highly related to body mass, particularly the amount of muscle you have. Skeletal muscle is a highly active tissue that contributes a great deal to resting metabolism. The quantity of skeletal muscle in your body is something that you can control to some extent through resistance training, which is discussed further in the section on physical activity.

A second component of TEE encompasses all the activities that occur in the body after eating food, including digestion, absorption, and the transport and storage of nutrients throughout the body. This incremental energy cost of eating, also known as the thermic effect of food, is a relatively small (5%–10%) component of TEE. It is not something you can control to any significant extent for the purpose of weight management. Some diet books claim to increase the thermic effect of food by exploiting the fact that more energy is required to digest and metabolize carbohydrates and proteins than fats, but the total number of extra calories burned using these techniques is not very high and probably not worth the effort to attain.

The third component of TEE includes all energy burned off during physical exercise. This is also known as the thermic effect of activity. This represents any movement your body performs above the resting level and includes fidgeting, doing chores, and participating in formal exercise. This component makes up 15% to 30% of the TEE in most people; however, it is the most variable. For example, it may be lower than 15% in a very sedentary person and more than 50% in a marathoner. As long as you do not have a physical disability, this is the component over which you have the most control. You can choose how many calories you burn through various forms of physical activity.[6]

HEALTHY APPROACHES TO WEIGHT MANAGEMENT

The most successful fat losers are the ones who shed body fat and keep it off over the long haul. Many people have experienced remarkable short-term weight loss, only to see it all (or more) return in a few short months. For this reason, weight reduction programs need to be sustained efforts, rather than all-at-once approaches. You don't have to get back to your high school weight as fast as you can. In fact, attempting to attain your goal weight as fast as possible will most likely jeopardize your long-term prospects.

Research shows that losing as little as 10% of your current body weight can be beneficial to health. Once you have met this initial goal, you should try to maintain that weight loss for three to six months before deciding whether an additional 5% to 10% weight loss is warranted. Weight maintenance between cycles of weight loss is believed to allow the body to adjust to its new weight and gives you time to master the behaviors it took to achieve it. Of course 10% is not a magic number, but the general idea is that once you've maintained a modest weight loss for a lengthy period

A CLOSER LOOK

JoAnn

JoAnn is trying to determine how many calories she actually is consuming on a daily basis and is consulting food labels (see chapter 4 for more details). Food labels denote the serving size and the number of servings in the container, as well as the number of calories per serving. To determine the total calories in a container, JoAnn must multiply the number of servings she consumes by the number of calories per serving. For example, JoAnn drinks a bottle of soda that has 110 calories per serving and three servings in the bottle. Thus, she has consumed 330 (110 × 3) calories. If you would like a tutorial on how to read a food label, you can go to the U.S. Food and Drug Administration (FDA) Web site at www.fda.gov/ and enter *Understanding Food Labels* into the search box. You can be confident that the values listed on food labels on products sold in the United States are quite accurate because they are regulated by the FDA.[8]

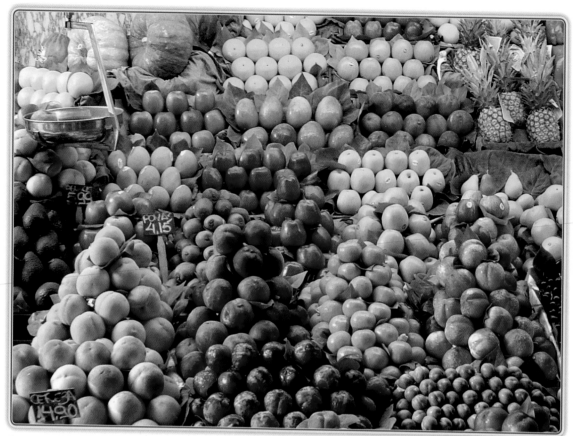

Fruits and vegetables are part of a healthy nutritional plan.

of time, you have likely made permanent lifestyle changes that will support your new lower weight and allow you to attempt further weight loss without overwhelming your resolve. A recommended amount of weight loss is 0.5 to 1 pound (0.23 to 0.45 kg) per week if your BMI is between 27 and 35 kg/m^2 and 1 to 2 pounds (0.45 to 0.9 kg) per week if your BMI is greater than 35 kg/m^2. It is desirable to achieve a moderate weight loss of 5% to 10% over approximately six months. This slow and steady approach may be the best way to sustain weight loss and prevent regain.[4]

Nutrition and physical activity together are important in weight management. The upcoming sections highlight how you can manage your body weight through dietary choices as well as exercise.

Focusing on Nutrition

Nutrition is an important part of the equation when managing weight. The foods and beverages you consume determine the calories you add to your body each day. Keeping the calories you consume in balance with the calories you expend will help you maintain your body weight.

As you learned in chapter 4, the macronutrients (carbohydrates, proteins, and fats) are required in the diet in relatively large amounts. On average, carbohydrates and proteins contain 4 calories per gram, whereas fats contain 9 calories per gram. As you can see, fats are more energy dense than carbohydrates and proteins, which is important to remember when thinking about fuel sources for different types of exercise. It is important also to keep in mind that all three macronutrients are required for optimal health. No single distribution of calories from carbohydrate, fat, and protein is widely accepted as the most effective for weight management.[4] This is reflected in the percentage ranges for each of the macronutrients that are presented in the upcoming sections.

Carbohydrate's Effect on Weight

The primary function of dietary carbohydrate is to fuel body activities. The simplest form of carbohydrate found in the human body is glucose (a sugar). Glucose is the sole fuel source for your brain and central nervous system, so it is absolutely critical in your diet. Glucose also powers skeletal muscle contractions, particularly during intense physical activity. Glucose essentially has three fates in the body: (a) it powers cellular activity, (b) it is stored in the muscles and liver in a different form of carbohydrate called glycogen, and (c) it is converted to fat and stored in adipose tissue throughout the body. Although all three fates occur simultaneously, the third tends to predominate only when carbohydrate ingestion exceeds the body's energy needs. Thus, it is possible to gain fat tissue by overeating carbohydrates.

Insulin also has a role in promoting fat storage in the body. Insulin is a hormone released by the pancreas (a small organ located in your abdomen) that helps to store carbohydrate in body cells in response to eating carbohydrates. The higher the concentration of carbohydrate consumed, the greater the amount of insulin secreted into the blood. If you consume a diet high in carbohydrate, but not in excess of your energy needs, you will not gain weight. However, a diet high in carbohydrate that exceeds your energy needs creates an environment in which insulin-facilitated fat storage is prominent. You should consume enough carbohydrates to allow your body to perform appropriate levels of physical activity, but not so much that it places you into positive EB and results in fat storage.[5]

The current adult recommendation for carbohydrate is 45% to 65% of total energy intake.[5] Relatively sedentary people do well at the low end of the range, and very active people require higher amounts of carbohydrate to support elevated energy demands. Many diet books promote a low-carbohydrate diet for weight loss, but current scientific evidence does not support this approach. Most research using low-carbohydrate diets shows significant short-term weight loss, but the long-term success rate is not well established.[4] The failure to exhibit sustained success probably is the result of a very restrictive diet coupled with insufficient lifestyle changes.

Protein's Effect on Weight

Normally, dietary carbohydrate and fat supply the body with virtually all the fuel it needs, thereby sparing protein for its other important functions. Protein contributes significantly as a fuel source only when blood glucose drops to very low levels, such as during the late stages of very long-duration exercises. Adults should consume protein equal to 10% to 35% of their total energy intake. Because dietary protein tends to keep you feeling fuller longer, you should consume protein with each meal to curb overeating.[5]

Fat's Effect on Weight

Similar to carbohydrates, dietary fat provides the body with fuel. The current recommendation for adults is to consume 20% to 35% of total energy intake in the form of dietary fat. Also like carbohydrate, fat consumed in the diet has three metabolic roles: (a) it is used to power body activities, (b) it is stored in adipose tissue as body fat, and (c) it is converted to an entirely different form called ketones, which some cells can use in place of glucose. The first two roles are the most common; the third tends to occur only when blood glucose levels fall below normal levels.

Because dietary fat is the most energy-dense macronutrient and is easily converted to body fat, consuming a low-fat diet seems to be an obvious approach to take to modify your body weight. Furthermore, reduced-fat diets may have beneficial effects on other health conditions such as high blood lipids.[4] A low-fat diet can be a useful strategy as long as you are not overconsuming other macronutrients. For example, it is easy to find fat-free foods at the grocer, but many of these foods contain an abundance of carbohydrates and calories. A word of caution about low-fat diets: low-fat does not mean no-fat! Some dietary fats are absolutely essential to human life; without them, body cells would literally break apart. This is why current recommendations set a floor at 20% of total energy intake.

Focusing on Physical Activity

Physical activity is important for overall health as well as for long-term weight management. This section highlights some differences from the general recommendations previously outlined in this book and points out specifically how much exercise is recommended as part of a weight management plan.

Precautions Before Exercise

Before starting an exercise program, refer to the health risk assessment process in chapter 2. Obesity is a risk factor for heart disease and is defined for this purpose as a BMI above 30 kg/m^2 or a waist girth greater than 40 inches (102 cm) for men or 35 inches (88 cm) for women.[1] Follow the process outlined in page 21 to assess your overall risk. Consult with your physician or health care provider as needed based on this risk assessment.

Physical Activity Prescriptions

For many years now, it has been widely accepted that physical activity is an important part of any weight management program; however, recent research suggests that more physical activity than previously thought may be required to modify body weight. In 2001 and again in 2009, the American College of Sports Medicine published landmark position stands that summarize the most scientifically supported strategies for weight loss, prevention of weight gain, and weight maintenance. Both publications stress the benefits of physical activity; the only question is *Precisely how much physical activity is needed?*

Aerobic Prescription   People desiring simply to prevent weight gain over the long term should engage in moderate-intensity physical activity roughly 150 to 250 minutes per week. This is equal to about 1,200 to 2,000 calories per week. From a practical standpoint, this means exercising at a moderate intensity for 30 to 50 minutes five days per week, burning 240 to 400 calories in each session. It must be noted that this level of physical activity prevents weight gain only if you are consuming the same amount of energy you are expending.

If your goal is to lose weight, then a dose-response relationship exists between the quantity of exercise and the amount of weight loss exhibited. This means that the more exercise you do and the higher the intensity, the greater will be your weight loss. Physical activity of 150 minutes per week provides some benefit, but additional benefits can be realized with physical activity levels of 225 to 420 minutes per week. This is equal to about 1,800 to 3,360 calories per week. From a practical standpoint, this means exercising at a moderate intensity for 45 to 90 minutes five days per week, burning 360 to 720 calories in each session. If you tolerate higher-intensity exercise well, then you can burn the same number of calories by working harder for a shorter period of time, but there are risks associated with very strenuous efforts and you should consult with a certified fitness professional before attempt-

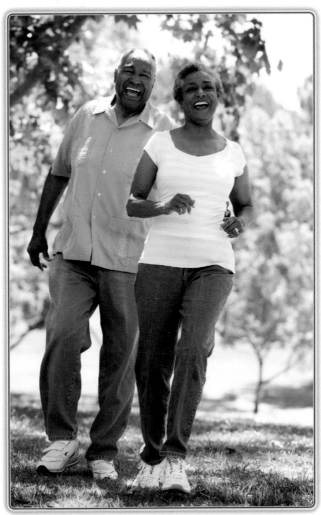

Physical activity is an important part of any weight management program.

ing such activities. Also, because weight loss requires that you be in a state of negative EB, your diet must provide fewer calories than you are expending. You can further enhance the rate of weight loss by combining physical activity with food restriction, but be careful not to consume too few calories, which will make it difficult to take in sufficient vitamins and minerals. As a general rule, you should never consumer fewer calories than required to fuel your resting metabolism.

Finally, if your goal is to maintain your body weight after weight loss, approximately 200 to 300 minutes per week of physical activity is probably sufficient. This can usually be accomplished by walking about 60 minutes per day at a brisk pace. Remember, you must maintain neutral EB by eating only as many calories as you expend.[3]

Resistance Training Prescription The physical activity guidelines discussed in this section pertain to aerobic activities, such as walking or cycling, but resistance training activities are a very important component of physical fitness that should not be ignored. Although a session of resistance training burns far fewer calories than a session of aerobic exercise does, resistance training has the potential to promote skeletal muscle growth, which contributes to resting metabolism. Because caloric restriction and subsequent weight loss usually lead to the loss of some skeletal muscle, resistance training activities are important to minimize this loss.[3] The recommended amount of resistance training is not unique for weight management, and so you should follow the guidance presented in chapter 7, performing resistance training two or three days per week.

Flexibility Prescription Flexibility training has more to do with daily functioning than with weight management. Thus, following the general stretching guidelines in chapter 8 will help you maintain or improve your level of flexibility. Include stretching activities a minimum of two to three days per week.

Weight Management Strategies

The most comprehensive research data on weight management comes from the National Weight Control Registry. This is an ongoing research study that has monitored over 5,000 people who have who have lost an average of more than 60 pounds (27 kg) and have kept it off for an average of five years. Successful fat losers in this registry tend to do the following:[10]

- Consume a low-calorie, low-to-moderate-fat diet.
- Limit consumption of fast food.
- Eat breakfast every morning.
- Have consistent food intake from day to day.
- Eat smaller meals four or five times per day.
- Weigh themselves regularly and take corrective action as needed.
- Watch TV less than 10 hours per week.
- Participate in moderate-intensity exercise for 60 to 90 minutes per day.

Two key points to take away from these findings are the importance of regular physical activity, which was discussed previously, and portion control. Portion control helps ensure that you do not consume excessive calories; this is actually more important than the relative distribution of carbohydrates, proteins, and fats in the diet.

To gain a better understanding of portion control, try to master the skill of reading food labels and translate that knowledge to the amount of food you normally eat. Learn how many calories there are in a typical serving of the foods that you eat most often. Actually visualize what a standard serving of your favorite food looks like on the serving plates you have at home. You may be surprised at how small a single serving appears on your plate or in your bowl and realize that you are more likely eating two or three servings instead of only one.

A couple of simple tips to help with portion control are to put food on your plate and bring only that serving to the table (box up the leftovers immediately for another day), and to serve meals on smaller plates or bowls. Both of these techniques will help you to consciously visualize the amount of food you consume.

Influence of Supplements and Medications

When you want to lose weight, it is easy to fall prey to quick fix promises. Evaluate any weight loss plan or supplement and use your common sense before implementing a program. If a diet seems too good to be true, it will likely not result in long-term success. Successful weight management includes not only weight loss, but also weight maintenance. A program that loudly proclaims rapid weight loss but mentions nothing about sustainability is probably one that you should avoid.

Like some diet plans, many dietary supplements promise easy weight loss. A dietary supplement is defined by the FDA as "a product (other than tobacco) added to the total diet that contains at least one of the following: a vitamin, mineral, amino acid, herb, botanical, or concentrate, metabolite, constituent, or extract of such ingredients or combination of any ingredient described above."[8] Dietary supplements are regulated by the FDA and are considered foods, not food additives or drugs. This means that the tests for efficacy and public safety are not as extensive as they are for food additives or drugs. Food additives and drugs must be tested for years to prove that they work and are safe before they are approved by the FDA. In contrast, supplements are not approved before they are placed on the market for sale.

Whereas nutrient content and health claims must be approved by the FDA, structure-function claims do not. But, how do you tell the difference between them? The only way to tell for sure is to read the label and package carefully. If the phrase "This statement has not been evaluated by the Food and Drug Administration. This product is not intended to diagnose, treat, cure, or prevent any disease" appears on the package, the claim has not been investigated and approved by the FDA. Be wary in this case because there may not be an extensive amount of research data to support the claims or promises made by the manufacturer.[8]

It would be amazing if body fat could be lost by simply swallowing a pill. If this were possible, the obesity epidemic would suddenly be solved, the pill would be acclaimed worldwide, and the manufacturer would likely win a Nobel Prize. Because none of this has happened to date, you should be skeptical when evaluating the merits of any weight loss supplement not approved by the FDA. Without providing an exhaustive review of every supplement on the market, it is pretty clear that no supplement currently exists that definitively produces significant weight loss and long-term safe weight maintenance. Until sound scientific evidence supports the use of a weight loss supplement, you would do better investing your money in healthy foods and a physically active lifestyle.

In addition, because weight loss medications have potentially serious side effects, they are generally used only by people who are obese or overweight with the presence of other diseases such as diabetes, cardiovascular disease, or hypertension. These medications are intended to be used in conjunction with permanent lifestyle changes including reduced calorie intake and physical activity, so that weight regain is less likely.[4]

One medication currently approved by the FDA for long-term use is Orlistat (the brand name is Xenical). Orlistat works at the level of the intestines to disrupt fat digestion, causing roughly one third of dietary fat to be excreted in the feces. This is a serious drug that should be taken only under the care of a physician. Possible side effects include gas, bloating, and an oily discharge. A lower-dose version of this drug is available as an over-the-counter option, but still requires lifestyle modification for maximum effectiveness.[4]

Dietary Supplement Claims

There are currently three types of claims that manufacturers can legally use to describe dietary supplements: nutrient content claims, health claims, and structure-function claims.

Nutrient Content Claims

Nutrient content claims must be approved by the FDA, are used on both foods and supplements, and include terms such as *excellent source of* or *low fat*. The FDA has approved these terms as defined:

- *Sugar-free*: Less than 0.5 grams of sugar per reference amount typically consumed
- *Reduced-calorie*: At least 25% fewer calories compared to a reference food
- *Low-fat*: 3 grams or less per 100 grams and not more than 30% of calories from fat

Health Claims

Health claims must also be FDA approved, apply to both foods and supplements, and include a statement of the relationship between a nutrient or substance and a disease or health-related condition. An example of an authorized health claim is "Diets low in sodium may reduce the risk of high blood pressure, a disease associated with many factors." For a health claim to be approved by the FDA, extensive scientific evidence must support the relationship. Following are FDA-approved health claims about relationships between nutrients and related diseases:

- A healthy diet with enough calcium may reduce the risk of developing osteoporosis later in life (calcium and osteoporosis).
- Diets low in sodium may reduce the risk of high blood pressure (sodium and hypertension).
- A diet low in total fat may reduce the risk of some cancers (dietary fat and cancer).
- Healthful diets with adequate folate may reduce a woman's risk of having a child with a brain or spinal cord defect (folate and neural tube defects).

Structure-Function Claims

Structure-function claims do not require FDA approval and are used only to describe dietary supplements. An example of a structure-function claim is, "Antioxidants maintain cell integrity." This is a somewhat vague statement whose veracity is not easily validated. The FDA has not evaluated any of the following claims:

- Calcium builds strong bones.
- Antioxidants help maintain cell integrity.
- Fiber maintains bowel regularity.

Facts About Fad Diets

If fad diets were as effective as they are advertised to be, then why do people tend to cycle from one fad diet to the next? Why with all the fad diets available does obesity continue to be such a large public health problem? Doesn't it seem logical that if fad diets really worked, they would be needed only a single time and everyone in our country would have a healthy body weight? The answers to these questions lead directly to the conclusion that fad diets do not offer effective long-term solutions to being overweight. But, how can you tell whether a weight loss program is actually a fad diet? In general, fad diet plans have the following characteristics:[9]

- They tend to advertise quick and easy weight loss.
- They have limited food selections or eliminate entire food groups altogether.
- They use testimonials instead of discussing and referencing sound scientific studies.
- They are promoted as a cure for many ailments.
- They recommend expensive supplements.
- They ignore the need to make permanent lifestyle changes.
- They criticize credentialed health professionals.

As mentioned previously, no single macronutrient distribution works best for everybody. If you find a plan that eliminates or severely limits one of the macronutrients, it is probably a fad diet that will likely fail in the long term. For example, one popular diet on the market advocates eating only foods that have a low glycemic index, which is basically a measure of how much a food causes blood insulin levels to rise after eating the food. The diet is based on the idea that insulin promotes fat storage, so eating only low glycemic index foods will minimize insulin's effect. This sounds reasonable except for the fact that it doesn't work.[4] This oversimplified explanation of insulin's action ignores many aspects, including whether the person is in positive or negative energy balance and the effect that food-combining has on glycemic index. Although baked potatoes have a high glycemic index, adding cheese or sour cream reduces their glycemic index. This is a great example of how restricting food choices actually has a negative effect on weight management.

Overweight and obesity is a growing problem. Both genetic and environmental factors contribute to body weight and body fat patterns. A key concept in weight management is energy balance—you must tailor your food intake to your energy expenditure to achieve your goals. No single macronutrient distribution is best for everyone when trying to lose or maintain body weight. Carbohydrates, fats, and proteins are all important nutrients that play a role in health and wellness. Based on the current scientific data, the best strategy for successful long-term weight management is food portion control and regular physical activity. It is easy to say that you are going to eat less and exercise more, but it takes quite a bit of effort to make this part of a long-term lifestyle. Behavior modification involves restructuring your environment to reduce actions and habits that contribute to weight gain. Registered dietitians with expertise and training in weight management and cognitive behavioral therapists are great resources to help you learn and use these strategies.

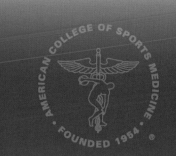

chapter 14

Diabetes

Diabetes is a common disease that is characterized by elevated blood glucose. More casually, this is often referred to as high sugar in the blood. Normally, after eating a meal, some of the food is broken down into glucose (a sugar) and is transported through the body in the bloodstream. This increase in blood glucose triggers the pancreas, a small organ in the abdomen, to release insulin. Insulin is a hormone needed to move the glucose into the body cells for energy. Diabetes results from an inability to produce insulin (type 1) or to use the insulin properly (type 2).

Diabetes affects approximately 24 million Americans, and another estimated 57 million people have higher-than-normal blood glucose levels (a condition referred to as prediabetes).[15] Approximately 90% of people with diabetes have type 2. The remaining 10% have type 1 diabetes, which tends to occur in younger people, ages 10 to 30. Other categories of diabetes do exist (e.g., gestational diabetes, which occurs during pregnancy), but they are less common.

If you are reading this chapter, you likely have diabetes—or someone important to you does. After diagnosis, you may have felt shocked, concerned, frustrated, sad, angry, or a combination of a number of emotions. Diabetes does not have to symbolize an end of life as you know it. Instead, you can take this opportunity to examine how you can take charge of your health. Although there is no magic wand to make diabetes disappear, exercise and attention to proper nutrition are two vital factors in managing diabetes. Exercise is the mainstay of treatment to improve insulin resistance and the effectiveness of medications. Diet along with exercise is also important in managing all type of diabetes and even potentially preventing type 2 diabetes.[11] This chapter provides general nutrition guidelines and addresses how to safely include physical activity in your life. Insulin and various oral medications are part of the treatment of diabetes and are reviewed as well.

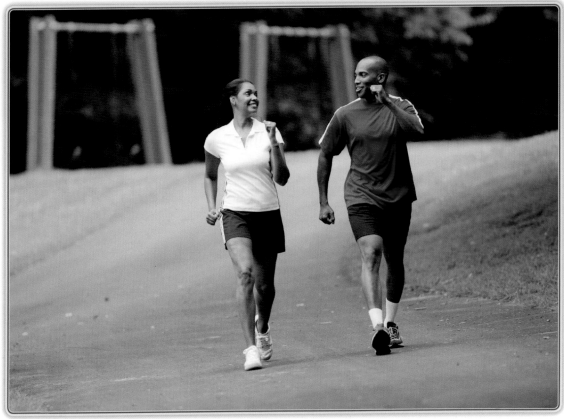

Risk factors for diabetes that you can control are your body weight and level of physical activity.

CAUSES OF DIABETES

The origin of type 1 diabetes differs from that of type 2 diabetes. Type 1 diabetes is an autoimmune disease.[3] This is a medical way of saying that the body attacks its own cells. There is no known way to prevent type 1 diabetes.[15] With type 1 diabetes, the cells in the pancreas that produce insulin are destroyed. Thus, insulin cannot be produced as it normally would in response to a meal. As a result, blood glucose is not able to enter the cells, causing glucose levels in the blood to become elevated. A high level of glucose in the blood is more technically referred to as hyperglycemia. *Hyper* means a high level and *glycemia* refers to blood glucose concentrations. As a result of the deficiency in insulin production, type 1 diabetes must be treated with insulin injections.

Type 2 diabetes occurs when body cells cannot properly use the insulin produced by the pancreas.[3] This is called insulin resistance (i.e., body cells are resistant to the action of insulin). Insulin normally allows glucose to enter cells in the body to provide energy, but with insulin resistance, the glucose cannot enter the cells and thus remains in the blood. The body's ability to produce insulin also decreases over time, which also contributes to hyperglycemia.

Obesity has a definite link with the development of type 2 diabetes, in particular upper-body fat stores (i.e., an apple-shaped physique).[3] In the past, type 2 diabetes was

The Slippery Slope of Prediabetes

Blood glucose exists on a continuum from normal to elevated (diabetes). Prediabetes is diagnosed when the fasting blood glucose is above normal (greater than 100 mg/dL) but below the cutoff for diagnosing diabetes (126 mg/dL).[3] Consider this a slippery slope toward fully realized type 2 diabetes. If your glucose level is in this range, you are at a higher risk for cardiovascular disease in addition to developing type 2 diabetes.[7] Although a diagnosis of prediabetes increases your risk, it does not mean that type 2 diabetes is unavoidable.[3] Losing weight and increasing your physical activity level will not only lower your risk for cardiovascular disease but also decrease your likelihood of progressing to fully developed type 2 diabetes. A weight loss of as little as 5% has been found to decrease the risk of developing type 2 diabetes and other obesity-related complications in people who are overweight.[13]

called adult-onset diabetes because of the typically older age of onset. Unfortunately, the increased incidence of obesity and a sedentary lifestyle has resulted in type 2 diabetes developing at earlier ages, thus exposing the body to elevated blood glucose for longer periods of time and increasing the risk of complications that can occur with diabetes such as kidney, eye, and heart disease in addition to nerve damage. Following are other factors in addition to excessive body weight and inactivity that increase the chances of developing diabetes:[6]

- Prediabetes (see *The Slippery Slope of Prediabetes*)
- Age (greater than 45 years old)
- Family history (parent or sibling)
- Other health concerns, including low HDL cholesterol, high triglycerides, high blood pressure
- Certain racial and ethnic groups, including non-Hispanic blacks, Hispanic Americans, Asian Americans and Pacific Islanders, American Indians, and Alaska natives
- Women who had gestational diabetes or have had a baby weighing 9 pounds (4 kg) or more at birth

Although a number of items cannot be changed (e.g., your race or age), you can control your body weight and physical activity level. These factors are the focus of this chapter.

HEALTHY APPROACHES TO MANAGING DIABETES

Physical activity and diet are two important lifestyle factors for anyone with type 1 or type 2 diabetes. Lifestyle factors are aspects over which you have control. This section describes how both nutrition and exercise can help you manage your diabetes as well as improve your health and fitness.

Focusing on Nutrition

Weight loss is very important for people with type 2 diabetes who are overweight.[9] Sustaining a weight loss of as little as 10% can lead to a decrease in insulin resistance and improvement in blood glucose control, and therefore allows for a reduction in the amount of medication taken.[13] Weight management is discussed in detail in chapter 13, and therefore the nutrition focus in this chapter is on the benefits of balancing carbohydrates, fats, and proteins in your diet to control blood glucose levels regardless of the type of diabetes you may be facing.

Recall from chapter 4 that the three marcronutrients that provide energy for activity and routine body functioning are carbohydrates, fats, and proteins. Everyone, including those with diabetes, will benefit from an appropriate balance of these three nutrients. Obviously, because diabetes results from a break in the link between food eaten and the body cells receiving energy, diet is a major consideration in managing diabetes. Food choices do not need to be a frustrating mystery—just giving your diet some extra attention will allow for better control of the disease. And, of course, you should exercise to keep blood glucose levels in check (you will learn more about exercise and medications later in this chapter). Working with your doctor, diabetes educator, or dietitian will result in an optimal individualized plan. This section addresses a couple of general ways to approach your diet.

The Plate Method of Meal Planning

The simplest way to promote a healthy diet is to take a look at your plate! By including foods in appropriate proportions, you will consume a good balance of nutrients. The American Diabetes Association recommends the following six steps to creating your plate at any given meal:[6]

1. Imagine a line down the middle of your plate, and then imagine one side cut in half again, as shown in figure 14.1.
2. For the largest section, select nonstarchy vegetables such as lettuce, spinach, green beans, broccoli, cauliflower, peppers, cabbage, bok choy, or salsa.

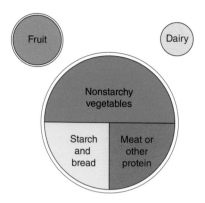

Figure 14.1   Meal planning using the plate method.

3. On the other half of the plate are two sections. In one, put starchy foods such as whole grain breads, whole grain high-fiber cereal, rice, pasta, potatoes, winter squash, low-fat crackers, snack chips, or pretzels.

4. In the final section, put your meat or meat substitute. Examples include skinless chicken or turkey, fish or other seafood, lean cuts of beef or pork, tofu, eggs, and low-fat cheese.

5. Then add an 8-ounce (227 ml) glass of nonfat or low-fat milk, or if you are not a milk drinker, grab a small serving of carbohydrate such as a container of light yogurt.

6. Add a piece of fruit or half a cup of fruit salad to complete your meal.

This plate plan helps to keep portion sizes in check (which is great if weight loss is a goal) and also helps you manage your blood glucose levels by providing a good balance of carbohydrates, fats, and proteins.

Counting Grams of Carbohydrate

Another common meal plan for those with diabetes is to count grams of carbohydrate.[6] Carbohydrates have three main forms—starches, sugars, and fiber. Of these three, starches and sugars have the greatest influence on blood glucose levels. Your first reaction might be to avoid carbohydrates as a way to keep your blood glucose levels in check. This is not a healthy option. Your body needs carbohydrate, especially to maintain an active lifestyle including regular exercise. The focus of this method of meal planning is to consume the right amount of carbohydrate for your personal activity level while also considering the medications you take.[9]

The exact amount of carbohydrate you need should be determined by your health care provider. In general, about 45 to 60 grams of carbohydrate per meal is a starting point.[6] Typically, starches and sugars are factored into this total, whereas fiber and nonstarchy vegetables are not. Examples of nonstarchy vegetables are salad greens, peppers, tomatoes, beans, carrots, cauliflower, and onions.

To determine the grams of carbohydrate in a given product, consult the package label. Be sure to check the serving size because serving sizes can be quite small— you may actually consume more than just one serving in a meal. For example, most cans of soup contain two servings. Thus, if you ate the contents of a whole can, you would need to double the amount of carbohydrate (as well as all the other nutrients listed) on the label. For more details on reading food labels, see chapter 4.

As you review food labels, you may note a special category under carbohydrate called sugar alcohol. Even though the name includes the term *alcohol*, the food does not contain alcohol; the term just refers to the chemical structure. Sugar alcohols are reduced-calorie sweeteners (usually about half the number of calories as sugar). Your blood glucose response to different products may vary, but in general, sugar alcohols will have less of an impact on your blood glucose level than other forms of carbohydrate. If a product has more than 5 grams of sugar alcohol, then you can subtract half the grams of sugar alcohol from the total amount of carbohydrate.[6] For example, consider a granola bar that has 15 grams of total carbohydrate, including 6 grams of sugar alcohol. When counting grams of carbohydrate, you can subtract half of the sugar alcohols (6 grams × 0.5 = 3 grams) from the total (15 grams of carbohydrate − 3 grams for the sugar alcohol = 12 grams). When calculating the grams of carbohydrate in your meal, you include only 12 grams of carbohydrate for the granola bar. Although low-calorie sweeteners are helpful in reducing calories and the effect on your blood glucose, these products are not calorie free and also may cause a laxative effect or other intestinal symptoms in some people.[6]

Although this method focuses on carbohydrates, do not forget to include proteins as well as fats to balance your meal (see chapter 4 for a refresher on the importance of fat and protein in your diet). Another factor you need to watch for in weight management is the number of calories you consume. As discussed in chapter 13, to lose weight, the calories you consume must be less than the calories your body uses for basic functions, daily activities, and exercise.

Focusing on Physical Activity

The benefits of exercise for those who have diabetes are well documented.[10] Health care providers often prescribe exercise for type 1 and type 2 diabetes in conjunction with medication, or exercise alone for type 2 diabetes.[11] Exercise can not only improve blood glucose levels, but also reduce blood pressure and cholesterol levels, decrease the risk of heart disease, promote weight loss, improve brain function, and enhance self-image. Exercise needs to be continued to be effective; once it is suspended, the physiological benefits related to the control of blood glucose are lost within days.[10]

Type 1 diabetes requires that glucose levels be controlled before exercise.[8] When glucose levels are poorly controlled, the liver production of glucose increases, which can result in higher blood glucose levels during exercise. This is because type 1 diabetes is characterized by a deficiency in insulin.[8] Higher blood glucose levels can also be observed after very intense exercise.[10] When blood glucose levels are controlled, moderate-intensity exercise can reduce blood glucose by increasing blood flow to the muscles, which increases the rate of glucose absorbed into the cells.[8]

Exercise is particularly important in improving A1c levels, an indicator of the three-month average of blood glucose.[16] (See *Blood Glucose Control and A1c*.) This is important in reducing the damage to blood vessels that can result from chronically elevated glucose levels. Exercise may also reduce the amount of oral diabetic medications or the amount of insulin you require.[8]

Exercise plays a major role in the control of type 2 diabetes.[14] Type 2 diabetes is a dual-defect disorder involving insulin resistance and impaired insulin secretion. Exercise significantly improves insulin sensitivity, which is the body's responsiveness to glucose; this can counteract insulin resistance and improve insulin secretion by the pancreas over time.[8] In insulin users, the improved insulin sensitivity can lead to decreases in the amount of insulin needed. Weight loss can also decrease abdominal fat, which can further reduce insulin resistance and improve glucose levels.

Exercise can also help prevent the onset of diabetes. People who have prediabetes and a family history of diabetes should focus on both diet and exercise to promote weight loss as a way to prevent type 2 diabetes.[11] In one well-known study, the Diabetes Prevention Program, people who had a high probability of developing diabetes reduced their risk by 58% as a result of lifestyle interventions including exercise, changes in diet, and weight loss of about 12 pounds (5.4 kg).[12] Weight loss decreases insulin resistance and improves the absorption of glucose in the body, both of which lead to better blood glucose control.

Blood Glucose Control and A1c

Hemoglobin is a protein found inside red blood cells whose main job is to carry oxygen around the body. When blood glucose levels are high (as with diabetes), hemoglobin links with glucose that enters the red blood cells. This is referred to as glycated hemoglobin or HbA1c (or commonly just A1c).[6] The higher the glucose levels in the blood are, the greater the A1c percentage is. Because red blood cells have a lifespan of about 120 days, looking at A1c levels can give a picture of the average glucose control for that time frame.[6] A1c cannot be used to check short-term glucose levels (you need to use your blood glucose meter for daily checks), but rather gives more of an overall picture. The A1c percentage for someone without diabetes would be 4% to 6%, but in those with diabetes this percentage can be elevated to 10% or higher if glucose levels are out of control. Your health care provider will help you establish a target value; generally, well-controlled glucose is evident by an A1c percentage of less than 7%.[5]

Improving your blood glucose control is of great benefit regardless of the type of diabetes you have. In general, for every 1 percentage point drop in A1c, you can reduce microvascular complications that affect the eyes, kidneys, and nerves by 40%.[15]

Precautions Before Exercise

Exercise plays a pivotal role in preventing as well as managing diabetes. Potentially of even greater importance is the role exercise can play in preventing the complications often associated with diabetes. Anyone with diabetes should be carefully evaluated before starting an exercise program.[8] In particular, if you have preexisting microvascular disease complications (eye, kidney, or nerve diseases) or macrovascular disease (disease of the large blood vessels, such as those of the heart), you should not start a vigorous exercise program without being evaluated by a health care professional first. Because diabetes is the leading cause of heart disease, you should have a cardiac stress test (i.e., treadmill test during which your heart rhythm is monitored) before exercising if you fall into any of the following categories:[2]

- Have previously been sedentary and are older than 35
- Have been sedentary at any age with diabetes for more than 10 years
- Have had type 1 diabetes for more than 15 years or type 2 diabetes for more than 10 years
- Have a major risk factor for heart disease (e.g., smoking, high cholesterol, obesity, sedentary lifestyle)
- Have peripheral vascular disease, kidney disease, heart or blood vessel disease, or nervous system disease

And, of course, if chest pain or discomfort occurs with exercise, the cause should be evaluated immediately.

Some medical conditions related to diabetes may also influence exercise choices, including diabetic retinopathy, peripheral neuropathy, and nephropathy. In addition to a stress test, eye examinations by an ophthalmologist should be considered before starting an exercise program.[4] Diabetic retinopathy is a disease affecting the retina of the eye. If this disease is present, certain activities should be avoided to prevent further damage.[4] If you have mild background retinopathy, most likely no major changes would be needed.[8] If you have moderate nonproliferative diabetic retinopathy, avoid exercises that affect blood pressure (e.g., heavy resistance training).[8] Avoid contact sports and heavy lifting if you have severe nonproliferative retinopathy.[8] Anyone with proliferative diabetic retinopathy should focus on low-impact cardiorespiratory exercises such as walking, swimming, and stationary cycling.[8]

Another potential concern is peripheral neuropathy, which is a nerve condition that alters the sensation of the hands and feet as well as proprioception (feedback to your brain from your limbs regarding body position).[4] Falls are more common with this condition, as are joint and soft tissue injuries.[8] Proper footwear is a must to prevent blisters or ulcers. Shoes and socks should be worn at all times to protect the feet. Inspect your feet both before and after exercise for blisters or ulcers. If a lack of flexibility makes seeing the soles of your feet difficult, use a mirror to get a complete view. Attention to your feet is important because diabetes can make you more prone to athlete's foot and fungal nail infections. Proper nail trimming should be done to prevent ingrown toenails. If you have had foot ulcers or foot deformities, schedule an appointment with a podiatrist to be measured for shoes with proper inserts. Lower-impact activities that are easier on the joints, such as swimming and stationary biking, are preferred in these cases to limit complications.[8]

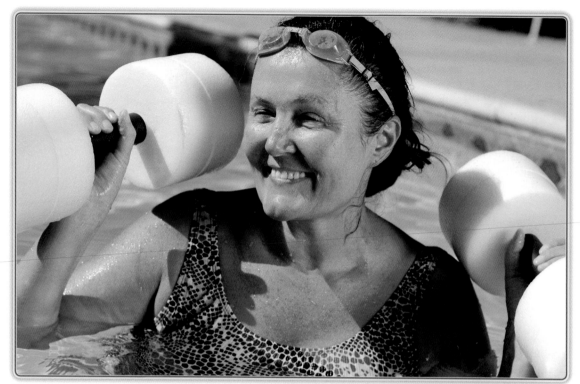
Water-based activities can provide low-impact aerobic conditioning.

Because diabetes may also result in nephropathy (kidney damage), a kidney evaluation before starting an exercise program is suggested. One sign of kidney damage is the presence of proteins in the urine. Kidney damage can be exacerbated by strenuous activity because of the sudden increases in blood pressure, leading to further damage to kidney function.[4, 8] Blood pressure medications called ACE inhibitors or angiotensin receptor blockers protect kidney function and may be considered when faced with the aforementioned conditions.

Although avoiding hypoglycemia is obviously optimal, at times your blood glucose levels may drop (see *Effects of Exercise on Blood Glucose: Hypoglycemia*). Always have some easily absorbed sources of glucose with you. When glucose levels are low (less than 70 mg/dL), consume a glucose-containing product that will rapidly become available in your blood (e.g., hard candies, juice, glucose tablets). Because fat and protein slow down the movement of glucose from the intestine into the blood, other snacks such as peanut butter and crackers or granola bars are better to use once glucose levels have risen, or to prevent a drop. To avoid overshooting and becoming hyperglycemic, the recommendation is to consume 15 to 20 grams of carbohydrate and then wait 15 minutes to see how much your blood glucose level rises.[6] If your glucose is still low, repeat the process. Letting those with whom you exercise know about your diabetes is important, just in case your glucose levels drop so low that you become unconscious. If this happens, they can call for emergency assistance.

To avoid hypoglycemia, be consistent with your carbohydrate intake with regard to meal timing and exercise. Maintaining a regular time of day for your exercise routine is also helpful, and monitoring your blood glucose before and after exercise is a good idea, especially if you take insulin or other oral medications that stimulate insulin release.[2, 8] If your exercise bout is prolonged, you may also want to check your blood glucose level during exercise, if possible. Keeping blood glucose between 100 and 250 mg/dL (and no higher) will optimize safety by helping you avoid both hypoglycemia and hyperglycemia.[2]

You should also take special care if you exercise later in the day. The concern is the potential of hypoglycemia occurring following the exercise session after you have gone to bed for the night. Exercise can affect blood glucose up to 12 hours or more after the exercise is completed. This underscores the need to monitor your blood glucose during that time and to eat an extra snack if necessary. If you need a snack, it should contain both carbohydrate (about 15 grams) and protein (7 to 8 grams).[8]

Effects of Exercise on Blood Glucose: Hypoglycemia

What you eat and when you eat are especially important for managing your glucose levels during exercise. Exercise itself will help to move glucose from the blood into the working muscles. This is helpful with regard to lowering blood glucose levels but also opens the possibility of blood glucose dropping too low. This is referred to as hypoglycemia (*hypo* means "low" and *glycemia* refers to blood glucose). Symptoms of hypoglycemia are as follows:

Shakiness	Headache
Weakness	Visual disturbances
Abnormal sweating	Mental dullness
Nervousness	Confusion
Anxiety	Amnesia
Tingling of the mouth and fingers	Seizures
Hunger	Coma

Checking your blood glucose on a regular basis is key to managing your diabetes and ensuring safety when exercising. Handheld glucose meters require only a small drop of blood and provide an immediate digital reading of your blood glucose level (see figure 14.2). Make a habit of checking your glucose before and after exercise.

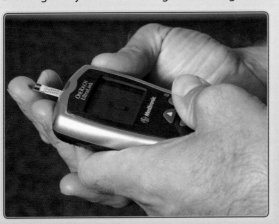

Figure 14.2 Glucose monitors provide quick feedback on blood glucose levels.

Diabetic Ketoacidosis

When diabetes is not controlled, the glucose needed for energy cannot enter your cells. As a result, fat, rather than glucose, is used for energy, resulting in the production of ketones (acids), which first build up in the blood and eventually also appear in the urine. You can check for ketones with a simple at-home urine test.

Situations that may result in ketones include insufficient insulin or insufficient food intake. Usually, ketoacidosis develops slowly, but if you become sick and are vomiting, it could develop within a few hours.[6] Early signs include thirst or a dry mouth, frequent urination, high glucose levels, and high ketones in the urine. Over time other symptoms may appear including constant feelings of tiredness, dry or flushed skin, nausea or vomiting, fruity-smelling breath, and confusion.[6] Diabetic ketoacidosis is a serious medical condition, and if you have these signs or symptoms, you should contact your health care provider immediately.

Consult with your health care provider to solidify your plan of action based on your type of diabetes as well as the medications you are taking.

If you take insulin or are on a medication that stimulates insulin release (e.g., sulfonylureas or meglitinides; see table 14.4 on page 296 for more information), be sure to check your glucose level before exercise. If your blood glucose level is low before an exercise bout (less than 100 mg/dL), consuming 20 to 30 grams of carbohydrate is one step you can take to avoid hypoglycemia.[1] Depending on the duration and intensity of your exercise session, you may need to take in additional carbohydrate during and after exercise as well.[8]

Delayed-onset hypoglycemia is a phenomenon that typically occurs 6 to 15 hours after exercise. It appears to be a result of the liver and muscles replenishing their glucose stores after exercise.[8] By eating regularly and monitoring your glucose, you can avoid delayed-onset hypoglycemia.

On the opposite end of the spectrum from hypoglycemia is hyperglycemia, or high blood glucose. With type 1 diabetes, if your blood glucose is elevated (greater than 250 to 300 mg/dL), you may need to postpone or at least decrease the intensity of the exercise session[2] (see figure 14.3 for a decision-making flow chart). You can base your decision on how you are feeling as well as whether you have ketones in your urine. Ketones make your blood more acidic potentially causing ketoacidosis, a condition that, if ignored, can cause coma and death (see *Diabetic Ketoacidosis* for more information). Ketoacidosis is more commonly found with type 1 diabetes than with type 2 diabetes.[6] The American Diabetes Association suggests the following general guidelines to help keep your glucose levels in check:[4]

- Avoid physical activity if your blood glucose is greater than 250 mg/dL and you have ketones in your urine.

- Use caution if your glucose is above 300 mg/dL even if ketones are not present.

If your blood glucose level is elevated but you find no ketones in your urine and you feel well, then moderate-intensity exercise is appropriate and may actually be helpful in lowering your blood glucose level.[10] However, if you have ketones in your urine, you should postpone exercise and contact your health care provider if

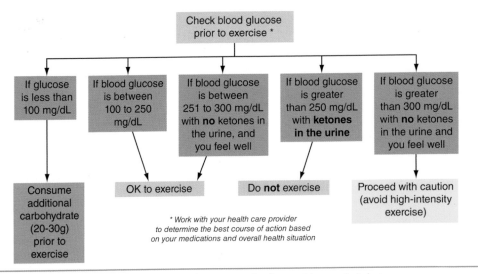

Figure 14.3 Decision-making flow chart for exercise for those with type 1 diabetes.

you have not already established a response plan for situations such as this. Often, treatment includes the administration of insulin to regain normal glucose levels.[2]

For type 2 diabetes, additional carbohydrate is not typically needed before exercise because hypoglycemia is not common, unless you are being treated with insulin or insulin-stimulating medications (see the previous recommendations on carbohydrate consumption if these medications are included in your treatment plan).[14] Other medications (e.g., metformin, thiazolidinediones, and alpha-glucosidase inhibitors) do not tend to cause hypoglycemia and thus do not require that you take in additional carbohydrate.[14] With regard to hyperglycemia and type 2 diabetes, when ketones are present, vigorous exercise should be avoided.[14] However, light to moderate exercise may actually help lower your blood glucose levels, especially if the high glucose level comes after a meal.[14] Blood glucose levels lower than 400 mg/dL typically indicate that it is safe for those with type 2 diabetes to engage in physical activity.[8] The American Diabetes Association suggests that as long as you feel well, are adequately hydrated, and have no ketones in your urine, it is not necessary to postpone exercise based on hyperglycemia alone.[14] To optimize your safety when exercising, discuss your medical situation, including the medications you are taking, with your health care provider so you will know what steps are most appropriate for you.

Physical Activity Prescriptions

Exercise comes in many forms, and your program should be tailored to your situation. Although age and type of diabetes may support different exercise programs, the goal is the same—to improve health outcomes. Following appropriate screening and armed with blood glucose monitoring skills, you are ready to get started. A complete exercise program should include aerobic activities, resistance training, and flexibility exercises.

Aerobic Prescription Aerobic activities, which help improve the efficiency of the cardiovascular system, typically are the most beneficial for regulating blood

Table 14.1 **Aerobic Training Recommendations for People With Diabetes**

	Type 1	Type 2
Frequency	Three to seven days per week	Three to seven days per week
Intensity	Level 5 or 6 on a 10-point scale	Level 5 or 6 on a 10-point scale
Time	20–60 minutes per session of moderate-intensity activity	At least 150 minutes per week of moderate-intensity activity or 90 minutes per week of vigorous-intensity activity
Type	Large-muscle-group activities such as walking, biking, jogging, and water aerobics	Large-muscle-group activities such as walking, biking, and water aerobics

Adapted by permission from American College of Sports Medicine, 2010, p. 605.

glucose levels.[8] Examples include walking, jogging, swimming, and biking. If you cannot do weight-bearing or high-impact activities, chair exercises, water aerobics, and recumbent biking can be beneficial.[8] Recommendations for type 1 and type 2 diabetes are found in table 14.1 following the FITT principle discussed in chapter 6, which addresses frequency, intensity, time, and type of activities.[2]

Daily aerobic activity has benefits for both type 1 and type 2 diabetes.[2] For those with type 1 who use insulin, daily physical activity helps maintain the balance between insulin doses and food consumed. For those with type 2 diabetes, the focus is typically on burning calories and weight management. To maintain weight loss, the amount of exercise is expanded by manipulating time, frequency, and duration (see chapter 13 for more information on weight management). Keep in mind that the recommendations in table 14.1 are targets, not initial levels. If you are just starting out, begin gradually because your body will need to adapt to the exercise, and you also have to monitor how your blood glucose levels are affected. Consult chapter 6 for suggestions on beginning or advancing in your aerobic training program.

A CLOSER LOOK
Cindy

On Cindy's 58th birthday, she learned that she has prediabetes. Although her physician had cautioned her about her gradually increasing weight, she had ignored him. Currently, she weighs about 200 pounds (91 kg). At 5 feet 4 inches tall (64 inches, or 163 cm), she is in the obese category for BMI. This diagnosis brings home the importance of the need for some lifestyle changes. Cindy is committed to turning her health crisis into a health celebration by increasing her activity and improving her diet. Her long-term goal is to lose 50 pounds (23 kg), which will bring her closer to a normal BMI classification. By combining daily walking in her neighborhood or cycling on her recumbent stationary bike along with cutting extra calories and using the plate plan to provide a more balanced diet, she continues to make weekly steps toward that goal. Prediabetes does increase the risk of developing type 2 diabetes, but lifestyle changes, such as the ones Cindy is pursuing, have the potential to prevent the development of type 2 diabetes.

Table 14.2 **Resistance Training Recommendations for People With Diabetes**

	Type 1	Type 2
Frequency	Two or three days per week	Two or three days per week
Intensity	Low to moderate (level 5 or 6 on a 10-point scale)	Lower intensity (level 4 to 6 on a 10-point scale)
Time	8–12 repetitions per exercise Two or three sets per exercise	8–20 repetitions per exercise Two or three sets per exercise
Type	All the major muscle groups	All the major muscle groups

Adapted by permission from American College of Sports Medicine, 2010, p. 607.

Resistance Training Prescription　Resistance training can lower A1c levels and confer other health benefits as well (see chapter 7 for more details on resistance training). Including both aerobic exercise and resistance training can optimize the benefits related to managing your glucose levels.[16] A few precautions do need to be mentioned. If you have microvascular disease, be aware of the potential concerns about damage to the eyes, kidneys, and joints. Straining while lifting weights can lead to an increased risk of bleeding and retinal detachment for those with proliferative and severe nonproliferative eye disease.[8] Resistance training may not be appropriate if you have diabetic retinopathy. Also, be careful if you have nerve involvement because you will be more susceptible to foot ulcers and bone damage because of the lack of sensation and weakening of the muscles and ligaments in the foot. If you have nephropathy, or kidney damage, related to diabetes, strenuous activity can increase protein excretion.[4]

With these precautions in mind, you can implement a safe and effective resistance training program.[2] Enlarged muscle mass increases the use of glucose. Increasing lean muscle while reducing fat tissue can decrease insulin resistance and improve blood glucose control. Increased muscle mass can also improve your balance, posture, ability to move, and daily functions.[8] The goal of resistance training is to focus on exercises involving the major muscle groups including the legs, back, chest, arms, shoulders, thighs, and abdominal area. Table 14.2 provides resistance training recommendations for type 1 and type 2 diabetes[2] based on the FITT principle. Details regarding the many exercise options for resistance training are found in chapter 7.

Flexibility Prescription　Flexibility is also an integral part of an exercise program for people with diabetes. Typically, static stretching is recommended. This involves placing the body into a position that creates tension in the muscles and then holding that position for 15 to 30 seconds. Table 14.3 provides flexibility recommendations for those with type 1 and type 2 diabetes[2] based on the FITT principle. Details regarding stretching are found in chapter 8.

Influence of Medications

Diabetes can be controlled with the appropriate use of medications including oral medications (for type 2) as well as insulin injections (for type 1 mainly but also for some with type 2). A general understanding of how these medications work will help you see how they can be part of your total treatment plan.

Table 14.3   **Flexibility Recommendations for People With Diabetes**

	Type 1 and Type 2
Frequency	Two or three days per week
Intensity	Stretch to the point of tightness (not pain)
Time	15–30 seconds per stretch Two to four repetitions per stretch
Type	Four or five exercises for both the upper and lower body

Adapted by permission from American College of Sports Medicine, 2010, p. 607.

Oral Medications for Type 2 Diabetes

Oral medications are the most common treatment for type 2 diabetes. In some situations, insulin, or a combination of insulin and oral medications, may be used depending on the severity of the disease.[11]

Several classes of oral medications are used to treat type 2 diabetes (see table 14.4). Some, such as the biguanides, help to decrease insulin resistance as well as decrease the release of glucose from the liver. Others focus only on decreasing insulin resistance (e.g., thiazolidinediones) or on stimulating insulin release after a meal (e.g., meglitinides) or when glucose levels are rising (e.g., sulfonylureas). The DPP-4 inhibitors, a relatively new class of medications, work by decreasing liver production of glucose and stimulating insulin release when blood glucose is elevated. A less commonly used class of medications is the alpha-glucosidase inhibitors, which slow the movement of glucose from the intestine into the bloodstream. GLP-1 agonists are a newer class of medication that can help with weight loss; they are given as a subcutaneous injection. When GLP-1 agonists are used with other medications that increase insulin levels (e.g., sulfonylureas), the other medications often must be decreased. As with all medications, there are side effects as well as situations in which certain medications may not be appropriate. Some of these issues are outlined in table 14.4.

Exercise should be employed for type 2 diabetes in conjunction with medication use. Exercise can contribute to weight loss, which can decrease insulin resistance and improve glucose tolerance. It also increases insulin sensitivity and makes the body work more efficiently. In most people with well-controlled type 2 diabetes, medications do not need to be adjusted for exercise. However, two classes of diabetes medications to watch closely are the sulfonylureas and the meglitinides, both of which can cause hypoglycemia.[14] Discuss your exercise program with your health care provider because these medications may need to be reduced on the days you exercise.

As mentioned previously, frequent monitoring of blood glucose levels before, during, and after exercising is important to avoid potential problems.[8] When you are exercising and losing weight, realize that medication doses may need to be decreased. Work with your health care provider to adjust oral medications (and insulin if that is part of your treatment plan). This is preferred over snacking to avoid hypoglycemia.[8] When you are trying to lose weight, increasing food consumption to balance your glucose level is not a good option. Instead, enjoy the benefit of

Table 14.4 Oral Medications for the Management of Type 2 Diabetes

Drug class	Primary mechanism	Possible side effects	Contra-indications	Comments
Biguanides	Decrease liver production of glucose	Diarrhea, stomach upset, lactic acidosis	Kidney disease as determined by creatinine in the urine of greater than 1.5 mg/dL in males or greater than 1.4 mg/dL in females; liver disease and severe congestive heart failure	May cause weight loss; typically do not cause hypoglycemia.
Sulfonylureas	Stimulate insulin release	Hypoglycemia	Be cautious with sulfa allergies	The elderly may need lower doses
Meglitinides	Stimulate insulin release after a meal	Hypoglycemia		Take before meals
DPP-4 inhibitors	Decrease liver production of glucose and stimulate insulin release	Rash; usually well tolerated	Reduce dose in renal disease	Should not cause weight gain
Thiazolidinediones	Improve insulin sensitivity	Edema, weight gain	Should not be used in people with congestive heart failure or liver abnormalities	Use lowest dose with insulin
Alpha-glucosidase inhibitors	Slow glucose absorption at the intestinal level	Diarrhea, abdominal pain, and flatulence	Avoid use in liver disease	Rarely used

exercise on your body and be pleased that you have taken positive steps to decrease your reliance on medications.

Insulin Options for Diabetes

A number of types of insulin are used to treat type 1 and type 2 diabetes. Insulin must be injected; it cannot be consumed orally. Periodic injections are required to provide background levels of insulin (referred to as basal insulin) and to cover the food in a meal or snack (referred to as bolus doses of insulin). One other option is an insulin pump.

Insulin pumps are small units that are either attached directly to the body or indirectly via a tube (see figure 14.4) to deliver insulin continuously throughout the day in a way that attempts to mimic the natural activity of the pancreas. Insulin levels can be adjusted up (when eating) or down (when being active) with a couple of button pushes. This provides more flexibility in timing meals as well as when you are active. For physically active people, the ability to more precisely administer insulin typically results in better glucose control and A1c values drop. In addition, the pump takes the place of separate insulin vials and syringes so it is much simpler to handle, especially for active, on-the-go people.

The types of insulin are grouped based on their onset of action, time of peak activity, and duration of activity in the body. Details on these characteristics and common brands are listed in table 14.5. In general, rapid-acting and short-acting insulins have a relatively quick onset and time of peak action. These types of insulin are given before meals and often need to be adjusted before exercise. How much insulin should be decreased depends on the intensity of exercise. If activity occurs within two hours of eating, pre-meal insulin should be decreased 5% to 30% (5% for low-intensity exercise and 30% for high-intensity and long-duration exercise).[8] Intermediate-acting

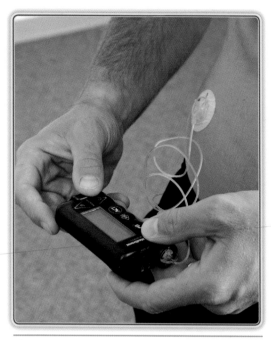

Figure 14.4 Insulin pumps help to regulate glucose levels and typically improve glucose control.

insulin has a longer onset of action as well as longer duration. Unless you are engaging in prolonged exercise, intermediate-acting insulin often does not need to be adjusted. Long-acting basal insulin does not have much of a peak; rather, it provides a low but constant level of insulin for up to 24 hours. Like intermediate-acting insulin, long-acting insulin usually does not need to be adjusted for exercise.

Exercise is not recommended at the point of peak insulin action.[1, 8] The combination of the high levels of insulin and the glucose-lowering effect of exercise can lead to hypoglycemia. If you are using rapid-acting insulin with meals, wait at least an hour after the meal before exercising.[8] By monitoring your blood glucose levels (before, during, and after exercise), you can make additional adjustments to your

Table 14.5 **Characteristics of Various Types of Insulin**

Insulin type	Brand names	Onset	Peak	Duration
Rapid acting: Insulin aspart analog Insulin glulisine analog Insulin lispro analog	NovoLog Apidra Humalog	10–30 minutes	0.5–3 hours	3–5 hours
Short-acting: Regular insulin	Humulin R Novolin R	30 minutes	1–5 hours	8 hours
Intermediate acting: NPH insulin	Humulin N Novolin R	1–4 hours	4–12 hours	14–26 hours
Long-acting (basal): Insulin detemir Insulin glargine	Levemir Lantus	1–2 hours	Minimal peak	Up to 24 hours

food intake and insulin. One other consideration with insulin injections is the site. You should avoid injecting insulin in an area that will be active during your exercise session.[10] Using an abdominal injection site is typically preferred to using a limb injection site when planning to exercise.[1]

— ▪▪▪▪ —

Exercise and a sound nutritional plan are the two cornerstones of managing and thriving with diabetes. Your diet is key whether you face type 1 or type 2 diabetes. With type 1, balancing your intake of carbohydrates, fats, and proteins will help you with blood glucose control. With type 2 diabetes, attention to calories consumed will be an asset for weight loss. A great complement to your diet is exercise. Your exercise program should include aerobic activity as well as resistance training and stretching. It is important to know that you can realize the benefits of exercise without losing control of your blood glucose. The most important strategy for exercise is individualizing your program. Your exercise program should improve health outcomes and blood glucose control but should not cause or worsen microvascular or macrovascular disease. A health care provider or diabetes educator can be helpful in making adjustments in medications and insulin when you are starting or expanding your exercise program.

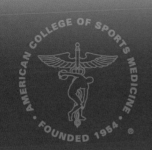

chapter **15**

High Blood Pressure

Unlike with other medical conditions, which typically have outward signs, you could have high blood pressure and not even know it. High blood pressure, also known as hypertension, has been called the silent killer because blood pressure can be abnormally elevated without any signs or symptoms.

Hypertension is the most prevalent cardiovascular disease. The American Heart Association estimates that approximately 73 million Americans age 20 and older (about one in three) and 1 billion people worldwide have hypertension.[6] Furthermore, the estimated direct and indirect costs of hypertension for 2010 equal $76.6 billion.[6] These numbers are quite shocking!

Taking action to prevent or treat hypertension is vital. Those with untreated hypertension have a much greater occurrence of heart attack, abnormal thickening of the heart muscle, stroke, kidney problems, and heart failure. Although outward signs aren't easy to identify, high blood pressure has a negative effect inside your body.

Blood pressure is reported as two distinct numbers: systolic blood pressure (top number) and diastolic blood pressure (bottom number). Both of these numbers are important, and they are expressed in millimeters of mercury (abbreviated as mmHg). At rest, the heart typically contracts between 60 and 80 times per minute. Every time the heart contracts, a pressure is generated that pushes against the major blood vessels. The pressure in the blood vessels during the heart's contraction phase is called systolic blood pressure, and the pressure during the relaxation phase is called diastolic blood pressure.

Hypertension is defined as abnormally high resting blood pressure. As noted in table 15.1, a normal resting systolic blood pressure is less than 120 mmHg, and a normal resting diastolic blood pressure is less than 80 mmHg. So, what exactly qualifies as hypertension? Any one of the following is considered abnormal and thus considered hypertensive:[4]

- Resting systolic blood pressure greater than or equal to 140 mmHg *or*
- Resting diastolic blood pressure greater than or equal to 90 mmHg

The overriding goal of this chapter is to provide information on exercise and nutrition related specifically to hypertension. As you will soon learn, regular exercise and healthy eating have clear benefits for anyone with hypertension. Lifestyle modifications, which include regular exercise and proper nutrition, are currently advocated for the prevention, treatment, *and* control of hypertension.

Table 15.1 **Classification of Blood Pressure for Adults**[4]

Blood pressure classification	Systolic blood pressure (SBP) in mmHg	Diastolic blood pressure (DBP) in mmHg
Normal	Less than 120	and less than 80
Prehypertension	120–139	or 80–89
Hypertension	140 or higher	or 90 or higher

Adapted from U.S. Department of Health and Human Services, National Institutes of Health, National Heart, Lung, and Blood Institute, 2004, p. 12.

A CLOSER LOOK
Joelle

Joelle, a 57-year-old female, made an appointment with her physician after what looked like a bruise appeared by her eye. Because no trauma had occurred to cause the darkening, she was concerned. Her response may have saved her life. Joelle had severely elevated blood pressure, which resulted in a small blood vessel above her eye bursting, thus causing the "bruise." According to her physician, if she had not sought treatment, she may have experienced a stroke as a result of her excessively high blood pressure. Medication, along with a recommended walking program, lowered Joelle's blood pressure back to a safe range. With no distinct signs or symptoms, Joelle's situation clearly shows why hypertension is potentially a silent killer.

CAUSES OF HIGH BLOOD PRESSURE

A fundamental question is: What causes blood pressure to be too high? Nine times out of 10 the cause of the elevation in blood pressure is not known. In less than 1 out of 10 cases of hypertension the cause of the elevation in blood pressure can be attributed to a known problem such as kidney disease. In these cases the hypertension is considered secondary to the known disease; the other 9 out of 10 cases are referred to as essential hypertension (meaning there is no known cause). Because of very complex interactions, the precise mechanisms underlying essential hypertension are not likely to be understood anytime soon.

Although the cause of most cases of hypertension is not known, risk factors for hypertension have been identified and include the following:[8]

- *Age.* Your risk for hypertension increases with age. Over half of all Americans age 60 and older have hypertension.
- *Race.* Hypertension is more common among African American adults than among Caucasian or Hispanic Americans. Also, African Americans tend to become hypertensive earlier in life and have more severely elevated blood pressure.
- *Family history.* Hypertension often runs in families.
- *Overweight or obesity.* Prehypertension or hypertension is more likely for anyone who is overweight or obese.
- *Lifestyle and nutritional factors.* Various lifestyle and nutritional factors can raise your risk, including diets with too much sodium and not enough potassium, excessive alcohol consumption, smoking, and insufficient physical activity.
- *Stress.* Long-lasting stress can increase the risk of high blood pressure.

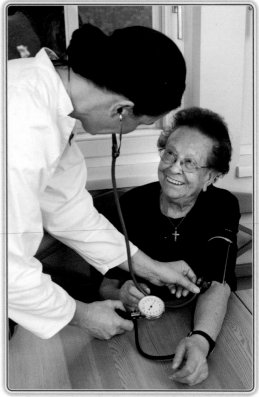

Resting blood pressure can easily be measured by qualified health care providers.

Consider the items on this list. Although some you cannot change (e.g., age, race, family history), there are a number that you can change or at least work to address. This chapter presents suggestions for increasing physical activity and improving nutrition to help lower your risk of developing hypertension.

The Slippery Slope of Prehypertension

As you saw in table 15.1, prehypertension is defined as a systolic blood pressure between 120 and 139 mmHg or a diastolic blood pressure between 80 and 89 mmHg. The term *prehypertension* is fairly new and replaced terms such as *high normal blood pressure*. The reason for this new designation is the evidence that people within this blood pressure range are at increased risk for developing heart and vascular problems. It is estimated that approximately 59 million Americans are within the prehypertensive blood pressure category.[6] People within this range who are otherwise healthy generally do not take blood pressure medications—although they should discuss this issue with their health care providers. It is critically important for those with prehypertension to adopt healthy lifestyle choices to avoid additional increases in blood pressure that could lead to hypertension and cardiovascular disease.

The risk of cardiovascular disease and stroke increases as resting blood pressure increases (see figure 15.1). Although those with hypertension are at greater risk than those with prehypertension, it is important to note that those with prehypertension are at a greater risk than those with normal blood pressure. Although it is convenient to have firm boundaries separating hypertensive, prehypertensive, and normal resting blood pressures (as listed in table 15.1), resting blood pressure is directly related to cardiovascular risk and mortality (i.e., death rate) across a wide range of resting blood pressures, spanning all the categories. Risk begins to increase once resting systolic blood pressure exceeds 115 mmHg and diastolic blood pressure exceeds 75 mmHg.[5]

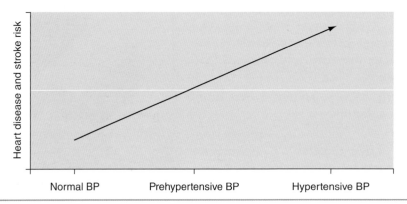

Figure 15.1   Risk of heart disease and stroke associated with blood pressure. Heart disease and stroke risk doubles for every 20/10 mmHg increase in resting blood pressure.

Adapted from Lewington, Clarke, Qizilbash, et al., 2002.

HEALTHY APPROACHES TO MANAGING BLOOD PRESSURE

Whether you are hypertensive, prehypertensive, or have normal blood pressure, you can benefit from adopting a physically active lifestyle that includes regular exercise. Exercise coupled with proper nutrition is strongly recommended by major organizations such as the American College of Sports Medicine[9] and the American Heart Association.[2] The influence of physical activity and various aspects of nutrition are listed in table 15.2. In addition, medications are often used to help lower blood pressure when physical activity and dietary changes are not enough.

Focusing on Nutrition

Nutrition has great potential to affect your blood pressure. In particular, you should thoughtfully consider the composition of your diet, including lowering your sodium intake and the calories you consume.

Low-Sodium Diet

Most Americans consume far too much dietary sodium. Recent estimates from the U.S. Department of Agriculture state that American men and women consume

Table 15.2 **Lifestyle Modifications to Lower Blood Pressure**[4]

Modification	Recommendation	Approximate range of systolic blood pressure reduction
Physical activity	Engage in regular aerobic physical activity such as brisk walking.	5–7 mmHg
Dietary salt reduction	Reduce dietary salt intake.	2–8 mmHg
DASH eating plan	Consume a diet rich in fruits, vegetables, and low-fat dairy products and reduce the intake of saturated and total fat.	8–14 mmHg
Weight reduction	Maintain normal body weight (body mass index 18.5–24.9 kg/m²).	5–20 mmHg per 20-pound (9 kg) weight loss
Moderation of alcohol consumption	Limit consumption to no more than two drinks per day (most men) and no more than one drink per day (women and lighter weight people).	2–4 mmHg

Adapted from U.S. Department of Health and Human Services, National Institutes of Health, National Heart, Lung, and Blood Institute, 2004, p. 26.

between 3,000 and 4,000 milligrams of sodium per day.[3] These values are very high, especially considering that most organizations such as the U.S. Departments of Agriculture and Health and Human Services as well as the World Health Organization recommend a daily sodium intake of less than 2,300 milligrams per day, and even lower (1,500 milligrams per day) for adults with hypertension.[16] More recently there has been a push to recommend the 1,500-milligrams-per-day level for most Americans. The American Heart Association also endorses dietary sodium reduction for most Americans.[2] These recommendations are based on research studies that have documented a decline in blood pressure with dietary sodium restriction, as discussed in table 15.2.[10]

A CLOSER LOOK
Jeffrey

Jeffrey is a 27-year-old chemistry graduate student who is currently working on his research dissertation. He is under a lot of stress, and other than working in the laboratory, he does little physical activity. At a campus health fair he had his blood pressure checked and was alarmed to find it was 142/88. Because the hustle and bustle of the health fair made it difficult to know if this accurately reflected his blood pressure, he arranged a follow-up visit with his physician, who found Jeffrey's blood pressure to be 138/86 on repeated assessments (when he was seated at rest in a quiet room, as is typically done to determine resting blood pressure with greatest accuracy). Although below the level for a diagnosis of hypertension, Jeffery *is* prehypertensive. His blood pressure is higher than would be desired and without some intervention may well progress upward to a diagnosis of hypertension. His physician recommends an on-campus stress management class and also a progressive increase in physical activity, focused on aerobic exercises such as walking and jogging.

In spite of these studies, one concept that has emerged over the last several decades is that of the sodium sensitivity of blood pressure.[15] Simply put, the sensitivity of blood pressure to dietary sodium varies among people; however, this is more of a continuous distribution across individuals than a question of either having or not having sodium sensitivity.[13] Estimates of sodium sensitivity of blood pressure range widely depending on the population studied. Among young healthy Caucasian adults with normal resting blood pressure, fewer than one in four have sodium-sensitive blood pressure. Among African American adults with hypertension, nearly three out of four may have sodium-sensitive blood pressure.[15] The sodium sensitivity of blood pressure increases as you get older. Research has shown that older adults and African Americans are especially responsive to the blood pressure–lowering effect of dietary sodium restriction.[2]

Recent data from the U.S. Centers for Disease Control and Prevention (CDC) suggest that the number of Americans with sodium-sensitive blood pressure may be even higher than initially thought. However, regardless of your sodium sensitivity status, keeping sodium consumption in check is a good idea. Researchers have found that populations with high dietary sodium consumption have a greater increase in blood pressure as they age.[7] New research suggests that dietary sodium may also damage blood vessels even if blood pressure does not rise.[11] These two points suggest that you can benefit from reducing the amount of sodium in your diet, even if you are not sodium sensitive.

You may be hoping to control your sodium intake by not adding table salt to your food. That is a great step, but you still need to check the rest of your diet. Keep in mind that a tremendous amount of sodium is hidden in foods, particularly highly processed foods, which include restaurant foods as well as canned and packaged goods. It is estimated that within industrialized societies, 75% of the sodium consumed comes from processed foods. Checking food labels, therefore, is as important as holding back on the salt shaker. Hints on cutting back on sodium are found in *Ways to Decrease Sodium Intake*.

Endurance athletes and those who exercise many hours per day have unique dietary sodium needs. Because sweat contains sodium,

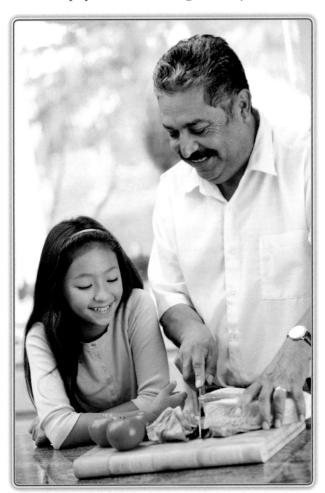

Work with family and friends to make good nutritional choices.

Ways to Decrease Sodium Intake[14]

- Choose low-sodium or reduced-sodium versions of foods when available.
- Select fresh, frozen, or canned vegetables that are low in sodium or have no salt added.
- Use fresh poultry, fish, and lean meat rather than canned, smoked, or processed options.
- Limit the use of condiments such as mustard, horseradish, ketchup, and barbecue sauce and especially typically high-sodium condiments such as soy sauce and teriyaki sauce.
- Cook without adding table salt. Also consider cutting back on instant or flavored pasta, rice, and cereal mixes, which typically already have a significant amount of salt added.
- Cut back on items that often contain a lot of sodium such as frozen dinners, canned soups, salad dressings, and packaged mixes.
- Consider using spices instead of salt, and use other items to flavor your food such as herbs, lemon, lime, vinegar, and salt-free seasoning blends.
- Replace salty snacks with fruits or vegetables.
- When eating out, avoid items that include the following terms in the meal description: *pickled, cured, smoked,* and *soy sauce.*
- When reading food labels (see chapter 4 for more details), check the sodium levels and the Percent Daily Values (%DV). Foods that contain less than 5% of the %DV for sodium are considered low. Watch out for items with 20% or more of the daily value for sodium—these are considered to be high.

Adapted from U.S. Department of Health and Human Services, National Institutes of Health, National Heart, Lung, and Blood Institute, 2006, p. 17.

high sweat rates cause these athletes to lose excess sodium when they exercise. For this reason, they should not drastically reduce their dietary sodium intake. Athletes should consult appropriate sources[12] that address their unique circumstances. For most people, however, the sodium intake guidelines outlined in this chapter can be a valuable tool for maintaining or controlling blood pressure.

Heart-Healthy Diet

Research studies suggest that a heart-healthy diet reduces blood pressure and is further enhanced when sodium content is also reduced. One study examined the effects of the Dietary Approaches to Stopping Hypertension, or DASH, diet on resting blood pressure.[10] The diet is plentiful in fruits, vegetables (potassium-rich foods), and whole grains, and low in fat. Several hundred people participated in this study that compared the DASH diet to a typical Western diet. Several dietary sodium levels were also investigated. The participants consumed each diet for 30 days. Resting blood pressure was highest when the participants consumed a normal Western diet with a lot of sodium (greater than 3,000 milligrams per day), and blood pressure was lowest when the participants consumed the DASH diet with less sodium (approximately 1,500 milligrams per day).

Of particular importance for those with hypertension, the DASH diet emphasizes consuming vegetables that are high in potassium. The *Dietary Guidelines for Americans* also highlights the importance of increasing dietary potassium intake to help lower blood pressure as well as to lessen the negative influence of sodium on blood pressure.[13] An adequate intake of potassium is 4,700 milligrams per day for anyone 14 years of age or older (it is somewhat less for children).[13] Food sources of potassium include milk, meat, fish, fruits (e.g., bananas, oranges, and other citrus fruit), and vegetables (e.g., potatoes, broccoli, carrots).

Information on the DASH diet, including sample menus, can be found on the American Heart Association website or the National Heart, Lung, and Blood Institute (of the National Institutes of Health) website (go to www.nhlbi.nih.gov and enter *DASH* into the search window). This site includes specific examples of healthful eating habits. In general, the recommendation is to eat several servings of fruit, several servings of vegetables, several servings of grains (with an emphasis on whole grains), and fat-free or low-fat milk products daily. You should limit fat, oils, and sweets and incorporate lean meats, poultry, and fish into your diet. The number of servings for each of these categories will depend on your overall caloric intake (see table 15.3 for some general guidelines for the number of servings from various food groups). The overall recommendation for hypertensive adults is to adopt the DASH eating plan, as mentioned in table 15.2.

Weight control is also important for managing blood pressure. Anyone who is overweight or obese should focus on reducing total calorie intake and burning more calories through exercise. Studies have reported that weight loss can lower blood pressure, as discussed in table 15.2, as well as improve overall cardiovascular health (for more details on weight management, see chapter 13). A critical review of your

Table 15.3 DASH Eating Plan for Various Calorie Levels

FOOD GROUPS	SERVINGS PER DAY			
	1,600 calories per day	2,100 calories per day	2,600 calories per day	3,100 calories per day
Grains (whole grains recommended)	6	6–8	10–11	12–13
Vegetables	3–4	4–5	5–6	6
Fruits	4	4–5	5–6	6
Milk and milk products (fat free or low fat)	2–3	2–3	3	3–4
Lean meats, poultry, and fish	3–6	6 or fewer	6	6–9
Nuts, seeds, legumes	3 per week	4–5 per week	1	1
Fat and oils	2	2–3	3	4
Sweets and added sugars	0	5 or fewer per week	2 or fewer	2 or fewer

Adapted from U.S. Department of Health and Human Services, National Institutes of Health, National Heart, Lung, and Blood Institute, 2006, p. 10.

own diet, and the decision to reduce sodium intake and consume fruits, vegetables, and whole grains in preference to high-fat, highly processed options, is very conducive to weight loss. In addition, alcohol intake can influence blood pressure. For those who consume alcohol on a regular basis, reducing alcohol intake has been shown to lower resting blood pressure, as mentioned in table 15.2.

Focusing on Physical Activity

A large number of scientific studies have established that regular exercise can lower blood pressure. On average, exercise can decrease blood pressure by approximately 5 to 7 mmHg.[9] These reductions in blood pressure translate into benefits for your health. Most, but not all, studies have examined the benefits of aerobic exercise such as walking, jogging, cycling, and swimming (see chapter 6 for more details on aerobic exercise). Fewer studies have focused on the benefits of resistance training; nonetheless, resistance training may also benefit people with hypertension, as part of a well-rounded fitness program (see chapter 7 for more details on resistance training).

Blood pressure does change with activity. It is normal for your blood pressure to increase *during* exercise when the heart is contracting faster and stronger. The blood pressure–lowering effect of exercise actually occurs *after* the exercise session and may last for up to 22 hours.[9] This effect reinforces the importance of regular exercise. The overall goal of the exercise program is to lower blood pressure during the times of the day when you are not exercising. The higher your resting blood pressure is, the greater the potential benefit of exercise is. Also, it is encouraging to note that even small declines in resting blood pressure reduce the risk of stroke and heart disease.

Precautions Before Exercise

If you are hypertensive, you should be evaluated by your health care provider before embarking on an exercise program. In some, but not all, cases your health care provider may recommend that you undergo an exercise test (i.e., stress test) before beginning an exercise program. The type of pre-exercise medical evaluation depends on your health status including your current blood pressure and the intensity of the exercise program you would like to adopt. If your resting blood pressure is uncontrolled (i.e., blood pressure greater than 200/110 mmHg), you should wait until it is in a safer range before initiating an exercise program.[1] Your health care provider can provide recommendations to ensure that it is safe for you to begin an exercise program.

Although people with hypertension derive an overwhelming benefit from taking medications to lower blood pressure, some of these medications may influence exercise responses (more information on medications is included toward the end of this chapter). For example, diuretics and beta-blockers may impair the ability to regulate body temperature.[9] This is a concern during hot weather, particularly if the humidity is also high. Therefore, you should be aware of the signs and symptoms of heat illness, which include headache, cramping, nausea, dizziness, and weakness. In hot and humid conditions, you should do the following:

• Wear lightweight clothing to facilitate evaporative cooling.

- Drink enough to avoid dehydration (e.g., dehydration is defined as a loss of body weight of more than 2% during a workout, as a result of sweating).
- Exercise during the coolest parts of the day—early morning or late evening.

An additional critical point is that you should decrease the intensity or duration of your workout in hot and humid conditions, especially when your body is not accustomed to the hot environment. However, frequent exercise in the heat will improve your ability to tolerate these conditions.[1] Consult an exercise professional if you have specific questions or concerns.

In addition, medications such as beta-blockers can cause blood glucose to drop too low.[9] This condition is called hypoglycemia and is an important concern for hypertensive adults who also have diabetes. At the very least, hypertensive people with diabetes should be aware of the symptoms associated with low blood glucose, which include shakiness, weakness, nervousness, anxiety, hunger, and abnormal sweating.[1] Additional details on hypoglycemia and diabetes are found in chapter 14. Needless to say, you should stop exercising if you experience any of these symptoms.

Some medications such as calcium channel blockers work by dilating (widening) the blood vessels, another very effective way to lower blood pressure. However, these medications can sometimes cause blood pressure to drop too much (referred to as *hypo*tension, or low blood pressure).[9] When blood pressure is too low, the most common symptoms are lightheadedness and dizziness. Regardless of medication intake, after exercise, blood pressure normally declines. However, if exercise is stopped suddenly, blood pressure may decline too quickly to the point where dizziness occurs. To avoid this, gradually cool down after the exercise session.[1] The specifics of a proper cool-down can be found in chapter 6.

Physical Activity Prescriptions

The exercise recommendations for people with hypertension are very similar to those for other adults. Recall the FITT profile for activities, an acronym for frequency (times per week), intensity (how hard), time (how long), and type (what kind of exercise).[1] The recommendations in the following sections are summarized from the most current research findings reviewed by experts in the field and put forth by the American College of Sports Medicine.[9] In general, aerobic exercise is the main focus for those with hypertension, although moderate-intensity resistance training and flexibility are also considered important supplements.[1]

Although regular exercise is an essential component of a healthy lifestyle for hypertensive adults, the best to way to think about this is to incorporate your exercise program *into an already active lifestyle*. An active lifestyle includes taking the stairs instead of the elevator, parking the car at the far end of the lot, and keeping the phone and TV remote control away from where you routinely sit at home. These are just a few examples of ways to increase habitual, daily physical activity. These minor suggestions may not necessarily lead to huge fitness gains (as your formal exercise program undoubtedly will), but they will help you burn more calories, thereby maintaining an optimal body weight.

Aerobic Prescription   Aerobic exercise is the most important fitness activity for lowering your blood pressure.[1] FITT recommendations for aerobic training are found in table 15.4.

Table 15.4 Aerobic Training Recommendations for Hypertensive Adults Based on the FITT Principle

FITT principle	Recommendation
Frequency	On most, preferably all, days of the week
Intensity	Moderate-intensity exercise (e.g., brisk walking)
Time	30 minutes or more (continuous or intermittent)
Type	Aerobic or endurance activities (e.g., walking, cycling)

Adapted from Pescatello, Franklin, Fagard, et al., 2004.

Ideally, you should exercise on most, preferably all, days of the week.[1] However, a training frequency of three to five days per week is also effective in lowering resting blood pressure.[9]

The recommendation for hypertensive adults is to exercise at a moderate intensity. This would correspond to brisk walking for an untrained middle-age or older adult. Extremely low exercise intensities (very slow walking) may not be as effective (although very low-intensity activity would be better than no activity at all!). In addition, engaging in very high-intensity exercise (e.g., sprinting) is not necessary to derive the blood pressure–lowering effects of regular exercise. Moderate-intensity exercise (e.g., brisk walking) may actually be more effective than high-intensity exercise, particularly given that compliance with an exercise program declines and injury rate goes up among people who engage in only very high-intensity exercise. Because sticking with a regular exercise program is vital, moderate exercise is best for most people.

Hypertensive adults should exercise for 30 to 60 minutes per day.[1] The time spent exercising can be continuous (without stopping) or intermittent (in shorter bouts of 10 minutes each spread throughout the day to total at least 30 to 60 minutes).

Experts recommend that hypertensive adults perform aerobic, or endurance, types of activities such as walking, jogging, running, cycling, and swimming. Aerobic activities are discussed in detail in chapter 6. Any activity that uses large-muscle groups can be beneficial and can help to lower blood pressure. Because long-term adherence is such an important issue, pick an activity that you find enjoyable and that is easily accessible.

Resistance Training Prescription   Although aerobic activities performed on most, preferably all, days of the week should be the focus of your exercise program, resistance training is an important part of a well-rounded fitness program and should also be included.[1] Blood pressure normally increases during any type of exercise, and often the increase is more pronounced during resistance training. An exaggerated increase in blood pressure during resistance training is a concern for everyone, but especially those with already elevated resting blood pressures. Because blood pressure goes up even more when you hold your breath during the lift (e.g., while straining), you should avoid doing so. Focus on exhaling during the lifting phase and inhaling during the lowering phase.[9] More safety pointers for resistance training are found in chapter 7. In general, resistance training should be performed two or three days per week and should include 8 to 10 different exercises targeting all of the major muscle groups at a moderate level of intensity.[1]

Flexibility Prescription   Although flexibility may not have a direct impact on your blood pressure, stretching after your warm-up or as part of your cool-down is recommended.[1] Chapter 8 includes guidance and examples of stretches that you can include in your activity program.

Influence of Medications

Health care providers use several classes of medications to lower blood pressure. More than two-thirds of adults with hypertension require two or more medications to control blood pressure. Following are the four commonly prescribed classes of medications that are very effective in lowering blood pressure:[4]

- *Diuretics,* which are often called water pills because they increase urine output
- *Beta-blockers,* which decrease the work of the heart
- *ACE inhibitors,* which block the production of a hormone that can elevate blood pressure
- *Calcium channel blockers,* which relax the blood vessels

This list is not exhaustive, but the important point is that different medications can lower blood pressure and reduce overall risk. How each medication works may vary for each person, so your health care provider will pick the most appropriate medication(s) for you. This is not an exact science; proper blood pressure control takes constant vigilance. You should not be surprised if your dosage or type of medication is changed based on how you are responding to the medication.

Taking blood pressure medication does not cure hypertension; rather, the medication gets blood pressure under control, thereby lowering your risk of developing cardiovascular disease. It is especially important to let your health care provider know if you are experiencing any adverse reaction(s) to medications, whether mild or severe. Your health care provider's role is to evaluate your blood pressure response to the medication as well as how you are tolerating it. Don't be discouraged if the first medication prescribed doesn't lower your blood pressure sufficiently, or if the medication causes you to experience a side effect. The important goal is to get blood pressure under control, and to do so often requires an ongoing dialogue with your health care provider.

Taking medications *does not* take the place of the lifestyle modifications discussed in this chapter (regular exercise, proper nutrition). Rather, taking medications and making lifestyle changes should be done together to lower resting blood pressure.

Hypertensive adults should adopt a physically active lifestyle and exercise on a regular basis. In addition, they should adopt healthy eating habits, which often involves reducing the amount of sodium in the diet and focusing on fruits, vegetables (potassium-rich foods), whole grains, and items low in fat. Research has shown that these healthy lifestyle behaviors can improve overall health and also help control blood pressure.

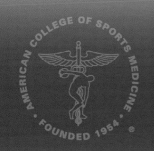

chapter 16

High Cholesterol

Research studies in the past 50 years have identified a number of factors associated with an increased risk of coronary heart disease (CHD). Heart disease has for many decades been the number one cause of death for both men and women in the United States; approximately 1.5 million Americans have a heart attack each year, and 500,000 of them die.[10] Moreover, CHD is not just a man's disease; heart attacks, strokes, and other cardiovascular diseases are just as devastating to women. Nearly twice as many women die from CHD and stroke than from all forms of cancer combined, including breast cancer.[10]

Unfavorable cholesterol levels and physical inactivity are two risk factors for CHD that are considered modifiable—in other words, you can change these! Physical activity and exercise, as well as healthy eating, are important initial interventions in the management of cholesterol. If cholesterol levels are still unfavorable after adopting these healthy lifestyle practices, then medications and the use of complementary or alternative therapies are typically considered.[4]

Cholesterol is one of several fats (also called lipids) found in the blood. Another lipid associated with heart disease risk is blood triglyceride.[9, 10] The following definitions of these lipids will help to explain the relationship between lipids and heart disease.

Cholesterol

This lipid is a soft, oily substance, also known as a fat, and in moderate amounts is essential for good health. For example, cholesterol is incorporated into all cell walls and membranes, is necessary for the body to properly make hormones such as testosterone and estrogen, and is vital in the formation of vitamin D. The body obtains cholesterol from two sources:[3, 4] the first and primary source is your own liver, which produces about 1,000 milligrams of cholesterol each day; the second source is food such as egg yolks, dairy products, and meat (primarily red meat).

It may seem confusing that your body actually produces cholesterol, but remember, a certain amount of cholesterol is necessary for proper body function. However, when the body has too much (as indicated when blood cholesterol is greater than 200 mg/dL),[10] CHD risk dramatically increases.

Triglyceride

Triglyceride is another body fat, or lipid, also related to CHD,[3] but this relationship is much weaker than the relationship between cholesterol and CHD. Like cholesterol, triglyceride has several bodily functions including being used as a source of energy in the body and in the construction of cell walls. As with cholesterol, some is needed, but too much becomes a concern. When triglyceride levels exceed 150 mg/dL, your risk of CHD is elevated.[6, 11, 12]

Both cholesterol and triglyceride do not mix well with water. Because the fluid portion of blood is mainly water, cholesterol and triglyceride need help moving around the body. Cholesterol and triglyceride must combine with proteins found in the body to form new particles, referred to as lipoproteins. The newly formed lipoproteins mix well with blood and other body fluids to allow for easy movement to all tissues. Because lipoproteins provide transport for cholesterol and triglyceride, the letters C or TG are associated with a lipoprotein's abbreviation. Four general lipoprotein classes exist; some are more beneficial whereas others are more detrimental to your health (see *Categories of Lipoproteins* on page 314 for more information on the various classes of lipoproteins). These include chylomicrons, very low-density lipoprotein (VLDL), low-density lipoprotein (LDL), and high-density lipoprotein (HDL). In general, higher levels of VLDL and LDL are a concern with regard to heart health. In contrast, HDL cholesterol is commonly referred to as good cholesterol, and thus higher levels are a plus. See table 16.1 for a list of lipids and lipoproteins and their relationships to heart disease.

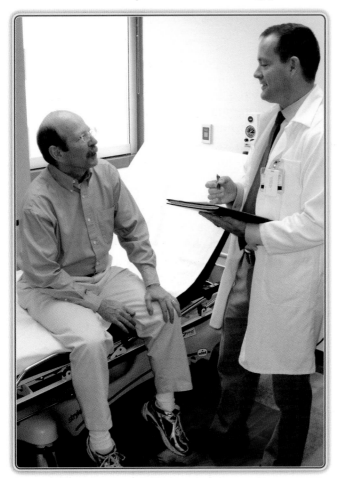

Ask your health care provider to review your blood test results for cholesterol and triglyceride with you.

Table 16.1 **Risk of Heart Disease Related to Lipids and Lipoproteins**

	Relationship to heart disease
Lipid	
Cholesterol	Strongly related to increased risk
Triglyceride	Associated with increased risk
Lipoprotein	
Chylomicron	Associated with increased risk
Very low-density lipoprotein (VLDL)	Somewhat related to increased risk
Low-density lipoprotein (LDL)	Strongly related to increased risk
Apolipoprotein(a) [Lp(a)]	Strongly related to increased risk
High-density lipoprotein (HDL)	Strongly related to reduced risk

CAUSES OF HIGH CHOLESTEROL

As mentioned, high cholesterol is associated with an increased risk of CHD, and as cholesterol levels increase, so does the risk of death from CHD. Although some cholesterol is necessary for many daily body functions,[3] when you have too much cholesterol, the risk for many diseases such as CHD is increased.[11, 12] As a simple example, consider laundry detergent. A certain amount is needed to clean your clothes, but too much results in soap suds all over the laundry room floor. The bottom line is that some cholesterol is needed in the body, but too much becomes bad.

Risk factors associated with elevated cholesterol include many of the factors associated with heart disease (see chapter 12):

- *Diet.* The impact of nutrition, especially the consumption of saturated fat, will be discussed later in this chapter in more detail.
- *Body weight.* Overweight and obesity tend to increase cholesterol levels.
- *Physical activity.* Inactivity is a concern, whereas regular physical activity, as discussed in this chapter, helps lower LDL cholesterol levels while raising HDL cholesterol levels.
- *Age.* Cholesterol levels tend to increase with age.
- *Family history.* High cholesterol levels tend to run in families.

Although age and family history are not under your control, the first three risk factors listed can be modified to decrease your risk. Cholesterol is one CHD risk factor that lifestyle interventions can address. An estimated 102.2 million American adults have total blood cholesterol values of 200 mg/dL or higher, and about 35.7 million American adults have levels of 240 mg/dL or higher.[10] The Framingham Heart Study (one of the longest-duration studies of heart disease) has been a leader in defining the critical blood cholesterol level for determining CHD risk. That critical level is 200 mg/dL (see table 16.2, page 316). In addition, if your blood cholesterol level exceeds 300 mg/dL, your CHD risk is three to five times higher than the risk for people with total blood cholesterol of 200 mg/dL.[3]

Categories of Lipoproteins

The term *total blood cholesterol* refers to the sum of all the cholesterol associated with the blood lipoproteins. Following are descriptions of the four general classes of lipoproteins.

Chylomicrons

Chylomicrons are formed in your body after a meal and are the main carrier for triglyceride. They are present in your blood for up to 10 hours immediately after a meal. The blood chylomicrons are normally removed during an overnight fast (when no food has been eaten for 10 hours). Elevated chylomicron levels after you have fasted are associated with a slight CHD risk.[3, 4]

Very Low-Density Lipoprotein (VLDL)

Very low-density lipoprotein (VLDL) particles are mainly found in your liver but also in your intestine after a meal. They help to move triglycerides around the body and are present for about eight hours after a meal. Normal VLDL-C is less than 30 mg/dL, and elevated fasted VLDL-C levels are associated with some increased CHD risk.

Low-Density Lipoprotein (LDL)

Low-density lipoprotein (LDL) particles are formed in your body when VLDL is naturally broken down. The LDL then picks up additional cholesterol and carries it out to the body tissues. The recommended LDL-C level is below 130 mg/dL for people of good health, or below 100 mg/dL for people who have been diagnosed with CHD. When cholesterol values exceed 130 mg/dL, CHD risk dramatically increases.[11, 12] As a result, LDL-C is typically referred to as bad cholesterol.

Also note that Lp(a), a unique LDL subclass containing a substance called apolipoprotein(a), is very similar to plasminogen (a blood protein that helps break up blood clots) in its chemical composition. As a result, high Lp(a) levels interfere with the work of plasminogen, so blood clot formation goes unchecked potentially contributing to a heart attack. Blood Lp(a) levels greater than 25 mg/dL are related to an increased risk for CHD. Elevated Lp(a) is a somewhat rare inherited trait and is only treatable with medications such as niacin or estrogen.

High-Density Lipoprotein (HDL)

High-density lipoprotein (HDL) particles are created in your liver and intestine. Their role is to pick up cholesterol from the body and transport the cholesterol back to the liver to be removed from the body. Thus, HDL is like the trash collector. HLD gathers up any excess cholesterol and gets rid of it. As a result, HDL-C is commonly known as the good cholesterol and is associated with a lower risk of heart disease.

HEALTHY APPROACHES
TO MANAGING CHOLESTEROL

Over the past 40 years, scientists have identified factors that affect cholesterol and the way cholesterol is carried by blood lipoproteins. Their work demonstrates that multiple factors affect blood lipids and lipoproteins, and that the best way to affect change is by concentrating on factors that are easiest to change, including those under your control. Modifying your diet, engaging in regular exercise, and reducing body weight are three of the initial recommendations. Additional factors such as smoking and stress negatively affect blood lipid and lipoprotein levels. By focusing on your diet (eating less saturated fat), becoming more physically active, stopping smoking, and reducing daily stress, you will be taking steps to optimize your blood lipid and lipoprotein levels.

Tackling one factor is good, but in many instances focusing on multiple factors at one time provides greater benefits than changing behaviors one at a time. One example is weight loss achieved by both making dietary changes and restricting calories. Weight loss by itself lowers blood cholesterol and LDL-C. Losing weight by reducing both caloric intake and dietary fat magnifies the beneficial blood lipid and lipoprotein changes, and both of these interventions are augmented by a third intervention of regular physical activity and exercise.

Most people can optimize blood lipid and lipoprotein levels by adhering to lifestyle changes. Unfortunately, in some instances, these changes are not sufficient or are too difficult to make. Also, genetic factors do exist that keep blood cholesterol levels high regardless of how good the person is at adhering to lifestyle changes. In these instances, medications, alternative and complementary therapies, or both, are required.

Focusing on Nutrition

Society's love affair with food and an excess in the amount of food consumed are pathways toward weight gain, obesity, and elevated blood cholesterol, increasing the likelihood of having many diseases such as CHD. The good news is that changing dietary patterns to prevent, stop, and even reverse the progression of heart disease is possible.

From a dietary point of view, the best way to favorably affect blood cholesterol and the cholesterol associated with lipoproteins is to reduce body weight, and this is best achieved by lowering the consumption of calories and saturated fat.

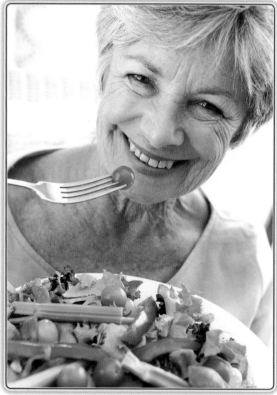

Keep a nutritional focus on reducing calorie intake, and in particular that of saturated fat.

Knowing Your Blood Cholesterol

Blood cholesterol, triglyceride, and lipoprotein values, including HDL-C and LDL-C, are easily obtained from a simple blood test completed in your physician's office. Blood is collected usually after a 10- to 12-hour overnight fast. An important point to remember is that a variety of circumstances affect blood cholesterol, triglycerides, and lipoproteins. Although fasting is not a requirement for total cholesterol or HDL-C measurements, an accurate triglyceride measurement is not obtained unless you have fasted. Recall that about 10 hours of fasting are needed to eliminate the triglyceride gained from your last meal from the blood. HDL-C and triglyceride are affected by alcohol consumption and even a single exercise session. A high-fat diet, the common cold, emotional stress, and the menstrual cycle all have different effects on blood lipid and lipoprotein values. Abstain from smoking during the fasting time if you smoke. Drinking water is permitted.

Once a blood test is completed, your physician will compare your results to known standards to determine your CHD risk.[3] The information in table 16.2, compiled by the National Cholesterol Education Program (NCEP), provides recommended lipid and lipoprotein values. Additional insight regarding CHD risk is gained by calculating some lipid and lipoprotein ratios. The most meaningful ratio related to CHD risk is the ratio of total cholesterol to HDL-C (total cholesterol/HDL-C). This ratio is easily calculated by dividing the total blood cholesterol value by the HDL-C value. The recommended range for this ratio is between 3.5 and 5.0.

Table 16.2 Classification of Blood Triglyceride, Total Cholesterol, Low-Density Lipoprotein Cholesterol (LDL-C), and High-Density Lipoprotein Cholesterol (HDL-C) Levels

Range	Classification
TRIGLYCERIDES	
Less than 150	Normal
150–199	Borderline high
200–499	High
Greater than or equal to 500	Very high
TOTAL CHOLESTEROL	
Less than 200	Desirable
200–239	Borderline high
Greater than or equal to 240	High
LDL CHOLESTEROL	
Less than 100	Optimal
100–129	Near or above optimal
130–159	Borderline high
160–189	High
Greater than or equal to190	Very high
HDL CHOLESTEROL	
Less than 40	Low
Greater than or equal to 60	High

Adapted from National Institutes of Health, National Heart, Lung, and Blood Institute, 2001, pp. 3, 16.

These beneficial diets are termed heart-healthy diets (see *Developing a Heart-Healthy Diet* for general guidelines).

At the start of a heart-healthy diet, most health professionals recommend consuming a proper mix of carbohydrates (approximately 50% to 60% of total calories), proteins (12% to 15% of total calories), and fats (no more than 30% of total calories). To achieve this mix, consume a variety of fruits, vegetables, grains, low-fat or nonfat dairy products, fish, legumes, and lean meats, including poultry.

Although most people have heard the recommendation regarding eating a low-fat and low-cholesterol diet, or a heart-healthy diet, before reading this chapter you may not have known about your body's ability to produce cholesterol. Limiting your body's production of cholesterol and reducing blood cholesterol are best achieved by reducing your dietary saturated fat intake. Health agencies such as the American Dietetic Association, the American Diabetes Association, and the American Heart Association recommend limiting dietary fat intake to less than 30% of your daily caloric intake for disease prevention. A diet of no more than 20% of calories as fat is wise for people with known CHD. By limiting dietary saturated fat intake, you can reduce your body weight and blood cholesterol levels and dramatically decrease your liver's production of cholesterol.[10]

Many dietary approaches are available for lowering blood cholesterol. One place to start is the U.S. Department of Agriculture (USDA) Food Guide Pyramid (www.mypyramid.gov) and *Dietary Guidelines for Americans*, as discussed in chapter 4. Related to this, the national program Fruits & Veggies—More Matters highlights the importance of fruits and vegetables in reducing the risk of many diseases including CHD. In general, women should have a target of 1.5 to 2 cups of fruit and 2.5 to 3 cups of vegetables per day. For men, 2 to 2.5 cups of fruit and 3.5 to 4 cups of vegetables are recommended (to see specific recommendations based on your activity level and age, see www.fruitsandveggiesmorematters.org/).

Developing a Heart-Healthy Diet

Here are a few ideas to keep in mind as you start a heart-healthy diet.

- *Eat only as much as you need.* Americans take in far more calories than they need. Reducing serving sizes and thus the total number of calories consumed is the first step in a lifestyle change that leads to lower body weight and lower total cholesterol.
- *Choose healthy options when eating out.* Many restaurants now have heart-healthy menus, so make choices from them. Because serving sizes are often much too large, remember to eat only as much as you need and not how much is given to you. Consider eating only half and taking the remainder home for lunch the next day.
- *Eat slowly.* Eating slowly gives your body and brain time to recognize the amount you have eaten and to begin to feel full.
- *Keep track of what you eat.* Knowing how much you have eaten can help reduce the amount of food you eat. Reviewing a record of all the food you consumed for a period of several days can help you identify foods too high in fat and develop strategies for exchanging undesirable food items for more desirable ones, and eliminating some entirely.
- *Visit a dietitian.* Now is a good time to visit a nutritionist or dietitian and get advice.

Several plans for developing a heart-healthy diet are described in the following sections. You may find that a combination of the plans works best.

Therapeutic Lifestyle Changes (TLC) Diet

The TLC diet was developed for people with high blood cholesterol or with known cardiovascular disease.[11, 12] Essentially, this diet emphasizes losing body weight and reducing saturated fat as a means to lower blood cholesterol (see *TLC Diet Recommendations* for more information). For additional information on this nutrition plan, go to www.nhlbi.nih.gov and enter *TLC Diet* into the search box.

DASH Diet

The Dietary Approaches to Stop Hypertension, or DASH, diet, like the TLC diet, contains large amounts of fruits and vegetables, is low in saturated fat and cholesterol, and is higher in fiber and lower in sodium. Though reductions in blood cholesterol and LDL-C are reported with this diet, unfortunately, so is the likelihood of reduced HDL-C. In addition, the levels of homocysteine, a substance in the body related to increased CHD risk, are lower.[1] For more information on the DASH diet, see page 305 of chapter 15.

Mediterranean Diet

The people from the Mediterranean region have a lower incidence of CHD than that found in most other parts of the world. Their diet has received much evaluation

TLC Diet Recommendations

The TLC diet is focused on lifestyle changes that promote weight loss as well as shifting to a lower-fat diet. Here are the diet's highlights:

Therapeutic Lifestyle Changes

- Total calories should be adjusted to help you reach and maintain a healthy body weight.
- Saturated fat intake should be no more than 10% of total calories.
- Polyunsaturated fat intake can be up to 10% of calories.
- Monounsaturated fat can be up to 20% of total calories.
- Total dietary fat intake should be adjusted to caloric needs. Overweight people should consume no more than 30% of total calories from fat.
- Dietary cholesterol intake should be less than 200 milligrams per day.
- Sodium consumption should be less than 2,400 milligrams per day, or about one teaspoon of sodium chloride (salt).

Healthy Food Choices

- Eat plenty of fresh fruits and vegetables rather than the juice forms.
- Eat the skin of clean fruit and vegetables.
- Eat bran and whole grain cereals and breads.
- As you consume more fiber, drink more water.
- Eat plenty of fresh food rather than processed food.
- Get fiber from foods instead of supplements because foods are more nutritious.
- Eat more legumes (red, black, pinto, and garbanzo beans) and dishes made with them, such as hummus.
- To avoid the mostly saturated fat in dairy foods, try nonfat or low-fat versions.

and is considered a factor in this lower CHD incidence, although the diet is not the only factor. Twenty-one countries border the Mediterranean Sea; the differences in culture, ethnic backgrounds, religions, economies, and agricultural production also contribute to the Mediterranean diet. Because of the differences that exist in these countries, no single diet exists, but the dietary intake from this area of the world has the following characteristics:

- Large amounts of fruits, vegetables, bread and other cereals, potatoes, beans, nuts, and seeds are consumed.
- Olive oil is an important source of monounsaturated fat.
- Little red meat is consumed, and dairy products, fish, and poultry are consumed in low to moderate amounts.
- Eggs are consumed fewer than four times a week.
- Red wine is consumed in low to moderate amounts.

Table 16.3 General Guidelines for the Mediterranean Diet

FREQUENCY*		
Daily	**Weekly**	**Monthly**
• Bread, pasta, rice, couscous, polenta, other whole grains, potatoes • Fruits • Beans, legumes, nuts • Vegetables • Olive oil • Cheese, yogurt	• Fish • Poultry • Eggs • Sweets	• Meat

*Note that foods are listed in order of dominance. For example, among daily foods, bread, pasta, rice, and so on, are in greater quantities, whereas cheese and yogurt are consumed in lesser amounts.[3]

Adapted from Willett, Sacks, Trichopoulou, et al., 1995.

The Mediterranean diet and the TLC diet are similar. People who follow the Mediterranean diet eat less saturated fat than the average American. Because the Mediterranean dietary fat is high in monounsaturated content (mainly from olive oil), people following this diet have lower total blood cholesterol. (See table 16.3 for general guidelines for the Mediterranean diet.)

Focusing on Physical Activity

Increasing the amount of daily physical activity and developing a planned exercise program yield many health benefits, including decreasing many CHD risk factors (e.g., blood lipid and lipoprotein levels).

Reduced blood triglyceride levels are associated with regular physical activity and exercise; cholesterol is not affected unless body weight, saturated fat consumption, or both, are reduced. If body weight and dietary intake of saturated fat are not changed, how does exercise training beneficially affect cholesterol levels? Exercise training increases the amount of cholesterol carried by the good lipoprotein HDL-C and decreases the amount carried by the other lipoproteins. Another point to understand is that different amounts of exercise are required for changing different lipids and lipoproteins. Most people must burn 1,200 to 1,500 calories each week to optimize blood lipid and lipoprotein changes. A good example of expending 1,200 calories per week is a brisk walk at 4 miles per hour (6.4 km/h) for 35 minutes, seven days a week. This equals approximately 2 miles (3.2 km) per day and 14 miles (22.5 km) per week.

Several exercise prescription modifications can impact blood lipid levels and the way cholesterol is carried by the various lipoproteins. Your exercise prescription should include aerobic activity, resistance training, and stretching. Although aerobic activity has the greatest impact on blood lipid and lipoprotein levels, improving your muscular fitness and flexibility provides a balanced program, benefiting you in many areas of your life. The following sections on the three exercise components address frequency, intensity, time, and type (FITT).

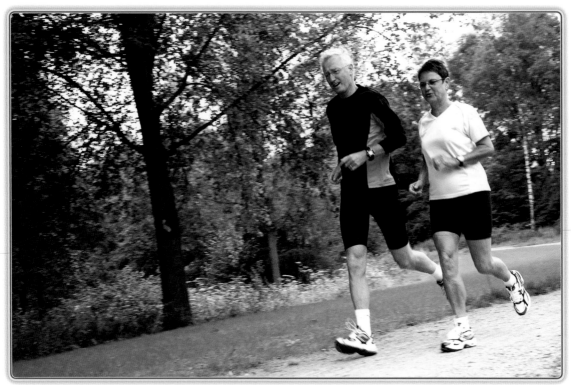

Regular physical activity can affect blood lipid and lipoprotein levels.

Aerobic Prescription

In 2008, the U.S. Department of Health and Human Services released the first *Physical Activity Guidelines for Americans.*[13] Two key guidelines incorporated into this statement are as follows:

- For substantial health benefits, adults should do at least 150 minutes (2 hours and 30 minutes) a week of moderate-intensity, or 75 minutes (1 hour and 15 minutes) a week of vigorous-intensity aerobic physical activity, or an equivalent combination of moderate- and vigorous intensity aerobic activity. Aerobic activity should be performed in episodes of at least 10 minutes, and preferably, activity should be spread throughout the week.

- For additional and more extensive health benefits, adults should increase their aerobic physical activity to 300 minutes (5 hours) a week of moderate intensity, or 150 minutes a week of vigorous intensity aerobic physical activity, or an equivalent combination of moderate- and vigorous-intensity activity. Additional health benefits are gained by engaging in physical activity beyond this amount.

The first guideline provides insight into the minimal amount of exercise needed to begin initiating blood lipid and lipoprotein change. Nonetheless, to optimize blood lipid and lipoprotein levels, especially if you have high cholesterol, the second guideline is more appropriate for a number of reasons. First, to positively optimize changes in blood lipid and lipoprotein levels, physical activity and exercise programming must exceed the 150 minutes outlined in the first recommendation. Second, the scientific studies for exercise support the concept that different levels of calories burned result in specific lipid and lipoprotein changes.

For example, a sedentary, or inactive, person just starting to exercise can expect to see some change in blood triglycerides within several weeks. This triglyceride change is directly related to the amount of exercise completed (burning as little as 800 calories each week would be required for a beginning exerciser). Decreases in triglyceride levels are related to the pre-exercise value as well as the exercise volume completed. If you have high triglyceride levels, you could see greater reductions.[3] In addition, greater exercise training volume will bring about greater triglyceride reductions.[3] On the other hand, to raise HDL-C levels, you would have to engage in several months of regular exercise, burning 1,200 to 1,500 calories per week. Most people will have greater increases in HDL-C levels with greater exercise volume completed each week.[2] LDL-C is lower after exercise training only if the person has also reduced dietary fat consumption, lost weight, or both.

Climbing stairs rather than taking elevators or parking at the farthest points in parking lots are good ways to incorporate more walking into your daily routine and burn more calories to meet the energy threshold levels needed for blood lipid and lipoprotein level changes. Because high cholesterol is a risk factor for CHD, you should progress to higher amounts of exercise in consultation with your health care provider, who will also be aware of any other risk factors or special circumstances you may be facing.

A beginning exercise plan should contain at least three sessions per week. The *Physical Activity Guidelines for Americans* recommends that a beginning exerciser work up to at least 150 minutes each week, and that exercise sessions be spread throughout the week.[13] As cardiorespiratory fitness increases, consider progressing to four, five, or more exercise days each week. People with high cholesterol should exercise five or more days each week.[12]

The *Physical Activity Guidelines for Americans* also recommends that adults wanting to positively alter blood lipid and lipoprotein levels (including those with high cholesterol) should progress their aerobic physical activity above the recommendation of 300 minutes (5 hours) a week of moderate intensity. They can perform aerobic activity episodes of at least 10 minutes several times a day or 30 minutes twice each day and progress to five or more days each week.

Either moderate-intensity and vigorous-intensity aerobic activities or some combination of both are recommended. Moderate-intensity aerobic exercise includes brisk walking at a pace of 3 to 4 miles per hour (4.8 to 6.4 km/h) or riding a bike at less than 10 miles per hour (16 km/h). Vigorous-intensity activities require greater energy expenditure. Examples of this type of activity are race walking, jogging, and running.[13] Remember, when doing vigorous-intensity activities, less time is needed during exercise to get the same benefit as that attained from moderate-intensity activities. Usually, two minutes of moderate-intensity activity equals one minute of vigorous-intensity activity.

Resistance Training Prescription

Aerobic, or endurance, training is the best type of exercise for improving blood lipid and lipoprotein profiles; resistance training will have less of an impact. Though the precise reasons for the lower impact with muscular fitness activities are not completely known, part of the answer is related to the amount of work completed during a resistance training session. In a set period of time, a greater volume of work is likely completed with aerobic exercise than with resistance training. Nonetheless, when designing an exercise program, muscular fitness activities should be included because they improve overall health (see chapter 7 for details).

The *Physical Activity Guidelines* recommends that adults do muscle-strengthening activities at least two days each week.[13] In general, resistance training should be performed two or three days per week (allow 48 hours between sessions for a given muscle group), and should include 8 to 10 different exercises targeting all the major muscle group at a moderate level of intensity. See chapter 7 for complete descriptions of resistance training programs. Because the energy expenditure associated with resistance training is much less than that associated with aerobic training, using similar times per session, little change in blood lipid and lipoprotein profiles are reported as a result of resistance training.[2]

Flexibility Prescription

Flexibility is an important component of physical fitness because increased flexibility allows you to perform activities requiring greater range of motion. Realize, however, that the time spent developing flexibility should not count toward meeting the aerobic or resistance training guidelines. See chapter 8 for a complete discussion of the proper steps to take to develop a flexibility program. In general, stretching the major muscle groups for 10 minutes two or three days per week is recommended.

A CLOSER LOOK
Bob

As part of a routine physical, Bob, age 46, had a blood test after an overnight fast. He was informed that his cholesterol and triglyceride levels were both borderline high (total cholesterol: 238; triglyceride: 187). His physician suggested that Bob start to incorporate exercise into his weekly schedule and also make some changes to his diet. Although Bob was occasionally active, he did not meet the goal of 150 minutes of physical activity a week, so reaching that level of activity was his first goal. As a beginning exerciser, Bob's initial intensity was light to moderate, done for short periods of time each day, with exercise sessions spread throughout the day and the week. By slowly increasing the amount of physical activity over a period of weeks to months, Bob reduced his risk of injury and gave his body time to adapt to the new exercise regimens. For example, Bob started his walking program with several minutes of slow walking several times each day, five or six days a week. Over a period of several weeks and months, he gradually increased the time he spent walking to 10 minutes per session, three times a day, and then increased his walking speed.

Once Bob reaches 150 minutes of moderate-intensity aerobic activity every week, he can consider increasing his weekly physical activity and exercise to gain additional health and fitness benefits.[13] Exceeding the minimum level of 150 minutes of aerobic activity and moving toward 300 minutes a week will enhance the likelihood of a positive effect on his blood lipid and lipoprotein levels. (Because each person has unique health circumstances, consult with your health care provider when creating your exercise plans.)

Influence of Medications

Lifestyle intervention programs that address exercise, diet, and weight loss are recommended as first steps in blood cholesterol and lipoprotein management. After three to six months of participating in such programs, if positive blood cholesterol and lipoprotein changes are not found or set goals are not reached, then medications for cholesterol and lipoprotein management are the next consideration. Several reasons exist for not being able to meet desired cholesterol and lipoproteins goals, including genetic factors. For example, some people's livers simply overproduce cholesterol, and starting lipid-lowing medications is the only means to curb this.

If you are considering using medications to manage blood cholesterol and lipoproteins, you need to keep several things in mind. First, having to take prescription medications to lower blood cholesterol because lifestyle interventions did not work does not mean that you have failed. Some people simply need additional help to optimize their blood cholesterol and lipoprotein profiles. Second, you need to continue your lifestyle interventions. These interventions have multiple health benefits that likely work with medications to optimize your overall health. Finally, if you stop taking the medication or stop exercising, the health benefits go away, which means a return to higher blood cholesterol and undesirable lipoprotein profiles.

Lipid-Lowering Medications

People starting lipid-lowering medications should do so under the direction of a physician who will choose the appropriate drug or drug combination. Lipid-lowering drugs are classified according to how they work. Remember, lipid-lowering drug classes work in different ways (see table 16.4).[1, 3, 4, 5, 12]

Unfortunately, most medications have side effects. Because many lipid-lowering drugs affect how the liver functions, damage to the liver is always possible. Though this rarely happens, precautions are initiated before starting any lipid-lowering medication regimen. Generally, liver function is routinely evaluated as long as the medication regime is continued. Another lipid-lowering side effect is muscle pain or discomfort. In some cases this discomfort is related to rhabdomyolysis, a condition in which large amounts of compounds (muscle proteins) are abnormally released from muscle cells into the blood. Normally, these substances are filtered by the kidneys and removed from the body. When abnormally large amounts of these proteins exist in the blood, the kidneys are not able to adequately perform their function, and kidney failure occurs. This condition can lead to death.

One class of lipid-lowering medications found in table 16.4, the HMG-CoA inhibitors (also called statin medications), in rare circumstances lead to rhabdomyolysis and death.[8] When someone who is exercising is taking a statin, muscle discomfort or pain may be a result of the medication and not the exercise. Report any uncommon muscle discomfort or pain to your physician.

An additional side effect to keep in mind is that one class of lipid-lowering medication may react adversely with another lipid-lowering medication, or with certain antibiotics or fibric derivatives. Keep accurate records of the medications you are taking and review this list with your physician. Finally, besides muscle discomfort or pain, many medications cause abdominal pain, constipation, or both. Niacin may give rise to headaches and itchy skin.

Table 16.4 **Lipid-Lowering Medications and Their Mode of Action, Follow-Up, and Effect**

Category	Generic name (brand name) examples	Mode of action	Follow-up	Effect
HMG-CoA reductase inhibitors	Atorvastatin (Lipitor), Simvastatin (Zocor), Rosuvastatin (Crestor)	Particularly blocks a liver enzyme called HMG-CoA reductase, which is involved in regulating the body's production of cholesterol.	Cholesterol profile and liver function test checked at 6 and 12 weeks after starting and then every 6 months.	Reduction in total cholesterol and LDL-C levels, small reduction in triglycerides, and slight increase in HDL-C.
Cholesterol-absorption inhibitors	Ezetimibe (Zetia)	Selectively inhibits the body's ability to absorb cholesterol from the intestine.	No liver function tests are required if used alone. When used in combination with a statin, follow statin recommendation.	Lowers triglycerides, plasma cholesterol, and LDL-C with increases in HDL-C.
Bile-acid sequestrants	Cholestyramine (Questran), Colesevelam (Welchol)	Binds with bile acid (made from cholesterol) in the intestines to be excreted in stool.	No follow-up necessary.	Increases special LDL-removing receptors in liver cells and so lowers LDL-C.
Niacin	Niacin (Niaspan, Nicobid)	Lowers the liver's production of VLDL particles.	Blood tests to evaluate cholesterol response, liver function, blood glucose, and uric acid.	Lowers triglycerides and LDL-C, and increases HDL-C.
Fibric acid	Clofibrate (Atromid), Gemfibrozil (Lopid), Fenofibrate (Tricor)	Increases the breakdown of triglycerides so they can be removed from the body. Also helps to slow down the production of triglycerides in the liver.	Tests for liver function and complete blood count within 6 weeks of starting the medication and 6 to 12 months thereafter.	Lowers triglycerides; raises HDL-C.

Adapted by permission from Roach.

Lipid-lowering medications can interact with foods and other non-lipid-lowering medications. Grapefruit, for example, enhances the positive effects of statin medications. Greater cholesterol-lowering effects are found when a grapefruit is consumed in conjunction with taking a statin medication. If grapefruit juice or grapefruit is a favorite food, consult with your physician to determine whether your statin dose may be reduced. Non-lipid-lowering medications such as beta-blockers, thiazine diuretics, oral antihyperglycemic agents (for diabetes), insulin, estrogen, and progesterone all have varying interactive effects with lipid-lowering medications, physical activity, and regular exercise. Physician consultation is not only recommended but imperative regarding these interactive effects.[3, 4, 7]

Complementary and Alternative Medicines

Many approaches to health care that do not fall within the realm of conventional medicine exist in the United States, and multiple reasons lead people to look at these for help in the management of high blood cholesterol. Complementary and alternative medicines (CAMS) are a group of diverse medical and health care systems, practices, and products that are not currently considered part of conventional medicine[2] but give people with high blood cholesterol other options for treatment. As the names imply, a complementary medicine is used in combination with conventional medication, and an alternative medicine is used in place of conventional medication.

The National Center for Complementary and Alternative Medicine (NCCAM) is an organization funded by the U.S. government that is responsible for furthering the knowledge and understanding of complementary and alternative medicine (http://nccam.nih.gov). The NCCAM works to accomplish this goal by encouraging thorough scientific investigations of CAMS and making this information available to the public. Before starting a CAM, a discussion with a primary care physician is recommended as an important part of the decision process, if not mandatory. Such a discussion accounts for personal needs and can prevent any harmful interactions between a CAM and medications currently being prescribed.

When choosing a lipid-lowering CAM such as an herbal product, nutritional supplement, or new food, find out as much as you can about the specific CAM,[3] so you can make an informed decision. Remember that some products have scientific data

Table 16.5 Lipid-Lowering Supplements and Functional Foods

Supplement or functional food	Mechanism	Lipid-lowering effect, average % change	Usefulness for lipid management
Vitamin E	Antioxidant	No significant change in TG/LDL; lowers HDL	May have harmful effect
Vitamin C, beta carotene	Antioxidant	No significant change in lipid profile	No clear benefit; may have harmful effect
n-3 fatty acids (fish oils)	Inhibit VLDL synthesis	Lower triglycerides; typical dose is 1–3 g per day	Useful as adjunct for high triglyceride; may be useful in diabetes
Garlic	Unknown	Lowers cholesterol-to-LDL ratio	No major role
Soy protein	May have phytoestrogen effect	Lowers cholesterol-to-LDL ratio; minor increase in HDL; typical dose is 25 g per day	Modest role; best used in place of high-saturated-fat foods
Plant sterols and stanols	Decrease dietary and biliary cholesterol absorption	Lower cholesterol-to-LDL ratio but do not change HDL; typical dose is 2 g per day	Moderate effect; may be useful adjunct
Fiber	Bile acid-binding action; decreases dietary cholesterol absorption	Lowers cholesterol-to-LDL ratio ; typical dose is 25–30 g per day of dietary sources of fiber	Modest role; best used in place of high-saturated-fat foods

Adapted from Fletcher, Berra, Ades, et al., 2005.

that are reliable and are consistent in showing a substantial health benefit, whereas others have contradictory or insufficient information that at best only suggests some health benefit.[3] Table 16.5 lists CAMs that have reported lipid-lowering effects.[3, 5]

One important concept to remember when using any lipid-lowering medication or CAM is that continued lifestyle interventions such as daily physical activity and exercise, following a well-balanced and heart-healthy diet, and continuing with weight loss programs remain essential parts of the lipid management program. These lifestyle modifications will likely enhance the effects of your lipid-lowering medications as well as provide other important and valuable health benefits.[3]

High cholesterol is associated with increased risk for heart disease. Adopting healthy lifestyle behaviors can optimize your cholesterol management. Although some cholesterol is needed in the body for normal functioning, too much cholesterol is a concern. To maintain cholesterol levels associated with good health, regular physical activity and exercise as well as healthy dietary habits work quite nicely together in optimizing favorable blood cholesterol and lipoprotein changes. Aerobic exercise is beneficial in many ways, and long-term maintenance of your exercise program will provide the greatest benefits. A nutrition plan focused on consuming adequate fruits and vegetables and reducing dietary saturated fat intake and body weight (if needed) will work along with your exercise plan to help you achieve your target cholesterol goals. When exercise and diet are not enough, various medications are also available to help keep your cholesterol levels in check.

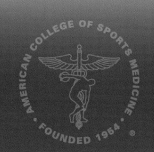

chapter 17

Arthritis and Joint Pain

Arthritis is a chronic disease affecting joints, muscles, and sometimes other body systems. Because of the resulting pain and disability, arthritis is the leading cause of impaired functioning in adults and affects more than 46 million Americans. There are more than 100 forms of arthritis, though the most common forms are osteoarthritis (OA), rheumatoid arthritis (RA), fibromyalgia, and the spondyloarthropathies (SA).[9] Although OA is primarily joint specific, the others are systemic and affect more than just the joints.

The most common symptoms of arthritis regardless of the type are stiffness and joint or muscle pain. Unfortunately, you may have stopped exercising when you started to have this joint or muscle pain, believing the activity would make your pain worse or speed up the degenerative process. However, this is just the opposite of the truth. Proper exercise will actually decrease your pain, it will not speed up the joint degeneration, and importantly, it will help you maintain normal function.

CAUSES OF ARTHRITIS

Trauma to a joint, abnormal biomechanics (movement), or repetitive joint stress can damage the articular cartilage (the special covering within the joint that absorbs stress and smoothes motion).[7, 27] As the damage progresses, the joint space narrows and the bone underlying the cartilage experiences abnormal stresses and deforms. However, for some people, there is no identifiable cause for their arthritis, and with the systemic forms of arthritis, an abnormal immune system response is often the cause of the joint destruction.

There are several risk factors for arthritis. Although some, such as age and sex, cannot be altered, addressing some of the other risk factors may help to control the discomfort of arthritis.

Risk factors include the following:

- *Age.* Your risk increases with advancing age.
- *Sex.* Females are at higher risk for RA.
- *Obesity.* Increases in body weight may result in increased stress on the joints and may alter biomechanics.
- *Previous joint injury.* Muscle strength may decrease after an injury and thus more force is transmitted through the joint. Also, changes in strength may also change the biomechanics of the joint.
- *Occupation.* Jobs that require sustained positions or repetitive motions place increased stress on the involved joints (e.g., butchers must use sustained grips, with repeated impact, and thus, they have a higher incidence of hand arthritis).
- *Smoking.* Smoking results in decreased oxygen to the tissues, contributing to delays in healing and reduced normal restoration of tissue.

Arthritis is often self-diagnosed during the initial stages. Most people do not go to the doctor until the pain, and perhaps loss of motion, limit their activity. Diagnosis of arthritis is done by correlating a health history and a physical examination to X-ray and various laboratory test results.[1, 4, 6] Some people have little joint damage, but significant pain, whereas others have significant damage and little pain. Regular activity appears to diminish the presence of pain. Laboratory tests are most helpful in diagnosing the systemic arthritis diseases.

Types of Arthritis

The two most common forms of arthritis are osteoarthritis and rheumatoid arthritis.[1] Osteoarthritis is most common (85% of arthritis is in this form). It is a local degenerative joint disease and as such most commonly affects the hands, hips, knees, and spine. One or more joints may be affected. Damage to the joint may be due to trauma, infection, mechanical stress, or often an unidentified cause.[21] For many with osteoarthritis, initial symptoms include aching within a joint or stiffness after prolonged sitting. Cartilage damage within the joint is the main problem with osteoarthritis, and over time the joint may become deformed and lose motion.

Rheumatoid arthritis is the second most common (1% to 2 % of the adult population, although it can occur at any age). The cause is unknown, but risk factors include age and being female. Unlike osteoarthritis, which is more localized, rheumatoid arthritis is bodywide (systemic) and affects tissues throughout the body. Symptoms develop slowly and include fatigue, weight loss, weakness, and general joint pain. Similar to osteoarthritis, joints become deformed and motion becomes difficult.

Two other common systemic conditions are fibromyalgia and spondyloarthropathy (a category). Fibromyalgia is an arthritis-related condition found more often in women than in men that causes widespread muscle tenderness. With fibromyalgia numerous "tender points" occur in various places (e.g., neck, shoulders, back, hips, arms, legs) when pressure is put on the area. Several forms of spondyloarthropathy exist, with ankylosing spondylitis being the most common. This condition causes back pain and eventually complete immobility in joints of the spine.

As noted previously, stiffness is the most common symptom of arthritis, and thus its presence is used to help diagnosis the disease. Generally, if morning stiffness lasts less than 30 minutes, it is osteoarthritis; most of the systemic forms result in stiffness that lasts at least an hour. Osteoarthritis is often limited to one or two distinct joints, whereas RA is diagnosed by the presence in multiple joints, and fibromyalgia has distinct muscle tenderness at points all over the body.

HEALTHY APPROACHES TO MANAGING ARTHRITIS

Physical activity and diet are two important lifestyle factors over which you have control. This section explains how both improved nutrition and regular exercise can help you manage your arthritis while also improving your health and fitness.

Focusing on Nutrition

Maintaining an appropriate body weight decreases the risk of developing arthritis; it also helps lessen pain if you already have arthritis.[21] Experts speculate that decreased weight results in less force to the joint. If you are overweight, you can use exercise and proper nutrition to control your weight. A loss of as little as 10 pounds (4.5 kg) has been shown to decrease the pain associated with arthritis.[20] Because obesity is a risk factor for arthritis, you may want to consult chapter 13, which focuses on weight management. The nutritional guidelines outlined in chapter 4 will provide you with a solid plan for ensuring optimal nutrition. Some nutritional supplements may be helpful and are discussed in the section, *Influence of Medications,* later in this chapter.

Focusing on Physical Activity

In general, the benefits of exercise are similar across all types of arthritis. A proper exercise program can diminish the pain and disability associated with arthritis. In fact, some studies have shown an immediate decrease in joint pain after gentle exercise, whereas participation in a regular exercise program results in more significant reductions in pain.[8, 22] In addition to reducing the associated pain of arthritis, you may also be able to reduce the amount of medication you take to control pain. As noted in the section on medications, many medications have some associated risks, so reductions in dosage are considered a very positive benefit.

Decreased muscle strength and joint motion often result in functional limitations and disability. Regular exercise improves strength and joint motion, thus improving function. Additionally, some studies have shown that even low-intensity exercise slows the progression of functional loss, although more intense exercise confers even more benefits.[13, 14, 23, 28] A common myth is that those with arthritis should participate only in low-intensity activities. In reality, more intense exercise does not speed the joint degeneration or worsen symptoms, as long as you have progressed your program gradually and are protecting your joints appropriately.

If you have one of the systemic forms of arthritis, such as RA, you have a higher risk of heart disease and other systemic complications. Participating in a regular exercise program will help decrease these risks as well.

Precautions for Arthritic Conditions Before Exercise

To maintain a safe and effective training program, you may have to make some modifications. One problem you may have is flare-ups—periods in which the joint swells more than normal and the pain is worse. These are more common with the systemic forms of arthritis. During a flare-up you may need to alter your program, reducing the intensity or temporarily eliminating a specific activity if it makes your symptoms worse. Balancing activity and rest is important, especially with systemic arthritis, because of the involvement of the immune system.

Another concern with arthritis is joint instability and laxity.[25] As the joint becomes more degraded and the joint space narrows, the tissues that normally stabilize the joint become slack. When this happens, they are no longer able to properly control the joint movement. In addition, the joint often becomes slightly deformed and out of alignment. Instability is the sensation of the joint giving way when you are active and is not necessarily related to laxity, though it is related to a decrease in function.

You may need a brace to provide stability and alignment if you are engaging in activities that stress a joint prone to laxity or joint instability. If joint alignment is the primary problem, especially for the lower extremity, you may benefit from an orthotic,[26] which is an insert placed in a shoe to correct the alignment of the foot. Correction of foot position has been shown to decrease knee pain.

If you are having any of these issues, consider consulting with a health professional with expertise in orthopedics or sports medicine. In particular, a professional evaluation is a good idea if you are experiencing your knee giving way with pain, clicking, or catching. Shoulders also are a joint at risk for being unstable.

If you have arthritis in the lower extremity, proper shoes are a must. Your shoes should provide support as well as cushioning. Good shoes can help with minor alignment problems, whereas worn shoes can turn minor problems into major discomfort.

Physical Activity Prescriptions

Exercise comes in many forms, and you should tailor your program to your current health status. A complete exercise program includes aerobic activities, resistance training, and flexibility exercises. In addition, to help with the joint instability associated with arthritis, neuromuscular training is recommended.

For the primary components of aerobic and muscular fitness, you can safely set up a program following the *Physical Activity Guidelines,* as endorsed by the American College of Sports Medicine, and as described in chapters 6 and 7.[3] If walking is difficult, biking is an excellent alternative that can be very effective.[18] You will require more flexibility activities than in a typical program (as described in chapter 8); depending on the severity of your arthritis, you should do range of motion activities on a daily basis, and perhaps several times a day.

Aerobic Prescription Aerobic fitness is often lower in people with arthritis than in those of the same age without arthritis. Much of this is likely due to decreased activity. Furthermore, some of the systemic forms of arthritis such as RA have a higher risk of heart disease, implying that aerobic activity is important to help to reduce the cardiac disease risk. Not only does aerobic exercise improve circulation to the muscles and joints, but the rhythmic nature of the activities also helps lubricate joints and get nutrition into them, thereby decreasing pain. Aerobic exercise is one of the easiest ways to reduce the stiffness associated with arthritis. You can safely follow the guidelines for aerobic activity outlined in chapter 6, though you may want to make a few modifications.[3]

If you have not been doing much physical activity, you should start at a lower intensity (e.g., two or three 10-minute sessions a day) until your joints get used to

A CLOSER LOOK
Tasha

Tasha is a 58-year-old who was recently diagnosed with rheumatoid arthritis. At the suggestion of her doctor, she began a walking program but is frustrated with how sore her feet are after her walks and is ready to give up on exercising. When she mentions this at a subsequent visit, her physician asks about her footwear. Tasha points to the canvas slip-on shoes she is wearing. Her physician quickly points out that the right shoes can have a major impact on Tasha's enjoyment of her exercise program. A good shoe does not have to be the most expensive. Following are some qualities to look for in a shoe:

- A sole that provides shock absorption and cushioning.
- Good arch support.
- A roomy toe box that accommodates toe deformities.
- A snug fit along the width of the shoe, especially in the heel counter. Her physician recommends that Tasha walk or jog around the store in them—the heels should not slip.
- Secure closure. Lace-up is preferable, but Velcro may be necessary because Tasha cannot manage laces because of arthritis in her hands.
- A design appropriate for the activity. Walking shoes are best for Tasha at this point. However, if she starts to participate in several types of activities, she may consider cross-trainers, which are multipurpose shoes.

Tasha doesn't have orthotics. If you do, be sure to bring them along when you shop for shoes so you can try them in the shoes before buying them.

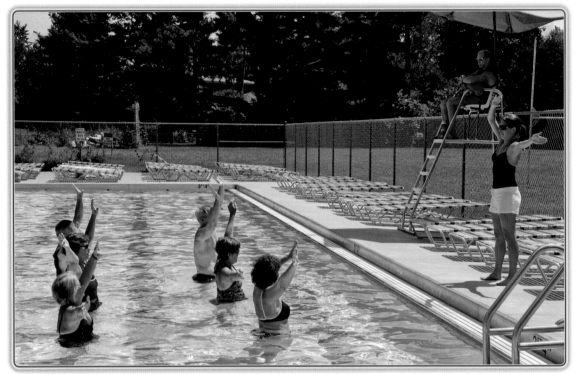

Aquatic activities are an excellent option for people with arthritis.

the increased activity. This will also allow you to develop your lower-extremity (thigh and leg) strength before doing higher-intensity or longer-duration sessions. Increased strength will help absorb forces around your joints, such as the knees, which should help decrease the stress through the joint and the pain.

Although walking is often the easiest and most functional aerobic activity, if you are a runner, there is no reason to give up running. Running will not increase the speed of joint breakdown; in fact, many regular runners report less pain with regular training. If you have severe joint instability (the sensation of the knee giving way or buckling), you might want to start with cycling or pool activities until you can decrease the instability. Some exercise ideas to address joint instability are found at the end of this chapter.

If your arthritis is more advanced and you have access to a pool, aquatic activities are an excellent option.[10] The buoyancy helps to unload your weight-bearing joints and allows you to work on joint motion as well. Because the shoulder joint is less stable, if you have arthritis in your shoulders, you should start stability exercises before swimming. Water activities in general are great for arthritis, but not everyone with arthritis in the shoulders tolerates swimming laps.

If you prefer group activities, many facilities have special classes for those with arthritis. Such classes may not be rigorous enough to build aerobic fitness, but they may be good for alternate training days. Tai chi can help improve lower-extremity strength, improve flexibility, and provide some aerobic benefits.[15] Aquatic classes are another alternative, especially if you are looking for something with reduced weight bearing. Other group aerobic classes can be good, as long as you make sure to modify movements that seem to stress your involved joint(s) and start at an appropriate intensity based on your level of fitness.

Warm-up activities are particularly important for those with arthritis, especially those who are very stiff. Before your exercise session, loosen up the joints and muscles that are stiff. A good way to warm up is to do some gentle rhythmic activities, starting with small movements and increasing the range of the movements as you loosen up. The objective is controlled movement with a slowly increasing range of motion.

Resistance Training Prescription   Resistance training may be one of the most important fitness activities that you can do to reduce symptoms and protect your joints.[5, 11] When there is pain around a joint such as your knee, the nervous system can also inhibit muscle contraction. For many, this results in a knee buckling unexpectedly, usually secondary to pain. After starting a strengthening routine, people with this concern have less pain and fewer problems with their knees giving way. Some have found that strengthening alone does not decrease their joint instability. In such instances, combining strengthening with some balance and movement activities has proven effective.[12, 25]

You can safely follow the guidelines for resistance training as outlined in chapter 7. A program of two or three days per week that emphasizes the major muscle groups is appropriate.[3] Start at a lower level of exertion and gradually work up to a moderate level of exertion in order to allow your body time to adapt. A resistance that allows you to do one set of 10 to 15 repetitions in a controlled manner is a good start and adequate for obtaining some strength benefits.

If you prefer to exercise at home, you can start with a few dumbbells and cuff weights, or use resistance bands. Many resistance bands have hand grips and cuffs so you can do upper-extremity or lower-extremity exercises (see figure 17.1 for an example of a shoulder-strengthening exercise using resistance bands). Resistance bands allow you to progress the resistance with the use of different densities of tubing (see chapter 7 for more information).

You can also do resistance training without equipment by simply using your own body weight. For example, the wall sit, as shown in figure 17.2, is an easy way to strengthen the front of the thigh, or the quadriceps. This exercise decreases the amount of pressure on the knee while still working the muscle. You can do the wall sit as a timed movement by holding the position for 15 seconds, returning to an upright stance, and then repeating three to five times (progressing the time as you get stronger).

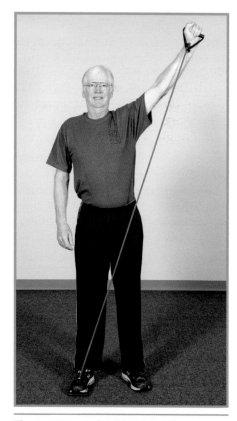

Figure 17.1   A shoulder-strengthening exercise using a resistance band.

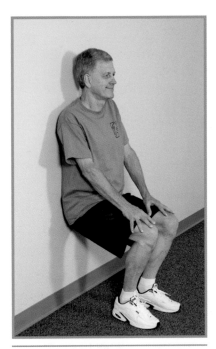

Figure 17.2 Wall sit for strengthening the quadriceps (thighs).

You can also do repetitions by using a towel (something that will allow your body to slide up and down against the wall) or a ball behind your back.

Flexibility Prescription Joint motion is usually lost as arthritis progresses, but regular stretching and range of motion activities can help slow this loss. Furthermore, if you do not move an involved joint, you may lose joint motion more quickly, with an associated increase in pain. Flexibility and joint range of motion can be restored if the loss is temporary, but the longer the impairment lasts, the more difficult it will be to regain your motion. Regular motion of each joint will decrease the stiffness and associated pain. Although the typical recommendation is to do flexibility exercises three days per week, you will benefit from daily stretching and range of motion activities.[3, 21]

Stretching focuses on increasing the extensibility of tight muscles. Stretching techniques include static and dynamic, as well as those that use assistive devices. You can use any of these safely, as long as you follow a few guidelines. You should never hold a stretch that is causing increased pain; rather, stretching should be gentle. Because arthritis can cause laxity in a joint, you should not stretch beyond what is considered normal for that joint. Several factors can affect your response to stretching. With age, muscles tend to lose elasticity, which means that the tissues do not respond as easily to stretching even though much of a stretching response is neural (i.e., the nervous system control of the resting tension in the muscle).

You can improve the response to stretching by warming your muscles, which improves elasticity. You can do this by increasing the blood flow to a muscle with a repetitive activity or by using external heat. Some people find that an elastic support not only provides a sense of stability to an affected joint, but also helps to keep the joint warm.

Staying hydrated is also important, because dehydration decreases the elasticity of your muscles. The use of a prolonged stretch (several minutes) may be helpful if you are extremely tight—just make sure to find a comfortable, supported position. For example, if you have tight hamstrings, you might lie on the floor with one foot on the wall (see figure 17.3). You should find a position that puts a gentle, but tolerable stretch on the hamstring.

Range of motion is simply moving a joint through its entire range without holding it at any one position. This type of activity may be even more important than stretching, because you can use it to prevent loss of motion and throughout the day to decrease stiffness. You should be moving every joint through its full range every day. If a joint stiffens with sitting or lack of activity, simply moving that joint through its range a few times will help decrease the pain and stiffness. For example, if you work at a desk and have arthritis in your knees, you might slide your feet back and forth (moving the knees) in the middle of a long session of work. Five to 10 repetitions will help to lubricate the joint and prevent discomfort. Most aquatic classes emphasize joint motion in the comfort of the water; thus, they are a nice way to work on flexibility.

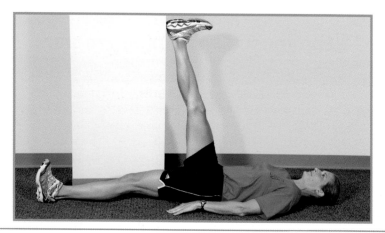

Figure 17.3 Hamstring stretch using a wall.

Neuromuscular Prescription   As noted earlier, if you have joint instability, you will need to do some specific activities to address the problem. Neuromuscular training addresses joint instability and includes agility, balance, and other types of activities that stimulate feedback between the muscles and the brain. Although general guidelines suggest two or three days per week, you will benefit from a more frequent program of five to seven days per week.[3, 12] Tai chi is an excellent activity to train the connection between the nervous system and the muscles; it addresses all of the necessary components.[15] Tai chi focuses on slow, controlled movements throughout the range of motion with limited impact on the lower extremities. Tai chi decreases pain, improves function, and has the side benefit of relaxation. If you don't want to take a class, you can get a DVD and learn it in the comfort of your home. Some people like starting their day with tai chi, because it helps reduce morning stiffness.

You can also design your own neuromuscular training program.[12] Because this is the most unique component of the training program, a sample is provided in figure 17.4, which includes both land- and water-based activities. Note that if your knees give way frequently, you might want to start balance and agility activities in the pool to remove the influence of gravity on the joint and decrease the chance of the knee buckling while doing the activity. Furthermore, if the knee does give way, you are protected against falling by the water. Once you are not having pain with the activities and can do them without your knee giving way, you can progress to land activities or alternate between water- and land-based activities.

Influence of Medications

Acetaminophen is recommended for people with mild to moderate pain due to arthritis. The most common, though still rare, side effects are upper gastrointestinal (GI) bleeding and liver damage. Nonsteroidal anti-inflammatories (NSAIDs) are the next type of medication taken to help control the pain of arthritis. The strength ranges from those that are available over the counter (aspirin and ibuprofen) to stronger forms that require a prescription and have different modes of action within the body. As with acetaminophen, GI bleeding is a possible side effect. Some of the prescription anti-inflammatories have a decreased risk of GI bleeding, but may have some cardiovascular-related risks.[17]

FIGURE 17.4

Neuromuscular Training Program

Land-based activities

Crossover walking	Bring your leg across the midline with each step for 10 feet (3 m), both forward and backward. Repeat three times in each direction.	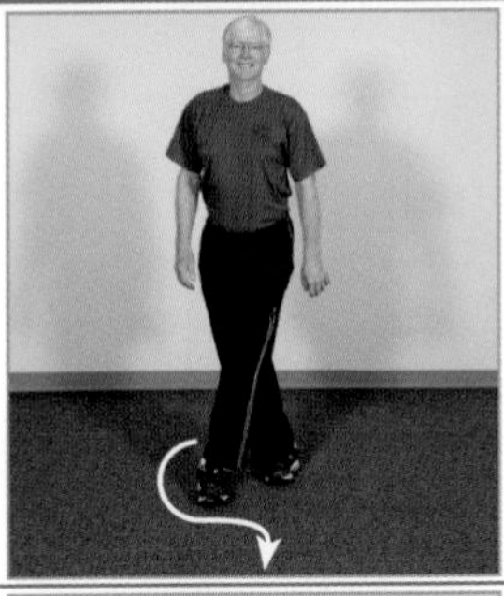
Braiding	Walk sideways, alternating placing your leg behind or in front of the other leg for 10 feet (3 m), both to the left and to the right. Repeat three times in each direction.	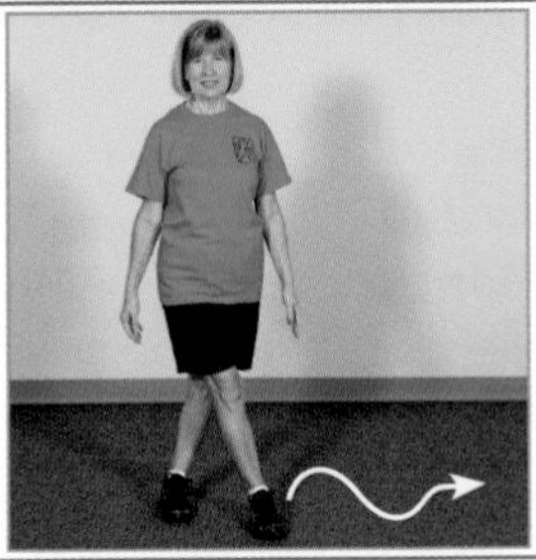
Double-leg stance on foam pad	Stand on a foam pad and shift from side to side, holding for 10 seconds. Repeat 10 times on each side.	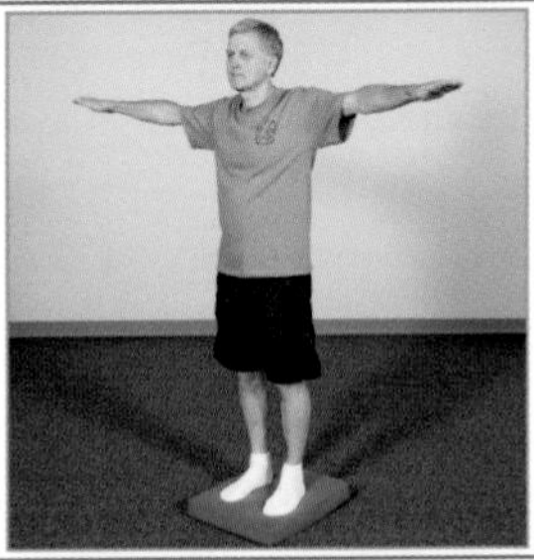
Single-leg stance	Shift to stand on just one leg (hold the other foot off the ground a couple of inches, or about 5 cm) holding for 10 seconds. Repeat five times on each leg. Increase to 30 seconds and repeat five times on each leg. Then, progress to a single-leg stance on a foam pad, holding for 10 seconds and repeat five times on each leg.	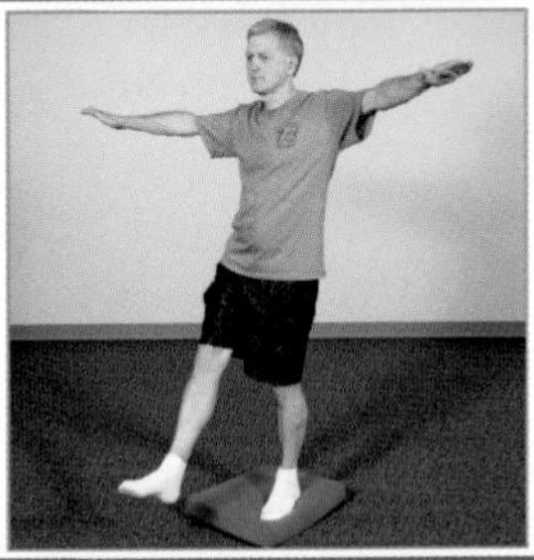

Water-based activities*

Braiding	Walk sideways, alternating placing your leg behind or in front of the other leg for 10 feet (3 m), both to the left and to the right. Repeat three times in each direction.
Crossover walking	Bring your leg across the midline with each step for 10 feet (3 m), both forward and backward. Repeat three times in each direction.
Leg raises	Raise your leg forward and backward as well as right and left for each leg. Repeat five times in each direction.

*Include water activities two or three times per week; start in chest-deep water and then progress to waist-deep water. Warm up by walking back and forth for 10 minutes.

Table 17.1 Benefits and Possible Side Effects of Common Arthritis Medications

Category	Example	Benefits	Possible side effects
Pain relievers	Acetaminophen	Decrease pain	GI bleeding, ulcers, liver damage
NSAIDs (nonsteroidal anti-inflammatory drugs)	Aspirin, ibuprofen, keto-profen, Naproxen	Decrease pain, decrease inflammation	GI bleeding, ulcers
DMARDs (disease-modifying antirheumatic drugs)	Gold, methotrexate	Decrease pain, decrease inflammation, slow pro-gression of joint destruc-tion	Liver damage, kidney damage, some cancers
Glucocorticoids	Prednisone, cortisone	Decrease pain, decrease inflammation	Increase risk of infection
Biologics	Etanercept	Decrease pain, decrease inflammation	Increase risk of infection

If you have a systemic form of arthritis, you are likely to be on a disease-modifying antirheumatic drug (DMARD), glucocorticoid (steroid), or biologic drug.[2] Possible side effects include liver and kidney damage and, with the steroids, a risk for infections. On the positive side, these drugs are the most effective for pain relief and slowing the associated joint deterioration. Because these drugs affect the immune system, you may need to slightly decrease the intensity of your program. A summary of the benefits and possible side effects of common arthritis medications is found in table 17.1.

A few nutritional supplements have been shown to decrease the pain associated with arthritis. A positive aspect of these supplements is that they do not have the health risks associated with some of the medications. For this reason, they could be worth trying. This section discusses glucosamine and chondroitin as well as fish oil and flaxseed. Although other supplements have been identified in the popular literature, the research is still lacking on many. See *Potentially Risky Supplements to Watch Out For* to read about supplements that you may want to avoid.

Glucosamine and Chondroitin

One of the most common nutritional supplement therapies is a combination of glucosamine and chondroitin. These compounds are normally found in body tissues, and it is thought that increased levels might protect and even improve the joint cartilage. Although the advertised promises are overwhelmingly positive, the research findings are varied. Some studies have shown decreased pain for those with OA, whereas others have not shown any benefit. Some of the studies reporting positive effects used supplements in addition to glucosamine and chondroitin, such as manganese ascorbate (a compound formed from ascorbic acid, or vitamin C, and the mineral magnesium).[16,19] Typical daily dosage recommendations are 1,500 milligrams for glucosamine and 1,200 milligrams for chondroitin. Benefits are typically found within a few weeks and may be related to the severity of the arthritis and your body's ability to respond to the supplement.

Watch Out For Potentially Risky Supplements

Dietary supplements are not tested as rigorously as medicines are, and thus may have harmful effects. They are not necessarily labeled properly, and they may interact with medications you take. Some have been linked to heart irregularities, increases in blood pressure, seizures, and even death. Steer clear of the following risky substances:

- Ephedrine or ephedra (used in weight loss or energy supplements)
- Kava (purported to produce relaxation and reduce sleeplessness)
- Prohormones or herbal anabolic supplements, such as androstenedione or yohimbine

Even vitamins and minerals can be toxic if taken in excessive quantities. Consider the following:

- Vitamins B_6 and B_{12} can cause liver damage.
- Vitamin C can cause stomach upset and interfere with copper and iron status.

Check with a knowledgeable person who is qualified to give you information about a supplement before you try it, such as a physician, pharmacist, or registered dietitian.

Also, the National Institute of Health's Office of Dietary Supplements provides summaries of many supplements at http://ods.od.nih.gov/HealthInformation/makingdecisions.sec.aspx.

Fish Oil and Flaxseed

Fish oil, which contains omega-3 fatty acids, has been shown to reduce the pain associated with arthritis.[16, 24] In several studies people were able to reduce the amount of NSAIDs or other medications they were taking when taking fish oil. Another positive side benefit of fish oil may be a reduced risk for heart disease and reductions in blood pressure that are associated with omega-3 fatty acids. The primary side effect is gastrointestinal discomfort, which can be addressed by reducing the dosage and taking the supplement with other foods. The recommended daily dosage varies between 3 and 8 grams per day, usually divided into two or three doses (2.6 grams two times per day for RA).

Flaxseed contains both omega-3 and omega-6 fatty acids, but research related to arthritis has been limited, and there are some side effects. Flaxseed can alter the absorption of some medications and thins the blood, so you should check with your physician if you are considering this supplement.

Exercise is important for those with arthritis. A balanced exercise program that includes aerobic activities, resistance training, stretching, and neuromuscular training (i.e., balance and agility) can help you maintain normal function. Medications used for arthritis can have side effects in addition to the intended benefits. Exercising may allow you to reduce the amount of medication you take to control pain. Although supplements are well advertised, few have proven to be beneficial. Some people benefit from a combination therapy of glucosamine and chondroitin or from fish oil (omega-3 fatty acids). In addition to physical activity, a healthy diet helps to maintain an appropriate body weight; overweight and obesity are concerns related to risk of developing arthritis as well as in pain associated with arthritis.

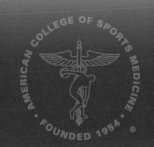

chapter 18

Pregnancy and Postpartum

Historically, pregnancy has often been thought of as a time requiring rest and limitations in activity, but today the majority of pregnant women in the United States choose to engage in at least some exercise.[20] If you are currently pregnant or thinking about becoming pregnant soon, the good news is that exercise can improve your health outcomes during pregnancy and postpartum (i.e., the first year after birth).[3] Even better, recent research also indicates that exercising during pregnancy may improve child health outcomes.

This chapter will touch on some nutritional areas to consider as well as highlight the benefits of various types of exercise during pregnancy, go over common concerns about exercise during pregnancy, and give tips about how to incorporate exercise into your life during pregnancy and the postpartum period.

GUIDELINES FOR PREGNANCY AND POSTPARTUM

The first U.S. guidelines for exercise during pregnancy were published in 1985 by the American College of Obstetricians and Gynecologists (ACOG).[1] Because of the lack of information at the time, these guidelines were conservative. They asked women to limit vigorous activity to no more than 15 minutes at a time and included the now infamous statement that "maternal heart rate should not exceed 140 bpm."[1] Using that upper heart rate limit excludes women from doing vigorous activities such as running or using a stair climber because heart rate almost always rises above 140 bpm during those types of activities. Since that time, researchers have found that exercise during pregnancy does not increase the risk of pregnancy complications such as low birth weight, preterm labor, or maternal conditions such as gestational diabetes or preeclampsia, and instead have found a broad range of health benefits related to exercise.[3, 26, 29] Further, exercise during the postpartum period does not appear to adversely affect breast milk volume or composition and has been linked to enhanced mood and fitness levels, as well as a decreased risk for postpartum weight retention.[3, 40] The current recommendation is that pregnant and postpartum women participate in at least 150 minutes per week of moderate-intensity exercise, with no heart rate limitations.[47]

What are some of the benefits of exercise? Exercise before and during pregnancy is associated with lower risk for gestational diabetes, preeclampsia, and preterm delivery.[3, 22, 26, 48] Exercise during pregnancy also appears to be a safe and effective treatment for controlling blood glucose in women who are already diabetic or who become so during pregnancy.[12, 16] As you might expect, exercise can help women avoid excessive weight gain during pregnancy as well. Specifically, women who engage in at least 30 minutes per day of moderate or vigorous aerobic activity during pregnancy are less likely to gain weight in excess of the recommended amount (see table 18.1 on page 345 for recommended weight gain during pregnancy).[42]

It now appears that exercise during pregnancy may reduce the risk of giving birth to a large infant without increasing the risk of giving birth to a small infant.[6, 27, 34] Giving birth to a large infant (i.e., greater than 10 lb, or 4.5 kg) increases the risk of birthing injuries for both mother and infant.[11] Children who are born large also have an increased risk of obesity, diabetes, and other health concerns later in life.[10, 24, 25] One small study has shown that children of women who exercised throughout pregnancy had less body fat at 5 years of age compared to children of women who did not exercise.[13] Thus, participation in aerobic exercise during pregnancy not only improves maternal health, but also may contribute to better child health outcomes.

The benefits of exercise don't stop at the end of pregnancy, but continue during the postpartum period. The 2002 ACOG guidelines recommend that women resume prepregnancy exercise routines gradually after birth as soon as it is physically and medically safe.[2] The exact amount of time needed for recovering after birth varies depending on the difficulty of labor, type of delivery (cesarean versus vaginal),

A CLOSER LOOK

Kayla

Kayla is the proud mother of a beautiful baby girl, now 4 months old. Kayla stayed active throughout her pregnancy with regular walking at a local park or swimming at a community center pool, in addition to a couple of yoga classes and regular stretching on a weekly basis. After the birth of her baby, Kayla started walking on her treadmill at home to maintain her aerobic fitness and used resistance bands for muscular fitness. After a while, though, Kayla got bored with her solo workouts and began to feel overwhelmed with trying to take care of her baby and herself. At a follow-up visit with her health care provider, she learned about an exercise program at a nearby mall specifically for mothers and their babies. With babies happily riding in their strollers, the moms power walk, resistance train with tubing and bands, and stretch in a continuous one-hour routine three mornings per week. Not only is the exercise session invigorating, but it also gives Kayla a chance to chat with other new mothers.

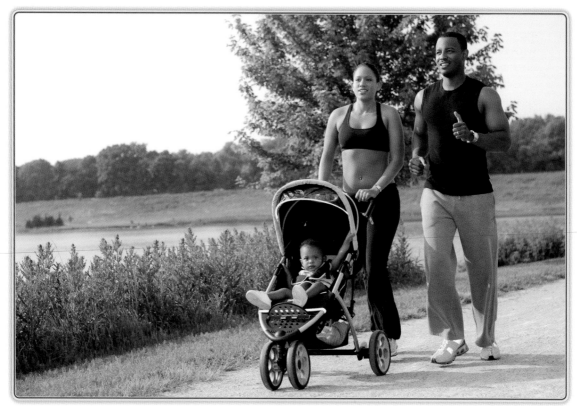
Exercise can be a great family affair.

pre-existing fitness level, and other medical complications. Typically, women can resume exercise within days of delivery if no complications are present, although women who experience cesarean deliveries should not start exercising before four to six weeks postpartum. Your health care provider can help you determine what is best for you and your situation.

Exercising during the postpartum period helps with weight loss and appears to have psychological benefits. Women reporting greater amounts of exercise have less weight retention at six weeks and one year postpartum compared to less active women.[33, 40] More active women report enhanced socialization as well.[40] Although being active during pregnancy or the postpartum period does not seem to reduce the occurrence of postpartum depression, exercise prescriptions have been effective at alleviating depressive symptoms among women with postpartum depression.[15, 18]

HEALTHY APPROACHES TO PREGNANCY

What makes a healthy pregnancy? Certainly, most pregnant women are primarily concerned with the appropriate growth and development of their babies. To ensure appropriate fetal development, mothers must optimize their health during pregnancy. Factors of particular interest to health care providers based on their importance during pregnancy include maternal weight and weight gain, fasting glucose levels, and blood pressure.

Starting pregnancy with a healthy weight (i.e., BMI between 18.5 to less than 25 kg/m²) and gaining an appropriate amount of weight helps to ensure a pregnancy with fewer complications.[38] Even if you start pregnancy underweight, overweight, or obese, gaining within the recommended weight ranges will improve your chances of experiencing a normal pregnancy and having a healthy baby.[38]

The most prevalent pregnancy complications are gestational diabetes, gestational hypertension, and preeclampsia. Gestational diabetes affects 5% to 9% of U.S. pregnancies and is diagnosed as glucose intolerance (i.e., abnormally high glucose levels in the blood) occurring for the first time during pregnancy.[41] Women with a family history of diabetes, who are overweight or obese, or who previously delivered a large infant (i.e., greater than 10 lb, or 4.5 kg) are at higher risk for developing gestational diabetes.[41] Gestational diabetes increases the risk of delivering a large infant, who then has a higher risk of being obese during childhood.[41] Women diagnosed with gestational diabetes should work closely with a health care provider or nutritionist to control their blood glucose levels while ensuring that optimal nutrients are available for the developing baby.

Gestational hypertension and preeclampsia affect 8% of U.S. pregnancies. Gestational hypertension is diagnosed as hypertension occurring for the first time during pregnancy, whereas preeclampsia is a more severe condition characterized by hypertension combined with excess protein in the urine.[39] Both conditions increase the risk of delivering a small or preterm infant.[39] Women who have a family history of hypertension, are African American, are overweight or obese, have gestational diabetes, or are carrying multiples are at higher risk for gestational hypertension or preeclampsia.[39]

Physical activity and good nutrition are two important lifestyle behaviors for pregnant women that can help them avoid or treat the pregnancy complications highlighted in this section. In addition, these behaviors also confer important health benefits.

Focusing on Nutrition

Nutrition during pregnancy takes on special importance because it affects both maternal and fetal health. The American Dietetic Association (ADA) outlines the following key components of a healthy pregnancy:[28]

Appropriate Weight Gain

The recommended amount of weight gain during pregnancy is based on the woman's prepregnancy weight. Keeping weight gain within the recommended amount optimizes the baby's birth weight, avoids excessive postpartum weight retention, and reduces the risk of later maternal chronic disease development. Gaining either less than or more than the recommended amount is associated with poorer birth outcomes.[38] To find out how much weight you should gain during a singleton pregnancy (i.e., resulting in the birth of one infant), first calculate your body mass index (BMI) from your weight and height before pregnancy (see chapter 2 for details on determining your BMI) and then check table 18.1. For multiple births (e.g., twins, triplets), higher weight gains are needed to improve birth weight and the length of the pregnancy: weight gain should be 40 to 54 pounds (18 to 25 kg) for normal weight women, more for underweight women (50 to 62 lb, or 23 to 28 kg), and less for overweight or obese women (as little as 29 to 38 lb, or 13 to 17 kg).[28]

Table 18.1 Recommended Ranges for Total Weight Gain During Singleton Pregnancy by Prepregnancy Weight Status

Prepregnancy BMI (kg/m²)	Recommended weight gain
Underweight (≤18.5)	28–40 lb (13–18 kg)
Normal weight (18.5–24.9)	25–35 lb (11–16 kg)
Overweight (25.0–29.9)	15–25 lb (7–11 kg)
Obese (≥30.0)	11–20 lb (5–9 kg)

Adapted by permission from Institute of Medicine and National Research Council of the National Academies, 2009, p. 2.

Consumption of a Variety of Foods

The *Dietary Guidelines for Americans*, as discussed in chapter 4, are appropriate during pregnancy. The energy needs of pregnant women do increase in the second and third trimester by 340 calories and 452 calories, respectively. Multiple births require additional calorie intake, but researchers have not precisely determined these energy requirements.[28]

Appropriate Vitamin and Mineral Supplementation

Many women of childbearing age do not maintain good nutrition, and this continues to be a concern during pregnancy. The ADA suggests that pregnant women consume 600 micrograms of folic acid (in natural foods as well as fortified foods or supplements) and supplement with 27 milligrams of iron (anemic women may need higher levels until the anemia is resolved).[28] A multivitamin and mineral supplement may be warranted for women with poor diets or who consume little to no sources of animal protein.[28]

A CLOSER LOOK

Amy

Amy was 5 feet 6 inches (66 in., or 168 cm) and 161 pounds (73 kg) before becoming pregnant. Her weight and height result in a BMI of 26 kg/m², which is considered overweight. Based on Amy's initial BMI, her physician recommends a weight gain over the course of her pregnancy of no more than 25 pounds (11 kg). Amy's exercise program has been an on-and-off endeavor. However, she realizes the benefits of exercise for her as well as her baby and now has a real incentive to make exercise a priority in her daily routine. At the suggestion of her physician, Amy purchases a simple pedometer to count her daily steps. Her target is 10,000 steps per day.

Amy gradually increases her activity and finds the feedback from the pedometer helpful. Even on days when she forgets to wear her pedometer, she retains the habit of increased activity. Her husband has joined Amy in a renewed commitment to better health, and they walk together at a local park on at least five evenings each week. Amy is surprised to find that she has more energy during the day and is finding it easier to stay within her recommended weight gain range because of her walking program.

Avoidance of Alcohol, Tobacco, and Other Harmful Substances

Pregnant women should not consume alcohol; drinking during pregnancy is associated with developmental and neurological birth defects.[28] Smoking should also be avoided because it limits the oxygen available for the baby and increases the risk of spontaneous abortion, preterm birth, and sudden infant death syndrome, among other concerns.[28]

Safe Food Handling

Pregnant women and their babies have a higher risk of developing food-borne illnesses. Therefore, pregnant women should avoid soft cheeses not made with pasteurized milk, cold smoked fish, and cold deli salads. Any deli meat, luncheon meat, bologna, or frankfurters should be reheated to steaming hot. Pregnant women should avoid any unpasteurized products or raw or undercooked eggs or meat. Because of the mercury levels in fish, pregnant women should not eat shark, swordfish, king mackerel, or tilefish. Lower-mercury-content seafood (e.g., shrimp, canned light tuna, salmon, pollock, catfish) is considered safe at 12 ounces (340 g) or less per week.

Thus, although good nutrition is always important for your health, it is especially important during pregnancy when your body needs extra energy and nutrients to ensure that both you and your baby stay healthy. In addition to the ADA recommendations regarding iron and folate supplements to ensure healthy birth outcomes, you should consume at least 8 cups of fluid per day to stay hydrated.[28] You can use MyPyramid for Moms (see www.mypyramid.gov/mypyramidmoms/index.html) to create a food plan that meets your energy needs (i.e., 2,200 to 2,900 calories per day for most pregnant women) while ensuring that all food groups are covered.[46]

When exercising during pregnancy, you should take additional care to make sure to balance your energy expenditure with your energy intake. In other words, eat extra calories to make up for the ones you burn while exercising—pregnancy is not the time to lose weight! Details on calculating the calories burned by particular activities based on your body weight are found in chapter 6. Recall that once you know the MET value (a unit of measure reflecting the amount of oxygen used), you can also determine the calories burned per minute during the activity using the equations on page 107 in chapter 6. The total number of calories you burn will depend on how long you exercise at a given intensity. If you choose to exercise vigorously during pregnancy or pursue athletic training for competition, you may wish to meet with a registered dietitian to make sure your and your developing baby's energy and nutrient needs are being met. For more information on general nutritional recommendations, see chapter 4, which includes details on the *Dietary Guidelines* recommendations.

Focusing on Physical Activity

The benefits of physical activity during pregnancy are well documented. It is encouraging that the ACOG guidelines now state that "recreational and competitive athletes with uncomplicated pregnancies can remain active during pregnancy and should modify their usual exercise routines as medically indicated."[2] Importantly, no heart rate constraints are included. The *Physical Activity Guidelines for Americans* recommends the following:[45]

- Healthy women who are not already highly active or participating in vigorous-intensity activity should get at least 150 minutes (2 hours and 30 minutes) of moderate-intensity aerobic activity per week during pregnancy and the postpartum period. Preferably, this activity should be spread throughout the week.
- Pregnant women who habitually engage in vigorous-intensity aerobic activity or are highly active can continue physical activity during pregnancy and the postpartum period, provided that they remain healthy and discuss with their health care providers how and when to adjust activity.

Although experts recommend that pregnant women get at least 150 minutes per week of moderate activity during pregnancy, more specific recommendations for aerobic fitness, muscular fitness, and flexibility training are not available.[47] Some women choose to continue running 50 miles (80 km) or more per week during pregnancy with no ill effects, whereas others choose to start walking or swimming during pregnancy. Women who already have an exercise program before pregnancy are advised to continue the same program until they feel the need to modify the program by decreasing the intensity, frequency, or duration of the exercise. Women who are not already active are advised to begin moderate exercise during pregnancy to improve their own health, as well as their child's. As discussed throughout this book, a balanced exercise program addresses aerobic and muscular fitness, along with flexibility. This section outlines some special considerations for pregnant women regarding exercise.

Precautions for Pregnancy Conditions Before Exercise

Because some pregnant women have contraindications to exercise, discuss physical activity with your health care provider if you are pregnant. Relative and absolute contraindications to exercise during pregnancy are as follows:

Absolute Contraindications to Aerobic Exercise During Pregnancy
- Hemodynamically significant heart disease
- Restrictive lung disease
- Incompetent cervix/cerclage
- Multiple gestation at risk for premature labor
- Persistent second- or third-trimester bleeding
- Placenta previa after 26 weeks of gestation
- Premature labor during the current pregnancy
- Ruptured membranes
- Preeclampsia/pregnancy-induced hypertension

Relative Contraindications to Aerobic Exercise During Pregnancy
- Severe anemia
- Unelevated maternal cardiac arrhythmia
- Chronic bronchitis
- Poorly controlled type 1 diabetes
- Extreme morbid obesity

- Extreme underweight (BMI<12)
- History of extremely sedentary lifestyle
- Intrauterine growth restriction in current pregnancy
- Poorly controlled hypertension
- Orthopedic limitations
- Poorly controlled seizure disorder
- Poorly controlled hyperthyroidism
- Heavy smoker

Reprinted by permission from American College of Obstetricians and Gynecologists, 2002.

If you have absolute contraindications, you should not exercise until those health conditions are resolved. If you have relative contraindications, you may participate in physical activities as long as you check with your health care provider first. You may require more intensive monitoring of your own or your baby's health, or both.

Pregnant women face unique barriers to exercise, including fatigue, lack of time, morning sickness, increasing physical or joint discomfort, and lack of child care for other children.[5, 21, 43, 44] Incorporating exercise into your daily life is one way to overcome these barriers. Break exercise sessions up into smaller bouts to ease fatigue and time constraints. If you experience low back or joint pain, you may wish to pursue non-weight-bearing activities such as swimming, water aerobics, or cycling. An abdominal support band can also help to support the pregnant belly during weight-bearing exercise and ease discomfort. In the postpartum period, you may choose to include your baby in your workout by using a jogging stroller. Exercising with a friend or a group is also a good idea, especially postpartum when many women encounter feelings of depression or feel shut off from the outside world.

Exercise prescription during pregnancy and postpartum does not differ from exercise prescription during any other time, except for the need to avoid or modify certain activities and monitor the baby's well-being (see table 18.2 on page 350). Keep in communication with your health care provider about your exercise program. Additionally, you can check on your baby's health by monitoring your weight gain to ensure that you are gaining the recommended amount, and by recording your baby's activity patterns, such as kicking or rolling, during the day. Knowing normal activity patterns can help you determine whether a change occurs with exercise. In general, the baby should move several times within the first half hour after exercise in the second and third trimesters.[14] If the baby stops moving or decreases the amount of usual activity throughout the day, you should contact your health care provider.

If you were already doing vigorous activities before becoming pregnant, you can feel good about continuing those activities throughout pregnancy, although you may choose to make some practical changes to your exercise routine later in your pregnancy. If you were not already an exerciser when you became pregnant, this can be a good time to start. Research confirms that starting a moderate aerobic exercise program during pregnancy, such as walking or swimming, is both safe and beneficial.

Women often ask, "How much do I need to exercise?" and "How much is too much?" during pregnancy. The guidelines suggest a minimum amount of exercise during pregnancy (i.e., 150 minutes per week of at least moderate activity), but they do not address an upper limit.[2, 47] If you were already active before pregnancy,

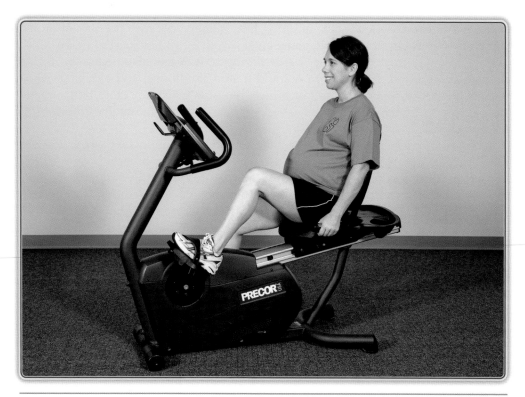

Figure 18.1 Exercise, such as cycling, during pregnancy provides many benefits.

continue your normal exercise routines until symptoms tell you to stop. Basically, if it feels good, it's probably OK to keep doing it while pregnant. ACOG provides the following list of warning signs; if you have any of these, you should terminate exercise during pregnancy:[2]

- Vaginal bleeding
- Severe dizziness or headache
- Preterm labor
- Amniotic fluid leakage
- Chest pain
- Muscle weakness or fatigue
- Decreased fetal movement
- Shortness of breath (before exercise)

Symptoms don't need to be dramatic. Because warning signs are unique to each woman, you should interpret them in light of your exercise and medical history. Many women simply report the need to decrease exercise intensity, duration, or frequency later in pregnancy. Now, more than ever, it is important to listen to your body!

Some women fear that exercise might hurt their baby and perceive that vigorous, high-impact activities as unsafe.[17, 31] Although such fears are unwarranted based on current research results, you should still take precautions. Specifically, do not perform exercises that have a high risk of blunt trauma, such as water skiing and contact sports. You should also be cautious about trying new activities that require balance and coordination, such as lifting free weights, because the risk of falling increases as a result of changes in your center of gravity and increases in joint laxity. Maintaining a normal body temperature during activity can also be harder during pregnancy, so avoid exercising in hot and humid conditions, and use a fan when exercising indoors on a treadmill or other exercising machine. Table 18.2 summarizes common exercise concerns during pregnancy and suggests modifications to lessen any risk.

In the postpartum period, many women are concerned about how exercise might affect breastfeeding. From a comfort perspective, enlarged breasts from lactation can pose a problem for exercise—coordinating breastfeeding and exercise may require some effort and planning. Breastfeeding mothers also require a lot of water, so drinking plenty of water before, during, and after exercise is important. Feeding or pumping immediately before working out can ease the discomfort associated with enlarged breasts. Also, many women choose to wear two sport bras or an ACE bandage wrap to give more support while exercising. Importantly, research shows that milk volume and nutrient content are not negatively affected by exercise.[3] So you can be active during the postpartum period and reap the many benefits associated with exercise, while knowing you are not depriving your infant in any way!

Physical Activity Prescriptions

Physical activity can provide benefits for you and your baby, with consideration given to the previously described precautions. This section offers recommendations for aerobic exercise, resistance training, and flexibility exercise.

Aerobic Prescription Much of the research on physical activity during pregnancy has focused on aerobic exercise. Among active women, the most commonly reported activity during pregnancy is walking for exercise (~50%), followed by swimming (~12%) and aerobics (~12%).[20] Fewer women choose to participate in more vigorous activities such as running (~6%) or team sports (~1%), and participation in vigorous exercise tends to decrease from the first to the third trimester.[19, 20]

Table 18.2 **Exercise Risks and Suggested Modifications During Pregnancy**

Exercise risk	Suggested modification
Fetal harm because of blunt trauma	Avoid activities such as water and downhill skiing and contact sports.
Falling because of changing center of gravity	Switch to weight machines rather than free weights; use a treadmill or track with even footing rather than a sidewalk.
Overheating during intense exercise	Do not exercise in hot and humid conditions; use a fan when exercising indoors; wear clothes that allow heat to dissipate; drink plenty of water.
Reduced blood return to the heart during supine exercise	Avoid prolonged exercises lying on your back; use an incline bench to do crunches with your head higher than your feet.
Feeling excessively tired or fatigued during or after exercise	Do not exercise to exhaustion; be sure to consume extra calories (pregnancy requires about 300 extra calories a day); have a snack right before exercising to avoid hypoglycemia.

Adapted by permission from Pivarnik and Mudd, 2009, p. 11.

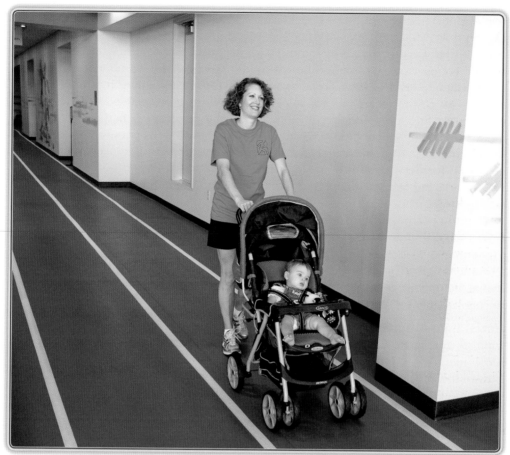

Exercise during the postpartum period is highly encouraged.

Importantly, even though most women do not choose to do vigorous activity, especially later in pregnancy, those who do so experience healthy pregnancies.[19]

Some active females may worry that their aerobic fitness levels will decrease during pregnancy. Actually, research shows that aerobic fitness declines very little during pregnancy when women continue to exercise, and their fitness rebounds quickly in the postpartum period to prepregnancy levels or better.[35, 37, 45] Part of the reason aerobic fitness does not decline too much may be related to changes in the body associated with pregnancy, which are further improved with exercise, such as greater blood volume.[36] Greater blood volume allows for better delivery of oxygen and nutrients to working muscles, a benefit during exercise as well as when performing daily activities. Active women also tend to gain less fat during pregnancy and instead preserve greater muscle mass.[37]

Aerobic exercise is described in detail in chapter 6. During pregnancy you can follow general adult population guidelines for exercise, with the caveat that you should monitor your symptoms, discomforts, and abilities and make any necessary adjustments. Regular aerobic activity is the target, so shoot for at least three days per week rather than sporadic exercise. If you are just starting to exercise, work up gradually to 30 minutes per day of accumulated activity with a weekly goal of 150 minutes. The most current ACOG guidelines recommend that pregnant women without obstetric complications accumulate 30 minutes or more of moderate exercise on most, if not all, days of the week.[2] Examples of these activities are found in chapter 6. If you are already doing more, that's great. Just continue to monitor your body's response to exercise and be willing to fine-tune the workout.

A moderate level of intensity is appropriate for most women. It is important to realize that resting heart rate tends to increase during pregnancy, so heart rate is not a good measure of exercise intensity during pregnancy. Rather, you should monitor intensity using your perception of effort.[4] An intensity corresponding to a level 5 or 6 on a 10-point scale is recommended for moderate-intensity activity (see chapter 6 for details on exercise intensity). The talk test also helps to ensure that you are staying at appropriate exercise intensities (you should be able to continue talking while exercising).

Walking is a popular form of exercise during pregnancy because it is low stress (physiologically) and easy to do at home or with friends. You may want to wear a pedometer to track the distance you walk each day and set goals for yourself. Pedometer-based programs (such as walking 10,000 steps per day) have been effective at helping overweight women stay within recommended weight gain ranges during pregnancy.[30]

Resistance Training Prescription   Very little research has considered resistance training and muscular fitness during pregnancy, which is reflected in the lack of recommendations for resistance training. In theory, heavy lifting could reduce blood flow to the developing baby and result in poorer growth; however, this has not been documented. Rather, the two research studies that compared women following a resistance training exercise prescription to women who did no exercise found no differences in length of gestation or birth weight.[7, 8, 23] Therefore, resistance training has not been found to be associated with preterm birth or low birth weight, at least among healthy pregnancies. Although one study found that muscular strength decreased during pregnancy, strength increased above prepregnancy levels by seven months postpartum among women who continued their resistance training routines.[45]

Past studies on resistance training during pregnancy involved light to moderate weightlifting programs that used machines, resistance bands, or body weight activities rather than free weights.[7, 8, 23] For details on the various methods of resistance training, see chapter 7. Typically, lifting free weights during pregnancy is not advised because of the increasing instability associated with changes in the center of gravity and increased joint laxity as pregnancy progresses. To avoid balance issues, you may want to use weight machines or resistance bands in place of free weights during pregnancy. Given the lack of documented research studies about possible benefits or adverse effects of resistance training during pregnancy, work with a health care provider or a fitness professional to develop an appropriate resistance training program.

In general, resistance training programs should include low-resistance, high-repetition exercises for the major muscle groups, rather than power-lifting activities, which are contraindicated during pregnancy. Completing 12 to 15 repetitions to the point of moderate fatigue is recommended.[4] Take extra care to avoid breath holding (called the Valsalva maneuver) while lifting. Instead, exhale during the exertion, or muscle-shortening, phase of each exercise. You should also modify exercises to avoid lying on your back (supine position), especially late in pregnancy when the weight and location of the baby may decrease the normal return of blood to the heart.[2] This can ultimately cause an unwanted drop in blood pressure. Although not traditionally thought of as strength training, Kegel exercises (voluntarily squeezing the muscles of the pelvic floor) are recommended during pregnancy and postpartum to reduce pregnancy-related urinary incontinence.[3]

Within the past decade, gyms across the country have begun offering prenatal yoga and Pilates classes. Although systematic research on the efficacy of yoga or Pilates to improve pregnancy outcomes is scarce, it is likely that evidence of any adverse effects would have shown up by now if the risk was high. Yoga and Pilates may improve pregnancy outcomes by helping to strengthen core muscles that help with labor and delivery, and by improving maternal mood and lowering stress. In fact, there is some evidence that participation in yoga during pregnancy lessens maternal stress, lowers anxiety, decreases low back and pelvic pain, and lowers the risk of delivering a preterm or low birth weight infant.[9, 32] More research is needed to determine what types of yoga stances have the best effects and which, if any, might be harmful during pregnancy.

As with aerobic exercise, general resistance training guidelines for adults hold true for pregnant women, with the considerations addressed previously in mind. As outlined in chapter 7, resistance training two or three days per week is recommended, including exercises for the major muscle groups.

Flexibility Prescription   It is well known that joint laxity (i.e., the feeling of joint looseness and flexibility) increases throughout pregnancy in preparation for labor and delivery. As a result, the risk of injury to joints and surrounding tissues (ligaments) is higher during pregnancy. For this reason, you should be cautious about rapidly changing direction during exercise to avoid ankle or knee sprains and other injuries. As with any exercise program, it is important to include proper warm-up and cool-down periods when exercising during pregnancy. All major muscle groups should be stretched during the cool-down when the muscles are warm.

As recommended for all healthy adults, pregnant women should stretch for at least 10 minutes a minimum of two or three days a week and include four or more repetitions of each stretch. Chapter 8 provides information on stretching programs.

Although these general recommendations on stretching are appropriate, some special considerations should be noted. Because of greater joint laxity, pregnant women should be especially careful not to stretch past the point of discomfort. Some stretching exercises, especially those for the lower body, might also need to be modified later in pregnancy to account for the "baby bump" and to avoid lying on the back for too long (see *Lower-Body Stretches for Pregnancy* for several suggested stretches). In addition to being an important part of an exercise routine, regular stretching may also help lessen low back pain during pregnancy.

Pregnancy is an exciting time of life, and it's the perfect time to make changes to nutrition and activity patterns not only to improve your own health, but also to ensure a healthy start for your infant. If you already exercise, there is no reason to make drastic changes to your routine as long as you talk with your health care provider. Use common sense, however, and listen to your body and modify your activities as needed. If you don't already exercise, you can begin at any time, but it's important to start slowly and progress as appropriate. As in any other time in life, consultation with your health care provider before starting an exercise program can help ensure that you are proceeding in the best manner possible.

Low Back Stretch 1

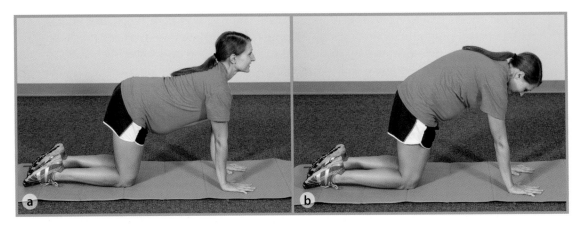

Begin on your hands and knees with your hands directly below your shoulders and your knees directly below your hips (*a*). Your back should be flat. Inhale, drawing your chin into your chest, pulling your abdomen into your spine, and rounding your back to make a hump (*b*). Exhale and return your back to a flat line. Slowly repeat several times.

Low Back Stretch 2

Stand up tall with your back against a wall. Exhale while pushing the small of your back against the wall. Inhale and relax. Repeat several times.

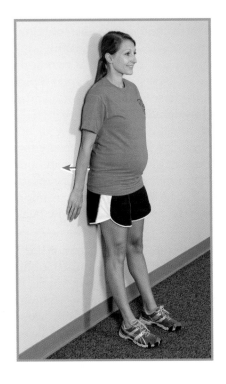

Low Back Stretch 3

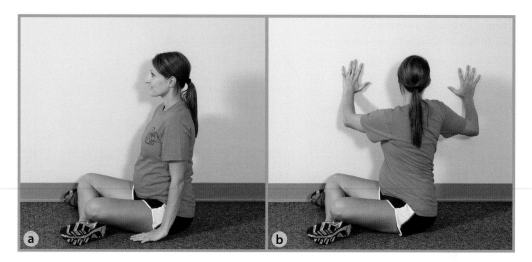

Sit up tall on your legs or cross-legged with your right side next to a wall (*a*). Maintaining good posture, slowly twist your upper body to face the wall (*b*). Press your palms or upper arms into the wall to support your body twist while keeping your legs on the floor. You should feel a stretch in your low back. Sit facing the opposite direction and repeat on the left side.

Hamstring and Buttock Stretch

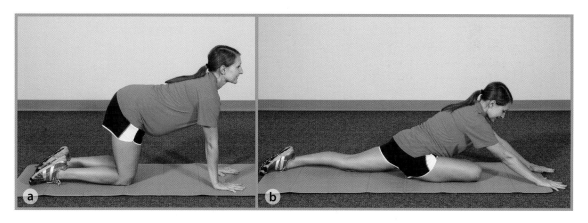

Begin on your hands and knees (*a*). Slide your right knee up so that it is on the floor under your right shoulder, and twist your lower leg so that your right foot is on the floor under your left hip. Exhale while slowly lowering your hips toward the floor and sliding your left knee back so that your left leg is extended and lying on the floor (*b*). Feel the stretch in the back of your right leg and buttock. For a deeper stretch once your back leg is extended, slowly lower your upper body to lie on top of your bent leg and place your arms on the floor. Repeat with your left leg bent under.

Inner Thigh Stretch

Sit on the floor with your back straight against a wall and your legs out in front. Slowly bend your knees out to the side while sliding your feet in toward your body until the soles of your feet touch. Keep sitting up tall and exhale while gently pushing down on your knees until you feel the stretch in your inner thighs.

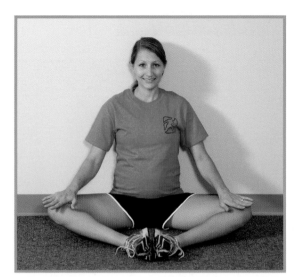

Calf Stretch

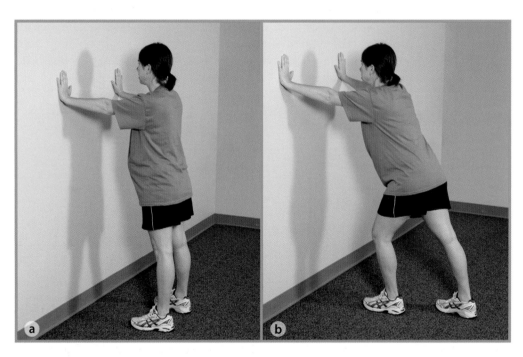

Stand an arm's length away from a wall and extend your arms until your palms are flat on the wall, slightly above shoulder height (*a*). Step back with your right foot, straighten your right leg, and bend your left leg toward the wall (*b*). Both feet should be flat and pointed toward the wall. Your weight should be balanced between your feet and your hands. You should feel the stretch in your right calf. Switch leg positions and repeat on the left side.

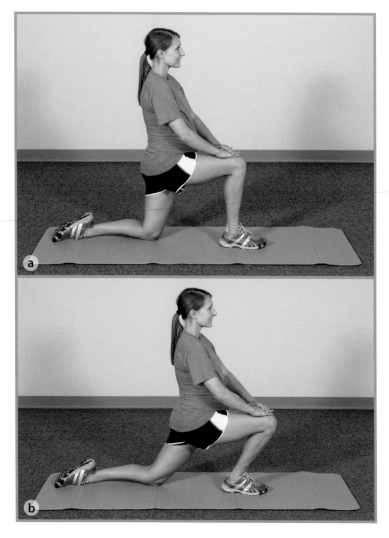

Begin kneeling on the floor with your body upright. Place your right foot in front of you, flat on the floor, with your knee bent directly over your ankle (*a*). Place your hands on top of your right knee and slowly shift forward, keeping your back straight, so that your right knee moves toward your right toe, and lean your hips forward (*b*). You should feel a stretch on the top of your left thigh (the hip flexor). Switch leg positions and repeat.

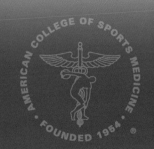
Osteoporosis and Bone Health

Imagine the internal structure of bone as being like the wood foundation of a house. The process of osteoporosis is similar to what happens during a termite infestation of a home's foundation, whereby termites slowly eat away at the wood supporting the structure. At some point, so much wood is consumed that the strength of the foundation is compromised and it begins to fail. This is not unlike the progressive nature of osteoporosis; over time, the internal architecture of bone is eroded as a result of a number of factors that eventually increase your risk for fracture (bone collapse). The term *osteopenia,* or *low bone mass,* refers to a condition of reduced bone density that has not yet progressed to osteoporosis. Those diagnosed with this condition should still be monitored to ensure that the condition does not get worse.

Osteoporosis is the most common disease affecting the skeleton and is one of the most important public health issues facing Americans. Consider the number of people affected by bone fracture: over 50% of women and 20% of men over the age of 50 will suffer an osteoporotic fracture at some time in their lives.[7] Sadly, one in six women will experience a hip fracture, the most devastating type of osteoporotic fracture.[2] Although an osteoporotic fracture can be devastating, the good news is that because this disease progresses slowly, you can take a number of steps throughout your lifespan to reduce your risk of developing it. Figure 19.1 shows a comparison of healthy bone and bone affected by osteoporosis.

CAUSES OF OSTEOPOROSIS

During growth and young adulthood, the skeleton is busy changing in size, shape, and density to ultimately support the physical needs of an adult. In adulthood, the skeleton remains relatively stable but is still constantly undergoing a process called

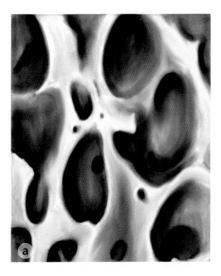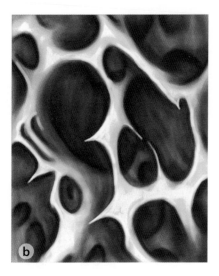

Figure 19.1 Comparison of *(a)* normal and *(b)* osteoporotic bone.

bone remodeling, in which bone repairs and renews itself. During bone remodeling, old bone cells are replaced with new bone cells in roughly the same amount. Many processes, however, can "uncouple" bone balance. With normal aging, bone breakdown outpaces buildup causing up to 1% of bone to be lost per year after around age 30. Certain conditions, such as estrogen loss from menopause or an overactive thyroid gland, may increase bone breakdown and slow down bone buildup, causing further overall loss of bone. On the other hand, pharmaceutical agents that stop the breakdown of bone, and physical activity, which causes bone to be built, can each cause a net bone gain.

Take a look at figure 19.2. On the left side of each scale are factors that have a *positive* influence on bone; the right side of the scales include factors that have a *negative* influence. When positive and negative factors are equal (scale in the middle) bone balance results and no change in bone mass occurs. This situation is typical over the period of middle adulthood. Bone loss (scale on the right) occurs where negative factors outweigh positive factors and bone mass is lost. This situation is typical of later life or when certain conditions shift bone balance in an unhealthy direction (i.e., disease or bedrest). Bone gain (scale on the left) occurs where positive factors outweigh negative ones and bone is gained. This situation is typical of the growing years or when certain conditions shift bone balance in a healthy way (i.e., exercise). The goal of any lifestyle strategy, such as exercise, is to achieve bone balance or bone gain.

Because bone is a dynamic tissue throughout life, however, strategies to slow down the breakdown of bone and to build new, stronger bone are useful at *any* life stage. Keep in mind, though, that many factors influence the state of your bones at any given time. The development of osteoporosis is complex, and no single factor can take the sole blame for the disease. Some of the factors you can control, and others you cannot (see *Risk Factors for Osteoporosis*). Uncontrollable factors that influence bone health include genetics, sex, race, age, and bone loss secondary to another

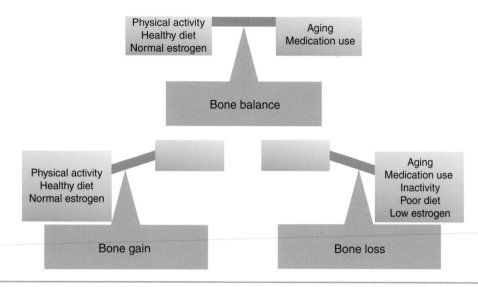

Figure 19.2 Factors that affect bone balance.

disease. Genes have already predetermined up to two-thirds of your bone mass, so a family history of osteoporosis, particularly with related fractures, is a significant risk factor. Women are at higher risk than men for osteoporosis because of their smaller frames and vulnerability to estrogen-related bone loss after menopause, but approximately 20% of cases are in men, and this percentage may increase as men live longer and awareness of the disease risk in men increases.

Osteoporosis is more prevalent among Caucasian and Asian women than it is among African American and Hispanic women, though these demographics may change over time as more data are gathered. Racial differences may be attributed to differences in bone size, muscle mass, or diet. Although you cannot change your genes, sex, race, or age, some influences on your bone health are under your control.

Smoking and alcohol consumption are two lifestyle factors you can manage. Avoid smoking and being in contact with secondhand smoke, and excessive alcohol consumption. Other controllable factors that affect the health of your bones include reproductive hormone levels, dietary adequacy (namely, of calcium and vitamin D), and physical activity. Near or at the onset of menopause, typically around age 50, women's bodies lose the ability to produce normal levels of estrogen. This loss of estrogen can cause bone to be lost two to five times more quickly than bone loss as a result of age alone. Although estrogen and hormone therapy (a combination of estrogen and progesterone; HT) has been shown to effectively stop menopause-related bone loss,[1] many women choose not to go on HT because of a history of breast cancer (HT is associated with a slight increase in risk for breast cancer) or other concerns, such as the potential link between HT and cardiovascular events.[4] Whether testosterone in men plays a similar role as estrogen in women is unclear. Adequate testosterone in men may be necessary to produce the small amounts of estrogen important for bone health in both sexes. Although some osteoporotic men also have low testosterone levels, low testosterone does not inevitably lead to osteoporosis.

Risk Factors for Osteoporosis

Your risk of osteoporosis is influenced by many factors, some of which you can control or modify, and others that are outside of your control.

Risk Factors You Cannot Control

- Being female
- Having a thin or small frame
- Being of advanced age
- Having a family history of osteoporosis
- Being postmenopausal, including early or surgically induced menopause
- Being male, with low testosterone levels
- Being Caucasian or Asian (although African Americans and Hispanic Americans are at significant risk as well)

Risk Factors You Can Control

- Having a diet low in calcium and vitamin D
- Being inactive
- Smoking, including exposure to secondhand smoke
- Excessive use of alcohol (more than three drinks per day)

Risk Factors You May Be Able to Control

- Abnormal absence of menstrual periods (amenorrhea)
- Anorexia nervosa (eating disorder characterized by low body weight)
- Prolonged use of certain medications, such as corticosteroids and anticonvulsants

A CLOSER LOOK
Lori

Lori is a 60-year-old postmenopausal woman who recently discontinued estrogen therapy. When browsing at a local shopping center, she saw a sign for bone density evaluations. The cost was minimal, and the sign explained that there was no exposure to radiation. Because she had her yearly physical scheduled for the next week, she proceeded with the evaluation, planning to share the result with her physician. The test involved an ultrasound of her heel, which provides an estimate of its bone density. Lori's physician was pleased to see that Lori was taking steps to check her bone health. However, her physician explained that the only test that can diagnose osteoporosis is a DXA test. Other bone density tests, such as the heel ultrasound, should only be regarded as screening tools that may indicate the need for further testing. Furthermore, these tests are not very reliable, and so results may vary as much as 5% to 10% on any given day. Lori's physician recommended that Lori schedule a DXA test considering the results of the ultrasound test along with other factors, including her age, her change in medication (discontinuation of estrogen therapy), and her prior history of smoking.

Most of the options for maintaining normal hormone levels are drug related and will be discussed later in this chapter, but some behaviors can also influence hormone levels. In particular, you should avoid very intense exercise training coupled with strict dieting. Women who exercise excessively and restrict their eating are prone to disturbances in their menstrual cycle as a result of low estrogen levels. The amount and type of exercise recommended in this book would not put someone at risk for such a problem. This chapter explains how to exercise your bones to keep them healthy while helping you better understand all the factors that influence your risk of osteoporosis so you can make the best choices for your bones.

Assessment and Diagnosis of Osteoporosis

The gold-standard technique for osteoporosis evaluation is called dual-energy X-ray absorptiometry, or DXA. You may have also heard this test called a bone density test, because it measures bone mineral density. Bone density tells us how much hard mineral is in a given bone, such as the spine or hip. Bone density is a very accurate index of bone strength and, therefore, how likely a bone is to fracture. Bone density is typically measured at the bones that are most often fractured—the hip, spine, and forearm. The test is very simple: you lie on a large, flat table while the measurement device passes over your body and takes the necessary readings.

Your risk of fracture is evaluated by comparing your bone density values to both age-matched and young-normal reference groups. Because bone loss is part of the aging process, you can be average for your age, but be at risk for or have osteoporosis. Therefore, the diagnosis of osteoporosis is based on a comparison of your bone density to the bone density of a young adult (20 to 29 years old). If your bone density is significantly less, then you are diagnosed with osteoporosis.

You may be asking yourself whether you should have a DXA screening. The National Osteoporosis Foundation (www.nof.org) suggests that people in the following categories be tested for bone density:

- Women age 65 and older and men age 70 and older, regardless of risk factors
- Younger postmenopausal women and men 50 to 69 years of age with risk factor profiles eliciting concern (see the list of items in *Risk Factors for Osteoporosis*)
- Women in the menopausal transition who have a specific risk factor associated with increased fracture risk (e.g., low body weight, prior low-trauma fracture)
- Adults with fracture after age 50 or with a condition (e.g., rheumatoid arthritis) or taking a medication (e.g., prednisone) associated with low bone mass or bone loss
- Postmenopausal women discontinuing estrogen (should be considered for testing)
- Anyone being considered for drug therapy for osteoporosis or who is currently being treated (to monitor the effect of treatment)

The decision to have a bone density assessment is thus based on your suspected fracture risk. Discuss your situation with your health care provider to determine whether an assessment would be beneficial.

HEALTHY APPROACHES
TO MANAGING OSTEOPOROSIS

Although many factors can influence bone health, this chapter focuses on the impact of diet and physical activity. These two lifestyle factors are under your control and can have a major impact on the strength of your bones.

Focusing on Nutrition

The quality of your diet can influence the health of your bones. A healthy, well-balanced diet as outlined in chapter 4 should provide the necessary building blocks for healthy bones. Even with the best efforts, however, your diet may fall short of meeting recommended levels. In this case, dietary supplements may help you meet the recommended dietary intake. In particular, calcium and vitamin D are two nutrients of importance for healthy bones.

Calcium

Calcium is a critical nutrient for bone health, and the body ardently defends its blood levels of calcium. If you do not replace daily losses through your diet, then your body keeps blood levels steady by taking calcium from your bones. In addition to inadequate dietary consumption of calcium, humans are not very good at moving calcium from the food eaten into the bloodstream. This poor absorption can also cause your skeleton to forfeit some of its stores to keep blood levels normal.

Why is calcium so important in your body? Calcium is the most essential building block for bones and combines with other minerals to form the hard crystals that give your bones their strength. Because humans cannot form calcium in the body, calcium *must* come from your diet. People who have greater milk and dairy consumption have fewer fractures. Because of the poor absorption of calcium, you will have to ingest a lot of calcium just to offset the small bodily calcium loss each day. With age, the ability to absorb calcium tends to decrease, so over time dietary calcium requirements increase (see table 19.1 for age-related calcium intake recommendations).

Table 19.1   **Recommended Dietary Intake of Calcium**

Age	Calcium (mg)
Birth to 6 months	210
6 months to 1 year	270
1–3 years	500
4–8 years	800
9–18 years	1,300
19–50 years	1,000
51+ years	1,200

Adapted from Institute of Medicine, National Academy of Science, 1997, pp. 94, 99, 105, 111, 115.

It is vital that growing children get as much calcium in their diets as they can because it may make a large difference in their bone health when they are adults. For adults, the role of dietary calcium is in preventing bone loss (i.e., maintaining the bone you have). Studies show that calcium intake at or above recommended levels cannot *increase* bone density, but is very important in preventing bone loss over time. Excessive calcium intake, on the other hand, could contribute to kidney stone formation in certain people, and taking more than 2,500 milligrams per day should be avoided.

As with all nutrients, calcium is most usable by the body when it is ingested in the form of food. Dairy products such as milk, yogurt, and cheese are high in calcium; other foods such as nuts, fish, beans, and some vegetables are less calcium dense, but can help you achieve your calcium requirement (see table 19.2 for examples of calcium-rich foods). Many nondairy foods are now fortified with calcium, such as orange juice, bread, cereals, and even margarine, but be sure to read the label because some foods contain more fortification than others.

When you cannot consume sufficient calcium in your diet, supplements may be warranted. Calcium supplements come in the form of calcium phosphate, calcium carbonate, and calcium citrate and can be an important addition to a diet low in calcium. Because the stomach can only absorb about 500 milligrams of calcium at a time, it is best to spread your supplements throughout the day. Supplements should be evaluated on the basis of their elemental calcium content (usually between 200 and 600 mg per tablet or chew), and not on the overall milligrams of calcium compounds. Some supplements made from bone meal, dolomite, or unrefined oyster shells may contain substances such as lead or other toxic metals and should be avoided.

Table 19.2 **Calcium Content of Select Foods**

Food	Amount	Calcium (mg)
Milk (reduced fat, 2%)	1 cup	270
Yogurt (nonfat, plain)	1 cup	450
Hard cheese (cheddar)	1 oz (28 g)	200
Cottage cheese (low-fat)	1 cup	150
Ice cream (vanilla)	1 cup	84
Tofu (soybean curd; firm)	1/4 block	130
Nuts (almonds)	1 oz (24 nuts)	70
Beans (navy)	1 cup cooked	130
Sardines with bones	3 oz (85 g) canned	325
Molasses, blackstrap	1 Tbsp	175
Spinach	1 cup raw	30
Broccoli	1/2 cup cooked	30
Orange	1 medium	50

One way to help ensure that the supplement you are taking is safe and effective is to look for products that have a USP symbol on the label, which stands for United States Pharmacopeia. USP is a nongovernmental, official public standards–setting authority. Unfortunately, testing of supplements is voluntary so not all suitable products will have this notation.

Vitamin D

Vitamin D is another nutrient important to bone health because it helps the body absorb and store calcium. Low vitamin D levels are related to low bone density and increased risk of fractures.[17] The recommended daily intake of vitamin D is between 400 and 800 international units (IU) for adults, which can be obtained from food and sunlight. Vitamin D–rich foods include eggs, fatty fish, and cereal and milk fortified with vitamin D (see table 19.3 for examples of foods rich in vitamin D). Based on recent research studies linking vitamin D supplementation to reduced risk of fractures and some chronic diseases, the Institute of Medicine is considering increasing the recommended intakes. Studies suggest that intakes in the range of 800 to 1,000 IU per day of vitamin D are associated with better health outcomes and are well below the 2,000 IU daily limit to avoid any harmful effects of excess vitamin D.

Vitamin D is sometimes referred to as the sunshine vitamin because when UV rays from the sun make contact with the skin, vitamin D is formed. Minimal sun exposure (to feet, hands, and face) of about 15 to 20 minutes per day is usually enough to get most of the needed daily vitamin D, although this ability does decline with age. Sunscreen can reduce vitamin D synthesis by the skin, and deficiencies may also occur in those who are housebound, reside in extreme northern latitudes, do not consume vitamin D–fortified foods, or have kidney or liver disorders that interfere with normal vitamin D metabolism.

Table 19.3 **Vitamin D Levels in Select Foods**

Food	Amount	Vitamin D (IU)
Eggs	1 hard cooked	20
Salmon	3.5 oz (99 g) cooked	360
Ready-to-eat fortified cereal	3/4 to 1 cup	40
Milk (nonfat, low-fat, or whole)	1 cup	98

Focusing on Physical Activity

Exercise can improve bone health by increasing bone mass or by slowing or preventing age-related bone loss. Researchers and scientists continue to examine what type and how much exercise is necessary to maintain or boost bone health. Though leisurely levels of physical activity are good starting points for beginning an exercise program, more moderate to vigorous levels of activity are necessary to challenge the bones to become healthier. Exercise is also important for fall prevention, and certain types of exercise have been shown to lower fall risk. To realize the potential benefits of exercise, some precautions should be considered.

Precautions Before Exercise

Specific exercise recommendations tend to be difficult for those diagnosed with osteopenia or osteoporosis because of the limited number of research studies. If you have been diagnosed with osteoporosis, even if you have not yet fractured, you should avoid activities that put higher stress on the bone, such as jumping activities or deep forward trunk flexion exercises (e.g., rowing, toe touches, and full sit-ups). A regular brisk walking program (with hills as tolerated) combined with resistance training to improve balance and upper- and lower-body muscle strength may improve muscle strength and coordination, thereby reducing fall risk. Exercise options may be limited for those with osteoporosis who are restricted by severe pain. It may be a good idea to begin exercise with a warm pool–based program, which, although non-weight-bearing, can improve flexibility and provide some muscle strengthening.

Exercise training after hip fracture and surgery has been found to significantly increase strength, functional ability, and balance as well as to reduce fall-related behavioral and emotional problems in elderly people.[6] Exercise plays a key role in reducing stiffness and increasing flexibility and muscle strength after hip replacement surgery. Recommendations for specific exercises should come from a physical therapist because the activity program will need to be individualized. Generally, these programs begin with safe range of motion activities and muscle-strengthening exercises for the muscles surrounding the hips, trunk, pelvis, and lower body. Progressing to more vigorous activities should come at the advice of your health care provider or physical therapist.

Typically, exercise recommendations include avoiding high-impact activities such as basketball, volleyball, soccer, jogging, and tennis. These activities can damage the new hip or loosen its parts. Resistance exercises that cause hip abduction or adduction (swinging the leg from side to side) should generally be avoided initially to prevent dislocation of the new hip. Recommended exercises often include walking, stationary bicycling, swimming, and cross-country skiing.

Rehabilitation after vertebral fracture should include exercises to maintain proper posture while moving (called dynamic posture training) and exercises specifically to strengthen the back extensor muscles (the muscles that help you stand up straight). Gentle yoga and tai chi are excellent activities to increase postural awareness and muscle strength and to improve balance. Specialized braces are also sometimes used under the supervision of a physician or physical therapist to improve back extensor strength and promote postural alignment. The goal of this type of program should be to reduce pain, improve mobility, and contribute to a better quality of life.

Physical Activity Prescriptions

You have probably heard that exercise must be weight bearing to benefit your bones. Some of the first evidence that weight bearing was important to the skeleton came from observations of bone loss in astronauts, which can be high as 1% every month. This is 12 to 24 times faster than the rate of bone loss due to aging! Bone can be lost very quickly when the invisible force of gravity on the skeleton is removed. Examples of this include immobilization (as when a leg is in a cast), long periods of bed rest (from prolonged illness), or being inactive. Unfortunately, the body quickly adapts to the reduced loads placed on it. Similarly, non-weight-bearing exercise, such as swimming and cycling, may not be an ideal exercise for bones because the body weight is supported by the water or the bike.

Studies of athletes have provided the basis for the design and testing of exercise interventions aimed to improve bone health. These interventions can better answer the question of what type and how much exercise strengthens bones. The Position Stand on Physical Activity and Bone Health from the American College of Sports Medicine[9] and the U.S. Surgeon General's National Report on Bone Health[16] recommend important lifestyle modifications (such as exercise) to improve bone health. This information forms the basis for the exercise recommendations and sample programs outlined in this chapter.

Researchers continue to work to answer questions about the best type and amount of exercise to both increase bone mass and slow bone loss with aging in order to reduce the risk of fracture. Currently, available information along with standard safety precautions will allow you to set proper exercise limits.

Traditional types of exercise have been studied for their bone benefits including weight-bearing aerobic exercise (e.g., walking, jogging, bench or stair stepping, aerobic dance), resistance (strengthening) exercises, and impact exercise (e.g., jumping). The good news is that *most* types of exercise can benefit your bones. However, some types are better than others, and the level of effort is also a factor.

The best program may be one that incorporates multiple types of activity and applies the principles of training with bone health in mind. With respect to bone, exercise is site specific. In other words, a particular bone must be directly stressed to receive benefits. A multimodal program can provide multiple benefits for musculoskeletal, cardiorespiratory, and metabolic health plus reduce the risk of injury. A sample program of bone health exercise that incorporates multiple types of activity is found in figure 19.3. Note that rest is included to allow bone to be responsive to the next loading bout. This program would be appropriate for a beginner exerciser who is otherwise healthy and with no known orthopedic problems. If you have any concerns about your readiness to begin exercise, consult with your health care provider.

As you can see, the sample program includes activities focused on aerobic and muscular fitness as well as flexibility. In addition, balance training is another consideration for fall prevention for anyone with osteoporosis. Each of these components is important to include in your exercise plans.

A CLOSER LOOK
Lynda

Lynda is a healthy 46-year-old office receptionist. Recently, her mother was diagnosed with osteoporosis. Lynda wants to do all she can to strengthen her own bones to avoid a similar diagnosis in the future. Her health care provider suggests that Lynda verify that she is consuming adequate calcium and vitamin D. After reviewing Lynda's activity program (including some walking a couple of days per week), her health care provider suggests some changes to provide a stimulus to strengthen her bones—a program similar to the sample one-month program shown in figure 19.3, which includes resistance training and jump training in addition to other activities.

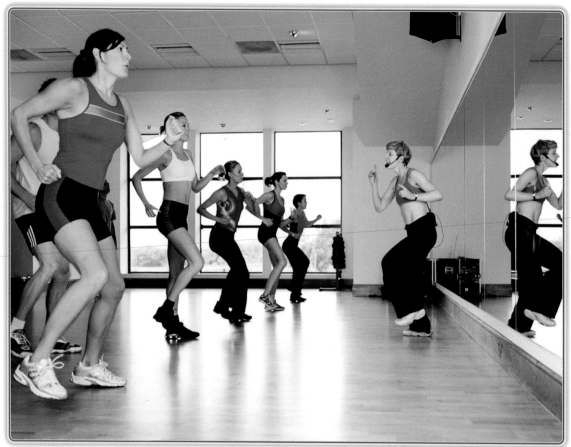

Weight-bearing aerobic activities can benefit your bones.

Aerobic Prescription   Moderate to vigorous aerobic exercise can improve or maintain bone mass of the hip and spine and has additional benefits to the cardiovascular, muscular, and nervous systems. To challenge the skeleton, the choice of aerobic exercise should be weight bearing, although rowing may have particular benefit to the spine. Examples of weight-bearing aerobic exercises that have been shown to build or preserve bone density when done at moderate to vigorous intensity include aerobic dance, fast walking (faster than 5 mph, or 8 km/h), jogging (may begin with walking and intermittent jogging), stair climbing or bench stepping, tennis, and rowing.

The general prescription for aerobic exercise aimed to improve bone health is to reach a minimum target of 30 minutes of continuous moderate-intensity exercise five days each week for a total of 150 minutes. Another option is 75 minutes of vigorous-intensity exercise per week (about 20 to 25 minutes three days each week), similar to the general public health recommendations for physical activity described in chapter 1. To see more improvement, you can increase the amount of exercise by increasing the intensity, duration, or frequency of the exercise. Generally, the upper range for effective aerobic exercise is 60 minutes of vigorous-intensity exercise five to seven days per week. Any more than this and your risk of injury or burnout increases.

FIGURE 19.3

Sample Multimodal Beginner Exercise Program*

	Mon.	Tues.	Wed.	Thurs.	Fri.	Sat.	Sun.
Week 1	Bench step** at slow, steady pace for 15–20 minutes	Three sets of 4 two-footed jumps from the ground; stretch	One or two sets of 12–14 reps of upper- and lower-body strength training exercises*** at a weight you can't lift more than 14 times	Three sets of 6 two-footed jumps from the ground; stretch	Walk at a steady pace (with short bursts of faster walking) for 15–20 minutes	Day off or stretch	See Wednesday
Week 2	*For week 2 note the increased time for aerobic activity and number of sets and repetitions for jumps and strength*						
	Bench step** at a slow, steady pace for 20–25 minutes	Four sets of 6 two-footed jumps from the ground; stretch	One or two sets of 14–16 reps of upper- and lower-body strength training exercises using the same weight as week 1	Four sets of 8 two-footed jumps from the ground; stretch	Walk at a steady pace (with short bursts of faster walking) for 20–25 minutes	Day off or stretch	See Wednesday
Week 3	*For week 3, note the increased intensity for aerobic and strength training and number of repetitions for jumps*						
	Bench step** for 20–25 minutes at a faster pace than week 2	Four sets of 8 two-footed jumps from the ground; stretch	One or two sets of 12–14 reps of upper- and lower-body strength training exercises, increasing the weight from week 2	See Tuesday	Walk at a steady pace (with bursts of faster walking or jogging) for 20–25 minutes	Day off or stretch	See Wednesday
Week 4	*For week 4, the time per session is increased*						
	Bench step** for 25–30 minutes at the same pace as week 3	Five sets of 8 two-footed jumps from the ground; stretch	One or two sets of 14–16 reps of upper- and lower-body strength training exercises, using the same weight as week 3	See Tuesday	Walk at a steady pace (with bursts of faster walking or jogging) for 25–30 minutes	Day off or stretch	See Wednesday

*Every exercise session should include a 5- to 10-minute warm-up before exercise and a 5- to 10-minute cool-down after exercise. The cool-down period is a perfect time to include flexibility exercises for good mobility and function.

**The bench step exercise can be substituted with any aerobic activity listed in chapter 6, including aerobic dance, walking (try adding intermittent jogging), tennis, or rowing.

*** Include exercises for the hips and legs, chest, back, shoulders, low back, and abdominals. Examples of exercises to target these areas begin on page 133 of chapter 7.

Why Walking May Not Be Enough

Walking is often advocated as a weight-bearing exercise that is good for bones. True, walking is weight bearing, but unfortunately, most research studies of inactive women who begin a moderate walking program fail to find any effect of walking on bone mass. Survey studies show that women who walk fracture less often than women who are inactive. However, because of the way these studies are designed, they cannot verify that walking *causes* a reduction in fractures, nor can they tell whether walking may lower fractures because of its effect on bone or through other means. These studies can only show associations between walking and fractures (i.e., those who walk also have fewer fractures). It is possible that walkers also engage in other healthy behaviors that could lower their fracture risk, such as better calcium intake or less smoking. These habits may be the reason for fewer fractures rather than the walking program. Perhaps habitual walking over many years provides a bone benefit that cannot be measured in research studies of short duration (one year or less).

Only two walking studies out of many showed a positive effect of walking on spine bone mass (but not the hip). In these studies, women walked at a very fast pace, similar to the speeds achieved by race walkers. These speeds are much faster than the average "brisk" walking pace reported by most women. Race walkers can walk 5 to 6 miles per hour (8 to 9.6 km/h), which is much faster than the usual 2 to 3 miles-per-hour (3.2 to 4.8 km/h) pace of most women. Because walking confers so many other benefits to the body, if you love walking, don't stop! Increasing the intensity of your walking program to include bursts of very fast walking or walking briskly up hills, however, will burn some extra calories and keep your heart healthy as well as help your bones.

If you already have been diagnosed with osteopenia or modest osteoporosis, a low- to moderate-intensity exercise program is recommended to improve bone mass or prevent or slow further bone loss. If you have advanced osteoporosis or have had a recent fracture, this type of program may be too rigorous. Consult your health care provider to determine the level of activity suitable for your circumstances.

Resistance Training Prescription   Resistance training, also called strength training, can have a positive effect on bone because the strong muscle contractions required to lift, push, or pull a heavy weight place stress on the bones. When your bone senses stress from regular resistance training, it responds by increasing in mass to better tolerate the strong muscle contractions. Resistance exercises can be done using resistance machines, free weights such as dumbbells and barbells, weighted vests, elastic tubing, or elastic bands. In general, strength training using any means of applying sufficient resistance will maintain or slightly improve hip and spine bone mass.[11, 12]

Resistance training has an added benefit of strengthening muscles that are important for fall prevention and to perform tasks that require some strength such as lifting groceries, rising from a chair, and climbing stairs. Strong leg muscles can also contribute to better balance and locomotion, which will reduce the risk of falls. When someone starts to fall, strong muscles are more likely to prevent a fall by moving the legs to counteract the downward movement. Strong back muscles can also be beneficial for bone density at the spine as well as in helping to prevent falls. Back muscles help to hold you upright (i.e., extend your truck) in good posture and thus protect your vertebrae (bones that make up the spine). In addition, resistance exercise can help to lower blood pressure, improve blood lipid levels (cholesterol and triglycerides), and aid in weight reduction. There are many good reasons to include resistance training in your exercise plan!

Resistance exercise, like aerobic exercise, must be slightly rigorous to affect bone. Low-intensity resistance training performed with light weights and for many repetitions generally does not help. Low-intensity resistance exercise, often called sculpting exercise or toning exercise, doesn't place enough force on the bones. Low-weight (weight that you can comfortably lift 15 to 20 times without stopping), high-repetition (three to five sets of 15 to 20 repetitions per set) resistance exercise may be a good starting point if you have never performed resistance exercise. This level provides an opportunity to become familiar with resistance training and start to build a base of strength.

Once you are comfortable with this level of activity, progress to heavier weights (weight that you cannot lift more than eight to twelve times) that you lift less often (two or three sets of 8 to 12 repetitions per set). Resistance exercise should be performed at least twice per week to be the most effective. If you are new to this type of training, one day a week may be a good starting point to get familiar with the activity, but you should then progress to two or three days per week. A particularly good regimen would include resistance training exercises while standing, which provides the added benefit of gravitational forces on bone. Standing exercises also promote good balance and translate into activities of daily living more directly than seated exercises do.

Resistance exercise is recommended for everyone, especially older adults who may have had some bone and muscle loss from age. Following proper guidelines, even 90-year-olds have safely performed resistance exercise. For complete details on resistance training, including specific exercises, see chapter 7. Resistance exercise may be new for you, but it could make a real difference in your life, so give it a try!

Flexibility and Balance Prescription   Stretching at least two to three days per week should be part of your exercise program to maintain or improve your flexibility (see chapter 8 for details). In addition to flexibility-promoting activities, balance exercises are also valuable. Because falls are a leading cause of fracture, along with weak bones, focusing on fall prevention is key. If you have osteoporosis, fall prevention should be a major focus of your exercise program. Fortunately, researchers now have pretty good ideas about what type of exercise and how much can help to prevent falls. Remember, though, that falls have many causes, and exercise may be one of several steps you can take to lower your risk. For a list of proactive steps you can take to prevent falls, see *Nonexercise Strategies to Prevent Falls* on page 375.

People with weak legs, poor balance, and difficult locomotion (gait problems) are much more likely to fall than those who are strong, stable, and move easily. Because muscle mass, strength, gait, and balance are all closely related, most exercise intervention programs include strengthening exercise along with balance training. Resistance training programs are largely successful at increasing muscle mass and dramatically improving muscle strength in people who are weak to begin with and can also improve balance and gait. Resistance training either with or without additional balance training has been shown to reduce the risk of falls. In contrast,

Exercise With Impact: Jumping!

Impact exercise, such as jumping, has been used for years by athletes to improve their muscular strength and power. Jump training may offer a quick and simple means to specifically improve bone mass at the hip, an area where fractures are particular debilitating. Jumping exercise works because it transmits forces up the skeleton and challenges bones in a way that they do not experience during normal daily activities. The skeleton perceives this force as a challenge and responds by laying down more bone to better tolerate the stress of regular jumping.

In general, studies have shown that women who perform jumping exercise either alone or added to a program of other exercise such as walking or resistance training, maintain or improve their hip and spine bone mass.[10] In one study, middle-aged and older women who regularly engaged in resistance exercise plus 50 to 100 jumps, three times per week, were able to increase or maintain hip bone mass; this even included women with low bone density.[15,18] Unfortunately, jumping exercise alone does not appear to improve the bone health of the spine because the forces generated from landing are quite small by the time they reach the spine. Remember, to improve a bone, you must challenge it.

People who have diagnosed orthopedic and joint limitations or are significantly overweight should discuss jump exercise with their health care provider before starting a program and may wish to consider other types of exercise first. Jumping exercise may not be for everyone, but some people love it and find it a quick way to exercise their bones. Jumping is a good exercise routine for people with limited time; it takes only about 5 or 10 minutes to do and so is easy to add to the end of a walk or jog.

Jump training has not been studied extensively. In most studies, women have performed a variety of jumping routines, including simply jumping straight up and down (see figure 19.4). When the height of the jump (jumping on and off small steps) or the weight of the person jumping is increased (jumping while wearing a weighted vest), the jump produces more force on the lower body. In general, doing 50 to 100 jumps in place three to five days per week is recommended based on current research. Jumps are usually done in sets of 10. However, if you have osteoporosis, do not perform jumping exercises without the recommendation of your health care provider, because the ability of fragile bone to tolerate the high impact of jumping remains unknown.

You may wonder how long you will have to exercise before your bones will start to benefit. Unlike other physiological systems such as the heart and muscles, which respond to exercise rather quickly, the process of building bone is slow. Rest assured that the bone-building process and structural changes begin as soon as you start to exercise regularly, but it will take at least six months to a year to detect that change through bone density measurements. Bone benefits from exercise are lost when you stop training, though, so you need to make a long-term commitment.

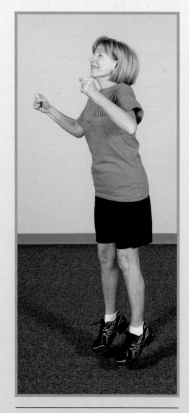

Figure 19.4 Jump training or bench stepping can be used to help stress your bones.

focusing on balance alone has not been found to prevent falls. Thus, combining resistance training with balance training appears to be the best prescription.

For specific suggestions on balance exercises, see chapter 8. Some nontraditional forms of exercise (such as tai chi) have also been shown to reduce the risk of falls, suggesting that both muscle strength and the ability to transfer weight while in motion can maintain stability, particularly while moving. Many research studies underscore how important strong muscles are for fall prevention.

Influence of Medications

If you have known osteoporosis, medical treatment that reduces your risk of fracture is important. New drugs continue to be developed, and new formulations of current drugs are being made to improve effectiveness while reducing dosage and side effects. It is important to remember, however, that although many of these drugs can effectively reduce fracture rates by up to 50%, none are 100% effective. Thus, it is important to consider all of the factors that contribute to fracture risk (i.e., exercise, nutrition, fall risk) to ensure that you follow a comprehensive program that may include drug management.

Most of the drugs currently approved by the U.S. Food and Drug Administration (FDA) for the management of postmenopausal osteoporosis are called antiresorptives. They increase bone density by rendering the cells that break down bone inactive, while leaving those cells that form bone alone. Drugs in this category include estrogens, calcitonin, bisphosphonates, and selective estrogen receptor modulators (SERMs). Two drugs have been shown to reduce fracture by actually stimulating bone-forming cells, parathyroid hormone (brand name, Forteo) and strontium ranelate (brand name, Protelos). The latter is still awaiting FDA approval in the United States.[13]

The class of drugs called bisphosphonates is currently the most widely used to reduce osteoporotic fractures. Several forms of bisphosphonates are currently available, alendronate (brand name, Fosamax), risedronate (brand name, Actonel), ibandronate (brand name, Boniva), and zoledronate (brand names, Reclast and Zometa), just to name a few. On average, these drugs cause bone density to increase by approximately 4% to 8% at the spine and 1% to 3% at the hip over the first three to four years of treatment,[1, 3] which may reduce the risk of vertebral fractures by 40% to 50% and nonvertebral fractures (including hip fractures) by as much as 20% to 40%.[5] Increases in bone density generally plateau at around the fourth year of use, so continued use of the drug maintains a higher level of bone density. Although these findings are positive, most long-term studies have followed patients for only three to five years into treatment, and so the optimum duration of therapy remains unclear.[8]

Despite the impressive potential of bisphosphonates to reduce fractures, new studies are questioning the long-term safety. These drugs remain in the skeleton for decades, and bone turnover can be affected for up to five years after the drugs are discontinued. Recall that bone remodeling is a natural process that allows the body to repair microdamage due to everyday wear and tear. If bisphosphonates prevent breakdown, resorption, and subsequent bone renewal, the concern is that bone could become brittle. Furthermore, the rare, but serious disorder called osteonecrosis of the jaw (a condition characterized by pain, swelling, infection, and exposure of bone) has been associated with bisphosphonate use, mainly in patients receiving

Nonexercise Strategies to Prevent Falls

Rather than dealing with the aftermath of a fall, you can make some simple adjustments to avoid a fall in the first place.

- Wear supportive, low-heeled shoes rather than walking in socks or slippers.
- Ensure that rooms are well lit.
- Use a rubber mat in the shower or bathtub.
- Use the handrails when going up and down stairs.
- Avoid the use of area rugs, but if you do, use skid-proof backing and secure corners to the floor or carpet underneath.
- Keep floors and walkways clutter free.
- Keep phone and electrical cords away from walkways.
- If needed, keep glasses handy rather than moving about with impaired vision.
- Realize the potential influence of medications on balance and talk with your health care provider about any medications you are taking.
- Consider the fact that some hip fractures occur as a result of tripping over small pets.

high doses in combination with cancer treatment. More investigation is needed to understand the mechanism of this disease.

Hormone therapy (HT, combination of estrogen and progesterone) and estrogen therapy (ET) offset the estrogen-related bone loss associated with menopause and even cause a slight increase in hip and spine bone density that plateaus after three years of use. Studies show that HT and ET reduce the incidence of fractures of the hip and spine by 30% to 50%. Hormone therapies are currently approved to reduce postmenopausal bone loss as a means to prevent osteoporosis, but are ineffective at preventing bone loss in men. To be most effective at preventing bone loss, therapy should begin close to, if not a few years before, the menopausal transition. After the publication of the Women's Health Initiative study in 2002, the role of long-term postmenopausal HT and ET for the prevention and management of osteoporosis became controversial because of a suspected increased risk of cardiovascular events.

You may be wondering whether HT or ET is appropriate for you. The National Institutes of Health currently sponsors a website that addresses questions and concerns about the use of HT and ET based on the latest research findings (www.nhlbi.nih.gov/health/women/pht_facts.htm). As additional studies are conducted, more clarity will emerge regarding risks and benefits of HT and ET. Consulting with your health care provider, who has an understanding of your complete health picture, is best. The current recommendation is to avoid hormone therapy in favor of alternative antiresorptive agents; hormone therapy should be an option only for short-term, early use around menopause in women with menopausal symptoms or those at risk for fracture.[14]

Selective estrogen receptor modulators (SERMs) represent a class of agents that, although similar in structure to estrogen, exert their effects only on target tissues.

Table 19.4 Pros and Cons of Common Osteoporosis Medications

Drug class (examples)	Approved for	Pros	Cons
Bisphosphonates (Actonel, Fosamax, Boniva, Reclast, Zometa)	Postmenopausal osteoporosis; postmenopausal bone loss; male bone loss; glucocorticoid-induced osteoporosis	Large increase in bone density at hip and spine; reduction of spine and hip fractures by up to 50%	Inconvenient dosing regimen; small risk of upper gastrointestinal side effects
ET/HT (Estrace, Prempro)	Postmenopausal bone loss	Modest increase in bone density; reduction of spine and hip fractures by up to 30%	Increased risk of cardiovascular events; slight increase in breast cancer risk
SERMs (Evista, Nolvadex)	Postmenopausal bone loss	Modest increase in spine bone density; preservation of hip bone density; reduction of spine fractures by up to 50%; reduction of breast cancer risk and bad cholesterol	No effect on hip fractures
Synthetic hormone: calcitonin (Miacalcin, Calcimar)	Postmenopausal osteoporosis	Modest increase in spine bone density; reduction of spine fractures by up to 36%	No effect on hip bone density or fractures
Synthetic hormone: parathyroid hormone (Forteo)	Men and women with osteoporosis and high risk of fracture	Potentially large increase in spine bone density (8%-10%)	Little to no effect on hip bone density; ability to reduce hip or spine fractures not tested

The most studied is raloxifene (brand name, Evista). Its overall effect is more modest than that of bisphosphonates, and its effect on nonvertebral fractures such as those of the hip have not been marked. For this reason, it is recommended for women with milder osteoporosis or for those with osteoporosis primarily in the spine.

Because each person's health history is unique, your choice of medication should be made with your health care provider in light of your total health situation. Table 19.4 lists the pros and cons of common osteoporosis medications.

- - - -

Osteoporosis is a progressive weakening of the skeleton that makes bones more breakable. Osteoporosis is referred to as the silent disease because bone loss is not painful and produces no noticeable symptoms, but a bone density test can easily diagnose osteoporosis and also determine the risk of osteoporosis before it develops. Depending on the diagnosis, medication may be recommended. Many factors contribute to the health of the skeleton, and many of these are under your control, such as diet and physical activity. A bone-healthy diet includes sufficient calcium and vitamin D from dietary sources, brought up to recommended levels with supplements if necessary. Everyone should engage in bone-healthy exercise, but especially women and men who are concerned about their risk of fracture. Because bone benefits from exercise are lost when you stop training, your commitment to exercise that targets the bones must be lifelong.

References

Chapter 1

1. American College of Sports Medicine. *ACSM's Guidelines for Exercise Testing and Prescription*. 8th ed. Philadelphia (PA): Lippincott Williams & Wilkins; 2010. 380 p.

2. American College of Sports Medicine. *ACSM's Resource Manual for Guidelines for Exercise Testing and Prescription*. 6th ed. Philadelphia (PA): Lippincott Williams & Wilkins; 2010. 868 p.

3. Blumenthal JA, Hart A, Sherwood A, et al. Depression and vascular function in older adults. Evaluating the benefits of exercise in a new study at Duke University. *North Carolina Medical Journal*. 2001;62(2):95-8.

4. Centers for Disease Control and Prevention Web site [Internet]. United States: Centers for Disease Control and Prevention; [cited 2010 February 1]. Available from: http://www.cdc.gov

5. Christmas C, Andersen RA. Exercise and older patients: guidelines for the clinician. *Journal of the American Geriatrics Society*. 2000;48(3):318-24.

6. Landers DM. The influence of exercise on mental health. [cited 2009 December 9]. *President's Council on Physical Fitness and Sports*. Available from: http://www.fitness.gov/mentalhealth.htm.

7. Long BC, Van Stavel R. Effects of exercise training on anxiety: a meta-analysis. *Journal of Applied Sport Psychology*. 1995;7:167-189.

8. Milani RV, Lavie CJ. Reducing psychosocial stress: a novel mechanism of improving survival from exercise training. *American Journal of Medicine*. 2009;122(10):931-8.

9. Mosca L, Manson JE, Sutherland SE, Langer RD, Manolio T, Barrett-Conner E. Cardiovascular disease in women: a statement for healthcare professionals from the American Heart Association. *Circulation*. 1997;96:2468-2482.

10. National Association for Sport and Physical Education. *Physical Activity for Children: A Statement of Guidelines*. 2nd ed. Reston (VA): AAHPERD Publications; 2004. 26 p.

11. National Institute of Mental Health Web site [Internet]. United States; [cited 2010 February 10]. Available from: http://www.nimh.nih.gov.

12. National Institute on Aging. *Exercise: A Guide from the National Institute on Aging*. Washington DC; National Institute on Aging; 2001; NIH Publication No. 01-4258.

13. Paluska SA, Schwenk TL. Physical activity and mental health: current concepts. *Sports Medicine*. 2000;29(3):167-80.

14. Penedo FJ, Dahn JR. Exercise and well-being: a review of mental and physical health benefits associated with physical activity. *Current Opinion of Psychiatry*. 2005;18(2):189-93.

15. Trivedi MH, Greer RL, Grannemann BD, Chambliss HO, Jordan AD. Exercise as an augmentation strategy for treatment of major depression. *Journal of Psychiatric Medicine*. 2006;12(4):205-13.

16. U.S. Department of Health and Human Services Web site [Internet]. *Healthy People 2010*; [cited 2010 January 15]. Available from: http://www.healthypeople.gov.

17. U.S. Department of Health and Human Services Web site [Internet]. *Physical Activity and Health: A Report of the Surgeon General*. Atlanta (GA): U.S. Department of Health and Human Services; 1996. [cited 2010 January 1]. Available from: http://www.cdc.gov/nccdphp/sgr/index.htm.

18. U.S. Department of Health and Human Services Web site [Internet]. *2008 Physical Activity Guidelines for Americans*. Atlanta (GA): USDHHS; [cited 2010 January 1]. Available from: http://www.health.gov/paguidelines.

Chapter 2

1. American College of Sports Medicine. *ACSM's Guidelines for Exercise Testing and Prescription* (8th ed). Baltimore MD: Lippincott Williams & Wilkins; 2010, 380 p.

2. Beam WC, Adams GM. *Exercise Physiology Laboratory Manual* 6th ed. New York NY: McGraw-Hill, 2011, 306 p.

3. Cooper Institute. *FITNESSGRAM/ACTIVITYGRAM Test Administration Manual*. 3rd ed. Meredith MD, Welk GJ, editors. Champaign, IL: Human Kinetics; 2004, 134 p.

4. Rikli RE, Jones CJ. *Senior Fitness Test Manual*. Champaign, IL: Human Kinetics; 2001. 161 p.

Chapter 3

1. American College of Sports Medicine. *ACSM's Guidelines for Exercise Testing and Prescription*. 8th ed. Philadelphia (PA): Lippincott Williams & Wilkins; 2010. 380 p.

2. American College of Sports Medicine. *ACSM's Resource Manual for Guidelines for Exercise Testing and Prescription*. 6th ed. Philadelphia (PA): Lippincott Williams & Wilkins; 2010. 868 p.

3. American College of Sports Medicine. *ACSM's Resources for the Personal Trainer*. 3rd ed. Philadelphia (PA): Lippincott Williams & Wilkins; 2010. 544 p.

4. American College of Sports Medicine Strategic Health Initiative on Aging. *Five Easy Steps to Beginning Strength Exercises*. [Internet] Indianapolis (IN): American College of Sports Medicine; [cited 2010 December 8]. Available from: http://www.agingblueprint.org/PDFs/Beginning_Strength_Exercise.pdf.

5. U.S. Department of Health and Human Services Web site [Internet]. *2008 Physical Activity Guidelines for Americans*. Atlanta (GA): USDHHS; [cited 2010 January 1]. Available from: http://www.health.gov/paguidelines

Chapter 4

1. American College of Sports Medicine. *ACSM's Resource Manual for Guidelines for Exercise Testing and Prescription*. 6th ed. Philadelphia (PA): Lippincott Williams & Wilkins; 2010; 868 p.

2. American College of Sports Medicine, American Dietetic Association, and Dietitians of Canada. Position Stand: Nutrition and athletic performance. *Med Sci Sports Exerc*. 2009;41:709-731.

3. American Heart Association Web site [Internet]. *Heart Disease and Stroke Statistics – 2007 Update At-a-Glance*. [cited 2010 May 26]. Available from http://www.americanheart.org/downloadable/heart/1166712318459HS_StatsInsideText.pdf.

4. Casa DJ, Armstrong LE, Hillman SK, et al. National Athletic Trainers' Association position statement: fluid replacement for athletes. *J Athl Train*. 2000;35(2):212–224.

5. Curhan GC, Willett WC, Speizer FE, Spiegelman D, Stampfer MJ. Comparison of dietary calcium with supplemental calcium and other nutrients as factors affecting the risk for kidney stones in women. *Ann Int Med*. 1997;126:497-504.

6. Curhan GC, Willett WC, Speizer FE, Stampfer MJ. Beverage use and risk for kidney stones in women. *Ann Int Med.* 1999;128:534-540.

7. Daily Weight Loss Tips. *High Carbohydrates Food Table.* [cited 2010 May 26]. Available from http://www.dailyweightlosstips.net/high-carbohydrate-foods-table/.

8. Flegal KM, Carroll MD, Ogden CL, Curtin LR. Prevalence and trends in obesity among US Adults, 1999-2008. *JAMA.* 2010;303(3):235-241.

9. Food and Nutrition Board of the Institute of Medicine. Dietary Reference Intakes for Water, Potassium, Sodium, Chloride, and Sulfate. Washington, DC: National Academy Press; 2005.

10. Food and Nutrition Board of the Institute of Medicine. Dietary Reference Intakes for Energy, Carbohydrate, Fiber, Fat, Fatty acids, Cholesterol, Protein, and Amino Acids. Washington, DC: National Academy Press; 2005.

11. Food and Nutrition Board of the Institute of Medicine Web site [Internet]. Dietary Reference Intakes. Washington, DC: National Academy Press; [cited 2010 May 29]. Available from: http://iom.edu/en/Global/News%20Announcements/~/media/Files/Activity%20Files/Nutrition/DRIs/DRISummaryListing2.ashx.

12. Hamada K, Doi T, Sakura M, et al. Effects of hydration on fluid balance and lower-extremity blood viscosity during long airplane flights. *JAMA.* 2002;287:844-845.

13. Harris J, Benedict F. A biometric study of basal metabolism in man. Washington, DC. Carnegie Institute of Washington. 1919. Publication no. 279.

14. Hulston CJ, Jeukendrup AE. No placebo effect from carbohydrate intake during prolonged exercise. *Int J Sport Nutr Exerc Metab.* 2009;19(3):275-284.

15. Jones JM, Anderson JW. Grain foods and health: a primer for clinicians. *Phys Sportsmed.* 2008;36(1):18-33.

16. Math MV, Rampal PM, Faure XR, Delmont JP. Gallbladder emptying after drinking water and its possible role in prevention of gallstone formation. *Singapor Med J.* 1986;27;531-532.

17. Maughan RJ, Dargavel LA, Hares R, Shirreffs SM. Water and salt balance of well-trained swimmers in training. *Int J Sport Nutr Exerc Metab.* 2009;19(6):598-606.

18. McGinnis JM, Foege WH. Actual causes of death in the United States. *JAMA.* 1993; 270(18):2207-2212.

19. Mifflin MD, St Jeor ST, Hill LA, Scott BJ, Daughterty SA, Koh YO. A new predictive equation for resting energy expenditure in health individuals. *Am J Clin Nutr.* 1990;51:241-247.

20. Minino A, Smith L. National Center for Health statistics, Centers for Disease Control and Prevention, U.S. Department of Health and Human Services. Deaths: preliminary data for 2000. *National Vital Statistics Report*, October 9, 2001, 49(12).

21. National Osteoporosis Foundation Web site [Internet]. *What is Osteoporosis?* Washington (DC):National Osteoporosis Foundation; [cited 2010 May 26]. Available from http://www.nof.org/.

22. Ogden CL, Carroll MD, Curtin LR, Lamb MM, Flegal KM. Prevalence of high body mass index in US children and adolescents, 2007-2008. *JAMA.* 2010;303(3):242-249.

23. Pereira MA, Kottke TE, Jordan C, O'Connor PJ, Pronk NP, Carreón R. Preventing and managing cardiometabolic risk: the logic for intervention. *Int J Environ Res Public Health.* 2009;6(10):2568-84. Epub 2009 Sep 30.

24. Sawka MN, Burke LM, Eichner ER, Maughan RJ, Montain SJ. Stachenfield NS. American College of Sports Medicine position stand: exercise and fluid replacement. *Med Sci Sports Exerc* 2007;39(2):377–390.

25. Slattery ML, Caan BJ, Anderson KE, Potter JD. Intake of fluids and methylxantine-containing beverages: association with colon cancer. *In J Cancer.* 1999;81:199-204.

26. U.S. Department of Health and Human Services Web site [Internet]. *Dietary Guidelines for Americans.* Atlanta (GA):USDHHS; [cited 2010 May 26]. Available from http://www.health.gov/dietaryguidelines/dga2005/default.htm#2.

27. U.S. Department of Health and Human Services Web site [Internet]. *How to Understand and Use the Nutrition Facts Label.* Atlanta (GA):USDHHS; [cited 2010 May 26]. Available from http://www.fda.gov/Food/LabelingNutrition/ConsumerInformation/ucm078889.htm.

28. U.S. Department of Health and Human Services and the U.S. Department of Agriculture Web site [Internet]. *Dietary Guidelines for Americans 2010* and *Report of the Dietary Guidelines Advisory Committee on the Dietary Guidelines for Americans 2010.* [cited 2011 February 1]. Available from: http://www.cnpp.usda.gov/DietaryGuidelines.htm.

29. Williams MH. *Nutrition for Health, Fitness, & Sport.* 8th ed. New York (NY): McGraw Hill; 2007. 574 p.

Chapter 5

1. American Association for Health/American Alliance for Health, Physical Education, Recreation and Dance. Report of the 2000 Joint Committee on Health Education and Promotion Terminology. *Journal of School Health.* 2000;72:3-7.

2. Anspaugh DJ, Hamrick MH, Rosato FD. *Wellness: Concepts and Applications.* 7th ed. New York: McGraw Hill; 2009, 537 p.

3. Baumeister RF, Heatherton TF, Tice DM. *Losing Control: How and Why People Fail at Self-regulation.* San Diego: Academic Press; 1994. 307 p.

4. Cohen S, Doyle WJ, Alper CM, Janicki-Deverts D, Turner RB. Sleep habits and susceptibility to the common cold. *Arch Intern Med.* 2009;169(1):62-7.

5. Deci EL, Ryan RM. *Handbook of Self-determination Research.* Rochester (NY): University of Rochester Press; 2002. 470 p.

6. Moyna NM, Robertson RJ, Meckes CL, Peoples JA, Millich NB, Thompson PD. Intermodal comparison of energy expenditure at exercise intensities corresponding to the perceptual preference range *Med Sci Sports Exerc.* 2001;33(8):1404-10.

7. National Sleep Foundation site [Internet]. Washington: National Sleep Foundation; [cited 2010 Apr 1]. Available from: http://www.sleepfoundation.org.

8. The Hormone Foundation site [Internet]. Chevey Chase (MD): The Hormone Foundation; [cited 2010 Apr 1]. Available from: http://www.hormone.org.

9. U.S. Department of Health and Human Services. *Survey on Drug Use and Health.* Ann Arbor, MI: U.S. Department of Health and Human Services, Office of Applied Studies; 2008. Available from U.S. GPO, Washington.

Chapter 6

1. American College of Sports Medicine. *ACSM's Guidelines for Exercise Testing and Prescription.* 8th ed. Philadelphia (PA): Lippincott Williams & Wilkins; 2010. 380 p.

2. American College of Sports Medicine. *ACSM's Resource Manual for Guidelines for Exercise Testing and Prescription.* 6th ed. Philadelphia (PA): Lippincott Williams & Wilkins; 2010. 868 p.

3. U.S. Department of Health and Human Services Web site [Internet]. *2008 Physical Activity Guidelines for Americans.* Atlanta (GA):USDHHS; [cited 2010 January 1]. Available from: http://www.health.gov/paguidelines.

Chapter 7

1. American College of Sports Medicine. *ACSM's Guidelines for Exercise Testing and Prescription.* 8th ed. Baltimore, MD: Lippincott, Williams and Wilkins, 2010. 380p.

2. Brill PA, Macera CA, Davis DR, Blair SN, Gordon N. Muscular strength and physical function. *Medicine and Science in Sports and Exercise.* 2000;32:412-416.

3. Chodzko-Zajko W, Proctor D, Fiatarone Singh M, Minson C, Nigg C, Salem G, Skinner J. American College of Sports Medicine postion stand. Exercise and physical activity for older adults. *Medicine and Science in Sports and Exercise.* 2009;41:1510-1530.

4. Guadalupe-Grau A, Fuentes T, Guerra B, Calbet A. Exercise and bone mass in adults. *Sports Medicine.* 2009;39:439-468.

5. Kraemer WJ, Ratamess NA. Fundamentals of resistance training: progression and exercise prescription. *Medicine and Science in Sports and Exercise.* 2004;36:674-688.

6. Kraemer WJ, Ratamess NA, French DN. Resistance training for health and performance. *Curr Sports Medicine Reports.* 2002;1:165-171.

7. Krieger J. Single versus multiple sets of resistance exercise: a meta-regression. *Journal of Strength and Conditioning Research.* 2009;23:1890-1901.

8. Mazzetti SA, Kraemer WJ, Volek JS, et al. The influence of direct supervision of resistance training on strength performance. *Medince and Science in Sports and Exercise.* 2000;32:1175-1184.

9. Myer G, Quatman C, Khoury J, Wall E, Hewett T. Youth vs. adult "weightlifting" injuries presented to United States emergency rooms: accidental vs. non-accidental injury mechanisms. *Journal of Strength and Conditioning Research.* 2009;23:2054-2060.

10. Ratamess N, Alvar B, Evetoch T, Housh T, Kibler WB, Kraemer WJ, Triplett T. Progression models in resistance training in healthy adults. *Medicine and Science in Sports and Exercise.* 2009;41:687-708.

11. Ratamess NA, Faigenbaum AD, Hoffman JR, Kang J. Self-selected resistance training intensity in healthy women: the influence of a personal trainer. *Journal of Strength and Conditioning Research.* 2008;22:103-111.

12. Rhea M, Alavar B, Burkett LN, Ball S. A meta-analysis to determine the dose response for strength development. *Medicine and Science in Sports and Exercise.* 2003;35:456-464.

13. Ruiz J, Sui X, Lobelo F, et al. Association between muscular strength and mortality in men: prospective cohort study. *British Medical Journal.* 2008;337:92-95.

14. Steib S, Schoene D, Pfeifer K. Dose-response relationship of resistance training in older adults: a meta-analysis. *Medicine and Science in Sports and Exercise.* 2010;42(5):902.

15. U.S. Department of Health and Human Services Web site [Internet]. *2008 Physical Activity Guidelines for Americans.* Atlanta (GA):USDHHS; [cited 2010 January 1]. Available from: http://www.health.gov/paguidelines.

16. Weinsier R, Schutz Y, Bracco D. Reexamination of the relationship of resting metabolic rate to fat-free mass and to the metabolically active components of fat-free mass in humans. *American Journal of Clinical Nutrition.* 1992;55:790-794.

17. Williams MA, Haskell WL, Ades PA, et al. Resistance exercise in individuals with and without cardiovascular disease: 2007 update. *Circulation.* 2007;116:572-584.

Chapter 8

1. Alter, M.J. *Science of Flexibility.* 2nd ed. Champaign, IL: Human Kinetics; 1996. 372 p.

2. American College of Sports Medicine. *ACSM's Guidelines for Exercise Testing and Prescription.* 8th ed. Baltimore (MD): Lippincott Williams & Wilkins; 2010. 380 p.

3. American College of Sports Medicine. *ACSM's Resource Manual for Guidelines for Exercise Testing and Prescription.* 6th ed. Baltimore (MD): Lippincott Williams & Wilkins; 2010. 868 p.

4. American College of Sports Medicine. *ACSM's Resources for the Personal Trainer.* 3rd ed. Baltimore (MD): Lippincott Williams & Wilkins; 2009. 544 p.

5. American College of Sports Medicine. Position stand: the recommended quantity and quality of exercise for developing and maintaining cardiorespiratory and muscular fitness, and flexibility in healthy adults. *Med Sci Sports Exerc.* 1998; 30:975–991.

6. Andersen JC. Flexibility in performance: foundational concepts and practical issues. *Athletic Therapy Today.* 2006;11(3):9-12.

7. Doriot N, Wang X. Effects of age and gender on maximum voluntary range of motion on upper body joints. *Ergonomics.* 2006;49(3):269-281.

8. Haff GG. Roundtable discussion. Flexibility training. *Strength and Conditioning Journal.* 2006;28(2):64-85.

9. Rose D. *Fallproof.* 2nd ed. Champaign (IL): Human Kinetics; 2010, 328 p.

10. U.S. Department of Health and Human Services Web site [Internet]. *2008 Physical Activity Guidelines for Americans.* Atlanta (GA):USDHHS; [cited 2010 January 1]. Available from: http://www.health.gov/paguidelines.

Chapter 9

1. Adolph KE, Joh AS. Motor development: how infants get into the act. In: Slater A, Lewis M, editors. *Introduction to Infant Development.* New York: Oxford University Press; 2007, p. 63-80.

2. American College of Sports Medicine. *ACSM's Guidelines for Exercise Testing and Prescription.* 8th ed. Philadelphia (PA): Lippincott Williams & Wilkins; 2010. 380 p.

3. American College of Sports Medicine. *ACSM's Resource Manual for Guidelines for Exercise Testing and Prescription.* 6th ed. Philadelphia (PA): Lippincott Williams & Wilkins; 2010. 868 p.

4. Behm DG, Faigenbaum AD, Falk B, Klentrou P. Canadian Society for Exercise Physiology position paper: resistance training in children and adolescents. *Appl Physiol Nutr Metab.* 2008;33:547-561.

5. Centers for Disease Control and Prevention. Youth risk behavior surveillance—United States, 2007. *MMWR.* 2008;57,SS-4.

6. Centers for Disease Control and Prevention Web site [Internet]. Atlanta (GA): Centers for Disease Control; [cited 2010 May 15]. Available from: http://www.cdc.gov/obesity/childhood/index.html.

7. Faigenbaum AD, Micheli LJ. Youth strength training. ACSM current comment [Internet]. [cited 3 June 2010]. Available at: http://www.acsm.org/AM/Template.cfm?Section=Current_Comments1.

8. Ferraro KF, Thorpe RJ, Wilkinson JA. The life course of severe obesity: does childhood overweight matter? *J Gerontol.* 2003:58B(2):S110-S9.

9. Freedman DS, Khan LK, Dietz WH, Srinivasan SR, Berenson GS. Relationship of childhood obesity to coronary heart disease risk factors in adulthood: the Bogalusa Study. *Pediatrics.* 2001;108(3):712-8.

10. Giddings SS, Dennison BA, Birch LL, et al. Dietary recommendations for children and adolescents: a guide for practitioners. Consensus statement from the American Heart Association. *Circulation.* 2005;112:2-61-2075.

11. Haskell WL, Lee I-M, Pate RR, et al. Physical activity and public health: updated recommendation for adults from

the American College of Sports Medicine and the American Heart Association. *Med Sci Sports Exerc.* 2007;39:1423-34.

12. MacKelvie KJ, Khan KM, McKay HA. Is there a critical period for bone response to weight-bearing exercise in children and adolescents? a systematic review. *Br J Sports Med.* 2002;36:250-57.

13. National Association for Sport and Physical Education. *Active Start: A Statement of Physical Activity Guidelines for Children from Birth to Five Years.* 1st ed. Reston (VA): National Association for Sport and Physical Education; 2002.

14. National Association for Sport and Physical Education. *Active Start: A Statement of Physical Activity Guidelines for Children from Birth to Five years.* 2nd ed. Reston (VA): National Association for Sport and Physical Education; 2009.

15. National Association for Sport and Physical Education. *Physical Activity for Children: A Statement of Guidelines* 2nd ed. Reston (VA): National Association for Sport and Physical Education; 2004.

16. Ogden CL, Carroll MD, Flegal KM. High body mass index for age among U.S. children and adolescents 2003-2006. *JAMA.* 2008;299(20):2401-5.

17. Telema R. Tracking of physical activity from childhood to adulthood: a review. *Obes Facts.* 2009;3:187-95.

18. Thune I, Furberg A-S. Physical activity and cancer risk: dose-response and cancer, all sites, and site-specific. *Med Sci Sports Exerc.* 2001;33(Supp 6):S530-50.

19. Strong WB, Malina RM, Blimke CJR, et al. Evidence based physical activity for school-aged youth. *J Pediatr.* 2005;146:732-7.

20. U.S. Department of Agriculture Web site [Internet]. Alexandria (VA): US Department of Agriculture; [cited 2010 June 2] Available from: www.mypyramid.gov.

21. U.S. Department of Health and Human Services Web site [Internet]. *2008 Physical Activity Guidelines for Americans.* Atlanta (GA):USDHHS; [cited 2010 January 1]. Available from: http://www.health.gov/paguidelines

22. U.S. Department of Health and Human Services and the U.S. Department of Agriculture Web site [Internet]. *Dietary Guidelines for Americans 2010* and *Report of the Dietary Guidelines Advisory Committee on the Dietary Guidelines for Americans 2010.* [cited 2011 February 1]. Available from: http://www.cnpp.usda.gov/DietaryGuidelines.htm.

Chapter 10

1. American College of Sports Medicine. *ACSM's Guidelines for Exercise Testing and Prescription.* 8th ed. Philadelphia (PA): Lippincott Williams & Wilkins; 2010. 380 p.

2. American College of Sports Medicine. *ACSM's Resource Manual for Guidelines for Exercise Testing and Prescription.* 6th ed. Philadelphia (PA): Lippincott Williams & Wilkins; 2010. 868 p.

3. U.S. Department of Health and Human Services Web site [Internet]. *Dietary Guidelines for Americans.* Atlanta (GA):USDHHS; [cited 2010 January 4]. Available from http://www.health.gov/dietaryguidelines/dga2005/default.htm#2.

4. U.S. Department of Health and Human Services Web site [Internet]. *2008 Physical Activity Guidelines for Americans.* Atlanta (GA):USDHHS; [cited 2010 January 1]. Available from: http://www.health.gov/paguidelines.

5. U.S. Department of Health and Human Services and the U.S. Department of Agriculture Web site [Internet]. *Dietary Guidelines for Americans 2010* and *Report of the Dietary Guidelines Advisory Committee on the Dietary Guidelines for Americans 2010.* [cited 2011 February 1]. Available from: http://www.cnpp.usda.gov/DietaryGuidelines.htm.

Chapter 11

1. Abbott RD, White LR, Ross GW, Masaki KH, Curb JD, Petrovitch H. Walking and dementia in physically capable elderly men. *JAMA.* 2004;292:1447-1453.

2. American College of Rheumatology. Recommendations for the medical management of osteoarthritis of the hip and knee: 2000 update. In *Arthritis Rheum*, edited by Guidelines. ACoRSoO. 2000, p. 1905-1915.

3. American Geriatrics Society. Exercise prescription for older adults with osteoarthritis pain: consensus practice recommendations. A supplement to the AGS clinical practice guidelines on the management of chronic pain in older adults. *Journal of the American Geriatrics Society.* 2001;49(6):808-823.

4. American Geriatrics Society. The management of persistent pain in older persons. *Journal of the American Geriatrics Society.* 2002;50(6 Suppl):S205-224.

5. Asia Pacific COPE Roundtable Group. *Global Strategy for the Diagnosis, Management, and Prevention of Chronic Obstructive Pulmonary Disease.* Edited by National Heart L, and Blood Institute, Bethesda, MD; 2001.

6. Beach LM, Tennant LK. Personal importance, motivation, and performance of older adults. *Perceptual and Motor Skills.* 1992;74:543-546.

7. Beattie BL, Whitelaw N, Mettler M, Turner D. A vision for older adults and health promotion. *Am J Health Promot.* 2003;18:200-204.

8. Bennett GG, McNeill LH, Wolin KY, Duncan DT, Puleo E, Emmons KM. Safe to walk? Neighborhood safety and physical activity among public housing residents. *PLoS Medicine.* 2007;4:1599-1607.

9. Brewer HB, Jr. New features of the National Cholesterol Education Program Adult Treatment Panel III lipid-lowering guidelines. *Clinical Cardiology.* 2003;26:III19-24.

10. Brignole M, Alboni P, Benditt D, et al. Guidelines on management (diagnosis and treatment) of syncope. *European HeartvJournal* 2001;22:1256-1306.

11. Brosse AL, Sheets ES, Lett HS, Blumenthal JA. Exercise and the treatment of clinical depression in adults: recent findings and future directions. *Sports Medicine* (Auckland, NZ). 2002;32:741-760.

12. Chobanian AV, Bakris GL, Black HR, et al. The seventh report of the Joint National Committee on prevention, detection, evaluation, and treatment of high blood pressure: the JNC 7 report. *JAMA.* 2003;289:2560-2572.

13. Chodzko-Zajko WJ, Proctor DN, Fiatarone Singh MA, et al. American College of Sports Medicine position stand. Exercise and physical activity for older adults. *Medicine and Science in Sports and Exercise.* 2009;41:1510-1530.

14. Doody RS, Stevens JC, Beck C, et al. Practice parameter: management of dementia (an evidence-based review). Report of the Quality Standards Subcommittee of the American Academy of Neurology. *Neurology.* 2001;56:1154-1166.

15. Fletcher GF, Balady GJ, Amsterdam EA, et al. Exercise standards for testing and training: a statement for healthcare professionals from the American Heart Association. *Circulation.* 2001;104:1694-1740.

16. Going S, Lohman T, Houtkooper L, et al. Effects of exercise on bone mineral density in calcium-replete postmenopausal women with and without hormone replacement therapy. *Osteoporos Int.* 2003;14:637-643.

17. Gordon NF, Gulanick M, Costa F, et al. Physical activity and exercise recommendations for stroke survivors: an American Heart Association scientific statement from the Council on Clinical Cardiology, Subcommittee on Exercise, Cardiac Rehabilitation, and Prevention; the Council on

Cardiovascular Nursing; the Council on Nutrition, Physical Activity, and Metabolism; and the Stroke Council. *Stroke.* 2004;35:1230-1240.

18. Haber D, Looney C. Health contract calendars: a tool for health professionals with older adults. *Gerontologist.* 2000;20(2):235-239.

19. Hagen KB, Hilde G, Jamtvedt G, Winnem MF. The Cochrane review of bed rest for acute low back pain and sciatica. *Spine.* 2000;25:2932-2939.

20. Keysor JJ. Does late-life physical activity or exercise prevent or minimize disablement? A critical review of the scientific evidence. *American Journal of Preventive Medicine.* 2003;25:129-136.

21. King AC, Oman RF, Brassington GS, Bliwise DL, Haskell WL. Moderate-intensity exercise and self-rated quality of sleep in older adults. A randomized controlled trial. *JAMA.* 1997;277:32-37.

22. Kunzmann U, Little T, Smith J. Perceived control: A double-edged sword in old age. *Journal Gerontology: Psychological Sciences.* 2002;57B(6):484-491.

23. Larson EB, Wang L, Bowen JD, McCormick WC, Teri L, Crane P, Kukull W. Exercise is associated with reduced risk for incident dementia among persons 65 years of age and older. *Annals of Internal Medicine.* 2006;144:73-81.

24. Locke GR, 3rd, Pemberton JH, Phillips SF. American Gastroenterological Association medical position statement: guidelines on constipation. *Gastroenterology.* 2000;119:1761-1766.

25. McDermott MM, Liu K, Ferrucci L, et al. Physical performance in peripheral arterial disease: a slower rate of decline in patients who walk more. *Annals of Internal Medicine.* 2006;144:10-20.

26. Neff K, King A. Exercise program adherence in older adults: the importance of achieving one's expected benefits. *Medical Exercise Nutrition and Health.* 1995;4:355-362.

27. Nelson ME, Rejeski WJ, Blair SN, et al. Physical activity and public health in older adults: recommendation from the American College of Sports Medicine and the American Heart Association. *Circulation.* 2007;116:1094-1105.

28. Oka R, King A. Sources of social support as predictors of exercise adherence in women and men age 50 to 65 years. *Women Health Research Gender Behavior Policy.*1995;1:161-175.

29. Penninx BW, Messier SP, Rejeski WJ, et al. Physical exercise and the prevention of disability in activities of daily living in older persons with osteoarthritis. *Archives of Internal Medicine.* 2001;161:2309-2316.

30. Pescatello LS, Franklin BA, Fagard R, Farquhar WB, Kelley GA, Ray CA. American College of Sports Medicine position stand. Exercise and hypertension. *Medicine and Science in Sports and Exercise.* 2004;36:533-553.

31. Pollock ML, Franklin BA, Balady GJ, et al. AHA Science Advisory. Resistance exercise in individuals with and without cardiovascular disease: benefits, rationale, safety, and prescription: An advisory from the Committee on Exercise, Rehabilitation, and Prevention, Council on Clinical Cardiology, American Heart Association; Position paper endorsed by the American College of Sports Medicine. *Circulation.* 2000;101:828-833.

32. Remme WJ, Swedberg K. Guidelines for the diagnosis and treatment of chronic heart failure. *European Heart Journal.* 2001;22:1527-1560.

33. Resnick B, Ory MG, Hora K, et al. A proposal for a new screening paradigm and tool called Exercise Assessment and Screening for You (EASY). *Journal of Aging and Physical Activity.* 2008;16:215-233.

34. Sigal RJ, Kenny GP, Wasserman DH, Castaneda-Sceppa C, White RD. Physical activity/exercise and type 2 diabetes: a consensus statement from the American Diabetes Association. *Diabetes Care.* 2006;29:1433-1438.

35. Singh MA. Exercise to prevent and treat functional disability. *Clinics in Geriatric Medicine.* 2002;18:431-462, vi-vii.

36. Singh NA, Clements KM, Fiatarone MA. A randomized controlled trial of the effect of exercise on sleep. *Sleep.* 1997;20:95-101.

37. Stewart AL. Community-based physical activity programs for adults age 50 and older. *Journal Aging Physical Activity.* 2001;9:S71-S91.

38. Stewart KJ, Hiatt WR, Regensteiner JG, Hirsch AT. Exercise training for claudication. *New England Journal of Medicine.* 2002;347:1941-1951.

39. Thompson PD, Buchner D, Pina IL, et al. Exercise and physical activity in the prevention and treatment of atherosclerotic cardiovascular disease: a statement from the Council on Clinical Cardiology (Subcommittee on Exercise, Rehabilitation, and Prevention) and the Council on Nutrition, Physical Activity, and Metabolism (Subcommittee on Physical Activity). *Circulation.* 2003;107:3109-3116.

40. U.S. Department of Health and Human Services Web site [Internet]. *2008 Physical Activity Guidelines for Americans.* Atlanta (GA):USDHHS; [cited 2010 January 1]. Available from: http://www.health.gov/paguidelines.

41. U.S. Department of Health and Human Services Web site [Internet]. *Administration on Aging: Evidence-Based Disease and Disability Prevention Program (EBDDP).* Atlanta (GA):USDHHS; [cited 2010 January 27]. Available from http://www.aoa.gov/AoARoot/AoA_Programs/HPW/Evidence_Based/index.aspx.

42. U.S. Department of Health and Human Services Web site [Internet]. *Be Active Your Way: A Guide for Adults.* Atlanta (GA):USDHHS. [cited 2010 January 1]. Available from http://www.health.gov/paguidelines/adultguide/default.aspx.

43. U.S. Department of Health and Human Services Web site [Internet]. *Dietary Guidelines for Americans.* Atlanta (GA):USDHHS; [cited 2010 January 27]. Available from http://www.health.gov/dietaryguidelines/dga2005/default.htm#2.

44. U.S. Department of Health and Human Services and the U.S. Department of Agriculture Web site [Internet]. *Dietary Guidelines for Americans 2010* and *Report of the Dietary Guidelines Advisory Committee on the Dietary Guidelines for Americans 2010.* [cited 2011 February 1]. Available from: http://www.cnpp.usda.gov/DietaryGuidelines.htm.

45. U.S. Preventive Services Task Force. Screening for obesity in adults: recommendations and rationale. *Annals of Internal Medicine.* 2003;139(11):930-932.

46. Weuve J, Kang JH, Manson JE, Breteler MM, Ware JH, Grodstein F. Physical activity, including walking, and cognitive function in older women. *JAMA.* 2004;292:1454-1461.

47. WHO. The Heidelberg Guidelines for Promoting Physical Activity Among Older Persons. Geneva: World Health Organization, 1996.

Chapter 12

1. American College of Sports Medicine. American College of Sports Medicine position stand: The recommended quantity and quality of exercise for developing and maintaining cardiorespiratory and muscular fitness, and flexibility in healthy adults. *Med Sci Sports Exerc.* 1998;30:975-91.

2. American College of Sports Medicine. *ACSM's Guidelines for Exercise Testing and Prescription.* 8th ed. Baltimore (MD): Lippincott Williams &Wilkins; 2010. 380 p.

3. American College of Sports Medicine. *ACSM's Resource Manual for Guidelines for Exercise Testing and Prescription.* 6th ed. Baltimore (MD): Lippincott, Williams & Wilkins; 2010. 868 p.

4. American Diabetes Association. Position statement. Standards of medical care in diabetes—2007. *Diabetes Care.* 2007;30:S4-S41.

5. American Heart Association Web site. [Internet]. Dallas (TX): American Heart Association; [cited 2010 June 16]. Available from: http://www.americanheart.org.

6. American Heart Association Web site. [Internet]. Dallas (TX): American Heart Association; [cited 2010 August 4]. Available from: http://www.heart.org/HEARTORG/.

7. Cucherat M. Quantitative relationship between resting heart rate reduction and magnitude of clinical benefits in post-myocardial infarction: a meta-regression of randomized clinical trials. *European Heart J.* 2007;28:3012-19.

8. Dalen JE. Aspirin to prevent heart attack and stroke: what's the right dose? *Am J Med.* 2006;119:198-202.

9. Dutcher JR, Kahn J, Grines C, Franklin B. Comparison of left ventricular ejection fraction and exercise capacity as predictors of two- and five-year mortality following acute myocardial infarction. *Am J Cardiol.* 2007;99:436-41.

10. Ernest CS, Worcester MUC, Tatoulis J, et al. Neurocognitive outcomes in off-pump versus on-pump bypass surgery: a randomized controlled trial. *Ann Thorac Surg.* 2006;81:2105-14.

11. Expert Panel on the Identification, Evaluation, and Treatment of Overweight and Obesity in Adults. Executive summary of the clinical guidelines on the identification, evaluation, and treatment of overweight and obesity in adults. *Arch Intern Med.* 1998;158:1855-67.

12. Falk E, Shah PK, Fuster V. Coronary plaque disruption. *Circulation.* 1995;92:657-71.

13. Ford ES, Ajani UA, Croft JB, et al. Explaining the decrease in U.S. deaths from coronary disease, 1980-2000. *N Engl J Med.* 2007;356:2388-98.

14. Franklin BA. What clients should know about the benefits—and risks—of aspirin therapy. *ACSM's Health & Fitness Journal.* 2001;5:19-22.

15. Franklin BA, Bonzheim K, Gordon S, Timmis GC. Snow shoveling: A trigger for acute myocardial infarction and sudden coronary death. *Am J Cardiol.* 1996;77: 855-8.

16. Franklin BA, Gordon NF. *Contemporary Diagnosis and Management in Cardiovascular Exercise.* Newtown (PA): Handbooks in Health Care, 2009.

17. Franklin BA, McCullough PA. Cardiorespiratory fitness: an independent and additive marker of risk stratification and health outcomes. *Mayo Clin Proc.* 2009;84:776-9.

18. Gao L, Taha R, Gauvin D, Othmen LB, Wang Y, Blaise G. Postoperative cognitive dysfunction after cardiac surgery. *Chest.* 2005;128: 3664-70.

19. Hausenloy DJ, Yellon DM. Targeting residual cardiovascular risk: raising high-density lipoprotein cholesterol levels. *Heart.* 2008;94:706-14.

20. Kodama S, Aaito K, Tanaka S, Maki M, Yachi Y, Asumi M, Sugawara A, Totsuka K, Shimano H, Ohashi Y, Yamada N, Sone H. Cardiorespiratory fitness as a quantitative predictor of all-cause mortality and cardiovascular events in healthy men and women. *JAMA.* 2009;301:2024-35.

21. Lichtenstein AH, Appel LJ, Brands M, et al. Summary of American Heart Association diet and lifestyle recommendations revision 2006. *Arterioscler Thromb Vasc Biol.* 2006;26:2186-91.

22. Little WC, Constantinescu M, Applegate RJ, et al. Can coronary angiography predict the site of a subsequent myocardial infarction in patients with mild-to-moderate coronary artery disease? *Circulation.* 1988;78:1157-66.

23. Lloyd-Jones D, Adams RJ, Brown TM, et al. on behalf of the American Heart Association Statistics Committee and Stroke Statistics Subcommittee. Heart disease and stroke statistics 2010 update: a report from the American Heart Association. *Circulation.* 2010;121:948-54.

24. Lloyd-Jones DM, Hong Y, Labarthe D, et al. on behalf of the American Heart Association Strategic Planning Task Force and Statistics Committee. Defining and setting national goals for cardiovascular health promotion and disease reduction. The American Heart Association's strategic impact goal through 2020 and beyond. *Circulation.* 2010;121:586-613.

25. Lloyd-Jones DM, Leip EP, Larson MG, et al. Prediction of lifetime risk for cardiovascular disease by risk factor burden at 50 years of age. *Circulation.* 2006;113:791-8.

26. McArdle WD, Katch FI, Katch VL. *Essentials of Exercise Physiology.* Vol. 1, 3rd ed. Baltimore: Lippincott Williams & Wilkins; 2005.

27. McCartney N, McKelvie RS, Martin J, Sale DG, MacDougall JD. Weight-training-induced attenuation of the circulatory response of older males to weight lifting. *J Appl Physiol.* 1993;74:1056-60.

28. Palmore EB. Predictors of the longevity difference: a 25-year follow-up. *Gerontologist.* 1982;22:513-8.

29. Sandmaier, M. United States Department of Health and Human Services. National Heart, Lung, and Blood Institute. Your guide to a healthy heart. NIH Publication No. 06-5269. December 2005. [Accessed June 16, 2010]. Available from: http://www.nhlbi.nih.gov/health/public/heart/other/your_guide/healthyheart.pdf.

30. Suaya JA, Stason WB, Ades PA, Normand S-LT, Shepard DS. Cardiac rehabilitation and survival in older coronary patients. *J Am Coll Cardiol.* 2009;54:25-33.

31. Thompson PD, Franklin BA, Balady GJ, et al. Exercise and acute cardiovascular events. Placing the risks into perspective. *Circulation.* 2007;115:2358-68.

32. U.S. Department of Health and Human Services. Your guide to lowering your blood pressure with DASH. NIH Publication No. 06-4082. Originally Printed 1998, Revised April 2006 [Accessed June 16, 2010]. Available from: http://www.nhlbi.nih.gov/health/public/heart/hbp/dash/new_dash.pdf.

33. U.S. Preventive Services Task Force. Aspirin for the prevention of cardiovascular disease: U.S. preventive services task force recommendation statement. *Ann Intern Med.* 2009;150:396-404.

34. Williams MA, Haskell WL, Ades PA, et al. Resistance exercise in individuals with and without cardiovascular disease: 2007 update. A scientific statement from the American Heart Association Council on Clinical Cardiology and Council on Nutrition, Physical Activity, and Metabolism. *Circulation.* 2007;116:572-84.

35. Williams PT. Physical fitness and activity as separate heart disease risk factors: a meta-analysis. *Med Sci Sports Exerc.* 2001;33:754-61.

Chapter 13

1. American College of Sports Medicine. *ACSM's Guidelines for Exercise Testing and Prescription.* 8th ed. Philadelphia (PA): Lippincott Williams & Wilkins; 2010. 380 p.

2. Centers for Disease Control and Prevention: Overweight and Obesity. 2010 [cited 2010 January 10]. Available from: http://www.cdc.gov/obesity/index/html.

3. Donnelly JE, Blair SN, Jakicic JM, Manore MM, Rankin JW, Smith BK. American College of Sports Medicine position stand. Appropriate physical activity intervention strategies for weight loss and prevention of weight regain for adults. *Med Sci Sports Exerc* 2009 Feb;41(2):459-71.

4. Seagle HM, Strain GW, Makris A, Reeves RS. Position of the American Dietetic Association: weight management. *J Am Diet Assoc* 2009;109(2):330-46.

5. Thompson JL, Manore MM, Vaughan LA. The role of nutrition in our health. In: *The Science of Nutrition*. San Fransisco: Pearson-Benjamin Cummings; 2008, p. 2-41.

6. Thompson JL, Manore MM, Vaughan LA. Achieving and maintaining a healthful body weight. In: *The Science of Nutrition*. San Francisco: Pearson-Benjamin Cummings; 2008. p. 526-71.

7. USDA. MyPyramid. 2010 [cited 2010 January 5]. Available from: http://www.mypyramid.gov.

8. United States Food and Drug Administration. 2010; [cited 2010 January 1]. Available from: http://www.fda.gov.

9. Wardlaw GM, Smith AM. Energy balance and weight control. In: *Contemporary Nutrition*. 7th ed. New York: McGraw-Hill; 2009. p. 234-79.

10. Wing R, Hill JO. National Weight Co*ntrol Registry*. 2010 [cited 2010 January 15]. Available from: http://www.nwcr.ws/.

Chapter 14

1. American College of Sports Medicine. *ACSM's Guidelines for Exercise Testing and Prescription*. 8th ed. Philadelphia (PA): Lippincott Williams & Wilkins; 2010, 380 p.

2. American College of Sports Medicine. *ACSM's Resource Manual for Guidelines for Exercise Testing and Prescription*. 6th ed. Philadelphia (PA): Lippincott Williams & Wilkins; 2010, 868 p.

3. American Diabetes Association. Position statement: diagnosis and classification of diabetes mellitus. *Diabetes Care*. 2010;33:S62-S69.

4. American Diabetes Association. Position statement: physical activity/exercise and diabetes. *Diabetes Care*. 2004;27:S58-S62.

5. American Diabetes Association. Position statement: standards of medical care in diabetes—2010. *Diabetes Care*. 2010;33:S11-S61.

6. American Diabetes Association Web site [Internet]. Alexandria (VA): American Diabetes Association [cited 2010 May 15]. Available from: www.diabetes.org/food-and-fitness.

7. Barr EL, Zimmet PZ, Welborn TA, et al. Risk of cardiovascular and all-cause mortality in individuals with diabetes mellitus, impaired fasting glucose, and impaired glucose tolerance: the Australian Diabetes, Obesity, and Lifestyle Study (AusDiab). *Circulation* 2007; 116:151-157.

8. Beaser R, Horton E, Mullooly C. Physical activity for fitness. In: Beaser RS, editor. *Joslin's Diabetic Deskbook,* 2nd ed. Philadelphia (PA): Lippincott Williams & Wilkins; 2007. p. 127-152.

9. Campbell AP, Beaser R. Medical nutrition therapy. In Beaser RS, editor. *Joslin's Diabetic Deskbook,* 2nd ed. Philadelphia (PA): Lippincott Williams & Wilkins; 2007, p. 81-125.

10. Horton E, Steppal J. Exercise in patients with diabetes mellitus. In: Kahn CR, Weir GC, King GL, et al. editors. *Joslin's Diabetes Mellitus*. Philadelphia (PA): Lippincott Williams & Wilkins; 2005. p. 649-657.

11. Jellinger RS, Davidson JA, Blonde L. Road maps to achieve glycemic control in type 2 diabetes mellitus: ACE/AACE Diabetes Road Map Task Force. *Endocrine Practice*. 2007;13:260-268.

12. Knowler WC, Barrett-Connor E, Fowler SE, et al. Diabetes Prevention Program Research Group. Reduction in the incidence of type 2 diabetes with lifestyle intervention or metformin. *N Engl J Med*. 2002;346(6):393-403.

13. Pasani F, Contaldo F, de Simone G, Mancini M. Benefits of sustained moderate weight loss in obesity. *Nutr Metab Cardiovasc Dis*. 2001;11:401-406.

14. Sigal RJ, Castaneda-Sceppa C, Kenny GP, White RD, Wasserman DH. Physical activity/exercise and type 2 diabetes: a consensus statement from the American Diabetes Association. *Diabetes Care*. 2006;29:1433-1438.

15. U.S. Department of Health and Human Services, Centers for Disease Control Web site [Internet]. United States: Centers for Disease Control and Prevention; [cited 2009 May 1]. Available from: http://www.cdc.gov/diabetes/pubs/pdf/ndfs_2007.pdf.

16. Zanuso S, Jimenez A, Pugliese G, Corigliano G, Balducci S. Exerciser for the management of type 2 diabetes: a review of the evidence. *Acta Diabetol*. 2010;47:15-22.

Chapter 15

1. American College of Sports Medicine. *ACSM's Guidelines for Exercise Testing and Prescription*. 8th ed. Philadelphia (PA): Lippincott Williams & Wilkins; 2010. 380 p.

2. Appel LJ, Brands MW, Daniels SR, Karanja N, Elmer PJ, Sacks FM. Dietary approaches to prevent and treat hypertension: a scientific statement from the American Heart Association. *Hypertension* 2006;47:296-308.

3. Bibbins-Domingo K, Chertow GM, Coxson PG, et al. Projected effect of dietary salt reductions on future cardiovascular disease. *N Engl J Med* 2010;362:590-599.

4. Chobanian AV, Bakris GL, Black HR, et al. The seventh report of the Joint National Committee on Prevention, Detection, Evaluation, and Treatment of High Blood Pressure: the JNC 7 report. *JAMA* 2003;289:2560-2572.

5. Lewington S, Clarke R, Qizilbash N, Peto R, Collins R. Age-specific relevance of usual blood pressure to vascular mortality: a meta-analysis of individual data for one million adults in 61 prospective studies. *Lancet* 2002;360:1903-1913.

6. Lloyd-Jones D, Adams RJ, Brown TM, et al. Heart disease and stroke statistics—2010 update. A report from the American Heart Association. *Circulation* 2010;121:948-954.

7. Meneton P, Jeunemaitre X, de Wardener HE, MacGregor GA. Links between dietary salt intake, renal salt handling, blood pressure, and cardiovascular diseases. *Physiol Rev* 2005;85:679-715.

8. National Heart, Lung, and Blood Institute Website [Internet]. Bethesda, Maryland.[cited 2010 July 17]. Available from: www.nhlbi.nih.gov.

9. Pescatello LS, Franklin BA, Fagard R, Farquhar WB, Kelley GA, Ray CA. American College of Sports Medicine position stand. Exercise and hypertension. *Med Sci Sports Exerc* 2004;36:533-553.

10. Sacks FM, Svetkey LP, Vollmer WM, et al. Effects on blood pressure of reduced dietary sodium and the Dietary Approaches to Stop Hypertension (DASH) diet. DASH-Sodium Collaborative Research Group. *N Engl J Med* 2001;344:3-10.

11. Sanders PW. Vascular consequences of dietary salt intake. *Am J Physiol Renal Physiol* 2009;297:F237-243.

12. Sawka MN, Burke LM, Eichner ER, Maughan RJ, Montain SJ, Stachenfeld NS. American College of Sports Medicine position stand. Exercise and fluid replacement. *Med Sci Sports Exerc* 2007;39:377-390.

13. U.S. Department of Health and Human Services and the U.S. Department of Agriculture Web site [Internet]. *Dietary Guidelines for Americans 2010* and *Report of the Dietary Guidelines Advisory Committee on the Dietary Guidelines for Americans 2010*. [cited 2011 February 1]. Available from: http://www.cnpp.usda.gov/DietaryGuidelines.htm.

14. U.S. Department of Health and Human Services, National Institutes of Health, and National Heart, Lung, and Blood Institute. Your guide to lowering your blood pressure with DASH. NIH Publication no. 06-4082, 2006. http://www.nhlbi.nih.gov/health/public/heart/hbp/dash/new_dash.pdf.

15. Weinberger MH. Salt sensitivity of blood pressure in humans. *Hypertension* 1996;27:481-490.

16. World Health Organization. WHO Forum on reducing salt intake in populations. Paris, France: World Health Organization, 2006.

Chapter 16

1. American College of Sports Medicine. *ACSM's Resource Manual for Guidelines for Exercise Testing and Prescription.* 6th ed. Philadelphia (PA): Lippincott Williams & Wilkins; 2010. 868 p.

2. Craddick S, Elmer P, Obarzanek E, Vollmer W. The Dash diet and blood pressure. *Current Atheroschlerosis Reports.* 2003;5(6):484-491.

3. Durstine, J.L. *Action Plan for High Cholesterol.* Champaign (IL): Human Kinetics; 2006. 195 p.

4. Dursine JL, Peel JB. Dyslipidemia. In: Durstine JL, Moore GE, Lamonte MJ, Franklin BA, editors. *Pollock's Textbook of Cardiovascular Disease and Rehabilitation.* Champaign: Human Kinetics; 2008. p. 219-228.

5. Fletcher B, Berra K, Ades, P, et al. Managing abnormal blood lipids: a collaborative approach. *Circulation.* 2005;112(1):3184-3209.

6. Grundy S, Cleeman J, Merz C, Brewer H, Clark L. Implications of recent clinical trials for the National Cholesterol Education Program Adult Treatment Panel III guidelines. *Circulation.* 2004;110(2):227-239.

7. Goraya T, Jacobson S, Kottle T, Frye R, Weston S. Coronary heart disease death and sudden cardiac death: a 20 year population-based study. *American Journal of Epidemiology.* 2003;157(9):763-770.

8. Hammer F, Stewar P. Cortisol metabolism in hypertension. *Best Practices & Research Clinical Endocrinology & Metabolism.* 2006;20(3):337-353.

9. Jeppesen J, Heins H, Saudicani P, Gyntelberg F. High triglyceride/low high-density lipoprotein cholesterol, ishemic electrocardiogram changes, and risk of ishemic heart disease. *American Heart Journal.* 2003;145(1):103-108.

10. Lloyd-Jones D, Adams R, Brown T, et al. Heart disease and stroke statistics—2010 update: a report from the American Heart Association. *Circulation.* 2010;121(7): 46-215.

11. National Institute of Health Web site [Internet]. National Cholesterol Education Program: detection, evaluation, and treatment of high blood cholesterol in adults final report. Bethesda (MD): USDHHS; [cited 2010 April 5]. Available from: http://www.nhlbi.nih.gov/guidelines/cholesterol/atp3full.pdf.

12. Pahan K. Lipid-lowering drugs. *Cellular and Molecular Life Sciences.* 2006;63(10): 1165-1178.

13. U.S. Department of Health and Human Services Web site [Internet]. *2008 Physical Activity Guidelines for Americans.* Atlanta (GA): USDHHS; [cited 2010 January 1]. Available from: http://www.health.gov/paguidelines.

Chapter 17

1. Altman R, Asch E, Bloch D, et al. The American College of Rheumatology criteria for the classification and reporting of osteoarthritis of the knee. *Arthritis and Rheumatism.* 1986;29: 1039-1049.

2. American College of Rheumatology Web site [Internet]. *Biologic treatments for rheumatoid arthritis.* American College of Rheumatology. [cited 2010 Jan 24]. Available from: http://www.rheumatology.org/public/factsheets.

3. American College of Sports Medicine. *ACSM's Guidelines for Exercise Testing and Prescription.* 8th ed. Philadelphia (PA): Lippincott Williams & Wilkins; 2010. 380 p.

4. Arnett FC, Edworthy SM, Bloch DA, et al. The American Rheumatism Association 1987 revised criteria for the classification of rheumatoid arthritis. *Arthritis and Rheumatism.* 1988;31:315-324.

5. Baker KR, Nelson ME, Felson DT, Layne JE, Sarno R, Roubenoff R. The efficacy of home based progressive strength training in older adults with knee osteoarthritis: a randomized controlled trial. *J Rheumatol.* 2001;28:1655-1665.

6. Barker K, Lamb SE, Toye F, Jackson S, Barrington S. Association between radiographic joint space narrowing, function, pain and muscle power in severe osteoarthritis of the knee. *Clin Rehabil.* 2004;18:793-800.

7. Brandt KD. *Osteoarthritis* (Rheumatic Disease Clinics of North America). Philadelphia: Elsevier Science Health Science; 2003.

8. Brousseau L, Pelland L, Wells G, et al. Efficacy of aerobic exercises for osteoarthritis (part II): A meta-analysis. *Phys Ther Rev* 2004; 9:125-145.

9. Centers for Disease Control and Prevention. 2001. Prevalence of Arthritis—United States, 1997. *Morbidity and Mortality Weekly Report* 50:334-336.

10. Cochrane T, Davey RC, Matthes Edwards SM. Randomised controlled trial of the cost-effectiveness of water-based therapy for lower limb osteoarthritis. *Health Technology Assessment.* 2005; 9:iii-76.

11. Ettinger WH Jr, Burns R, Messier SP, et al. A randomized trial comparing aerobic exercise and resistance exercise with a health education program in older adults with knee osteoarthritis. The Fitness Arthritis and Seniors Trial (FAST). *JAMA* 1997; 277:25–31.

12. Fitzgerald GK, Childs JD, Ridge TM, Irrgang JJ. Agility and perturbation training for a physically active individual with knee osteoarthritis. *Phys Ther.* 2002;82:372-382.

13. Häkkinen A, Sokka T, Kotaniemi A, Hannonen P. A randomized two-year study of the effects of dynamic strength training on muscle strength, disease activity, functional capacity, and bone mineral density in early rheumatoid arthritis. *Arthritis and Rheumatism.* 2001;44:515-522.

14. Häkkinen A, Sokka T, Hannonen P. A home-based two-year strength training period in early rheumatoid arthritis led to good long-term compliance: a five-year follow-up. *Arthritis and Rheumatism.* 2004;51:56-62.

15. Hall A, Maher C, Latimer J, Ferreira M. The effectiveness of tai chi for chronic musculoskeletal pain conditions: A systematic review and meta-analysis. *Arthritis & Rheumatism.* 2009;61:717-724.

16. Hauselmann HJ. Nutripharmaceuticals for osteoarthritis. *Best Pract Res Clin Rheumatol.* 2001;15:595–607.

17. Hochberg MC, Dougados M. Pharmacological therapy of osteoarthritis. *Best Pract Res Clin Rheumatol.* 2001;15:583–593.

18. Mangione KK, McCully K, Gloviak A, Lefebvre I, Hofmann M, Craik R. The effects of high-intensity and low-intensity cycle ergometry in older adults with knee osteoarthritis. *J Geront.* 1999;54(A): M184-M190.

19. McAlindon TE, LaValley MP, Gulin JP, Felson DT. Glucosamine and chondroitin for treatment of osteoarthritis: a systematic quality assessment and meta-analysis. *JAMA.* 2000; 283:1469–1475.

20. Messier SP, Loeser RF, Miller GD, et al. Exercise and dietary weight loss in overweight and obese older adults with knee osteoarthritis: The Arthritis, Diet, and Activity Promotion Trial. *Arthritis Rheum* 2004; 50:1501-1510.

21. Millar AL. *Action Plan for Arthritis.* Champaign (IL): Human Kinetics; 2003.

22. Minor MA, Hewett JE, Webel RR, et al. Efficacy of physical conditioning exercise in patients with rheumatoid arthritis and osteoarthritis. *Arthritis Rheum.* 1989; 32:1396–1405.

23. Munneke M, deJong Z, Zwinderman AH, et al. Effect of a high-intensity weight-bearing exercise program on radiologic damage progression of the large joints in subgroups of patients with rheumatoid arthritis. *Arthritis and Rheumatism.* 2005;53:410-417.

24. Proudman SM, Cleland LG, James JM. Dietary omega-3 fats for treatment of inflammatory joint disease: efficacy and utility. *Rheum Dis Clin North Am.* 2008;34:469-469.

25. Schmitt LC, Fitzgerald GK, Reisman AS, Rudolph KS. Instability, laxity, and physical function in patients with medial knee osteoarthritis. *Phys Ther.* 2008;88:1506-1516.

26. Sharma L, Song J, Felson DT, Cahue S, Samieyeh E, Dunlop DD. The role of knee alignment in disease progression and functional decline in knee osteoarthritis. *J Amer Med Assoc.* 2001;286:188-195.

27. Symmons DP. Epidemiology of rheumatoid arthritis: Determinants of onset, persistence and outcome. *Best Pract Res Clin Rheumatol.* 2002; 16:707-722.

28. Van den Ende CHM, Vliet Vlieland TPM, Munneke M, Hazes JMW. Dynamic exercise therapy for rheumatoid arthritis (Cochrane Review). In *The Cochrane Library,* Issue 1, Oxford: Update Software. 2002.

Chapter 18

1. American College of Obstetricians and Gynecologists. ACOG technical bulletin: *Exercise during pregnancy and the postnatal period.* Washington DC: American College of Obstetricians and Gynecologists, 1985.

2. American College of Obstetricians and Gynecologists. ACOG committee opinion. Exercise during pregnancy and the postpartum period. Number 267. American College of Obstetricians and Gynecologists. *Int J Gynaecol Obstet.* 2002;77(1):79-81.

3. American College of Sports Medicine Expert Panel. Impact of physical activity during pregnancy and postpartum on chronic disease risk. *Med Sci Sports Exerc.* 2006;38(5):989-1006.

4. American College of Sports Medicine. *ACSM's Guidelines for Exercise Testing and Prescription.* 8th edition. Philadelphia (PA): Lippincott Williams & Wilkins; 2010, 380 p.

5. Albright CL, Maddock JE, Nigg CR. Physical activity before pregnancy and following childbirth in a multiethnic sample of healthy women in Hawaii. *Women & Health* 2005;42(3):95-110.

6. Alderman BW, Zhao H, Holt VL, Watts DH, Beresford SA. Maternal physical activity in pregnancy and infant size for gestational age. *Ann Epidemiol.* 1998;8(8):513-9.

7. Barakat R, Stirling JR, Lucia A. Does exercise training during pregnancy affect gestational age? A randomised controlled trial. *Br J Sports Med.* 2008;42(8):674-8.

8. Barakat R, Lucia A, Ruiz JR. Resistance exercise training during pregnancy and newborn's birth size: a randomised controlled trial. *Int J Obes (Lond).* 2009;33(9):1048-57.

9. Beddoe AE, Paul Yang CP, Kennedy HP, Weiss SJ, Lee KA. The effects of mindfulness-based yoga during pregnancy on maternal psychological and physical distress. *J Obstet Gynecol Neonatal Nurs.* 2009;38(3):310-9.

10. Boney CM, Verma A, Tucker R, Vohr BR. Metabolic syndrome in childhood: association with birth weight, maternal obesity, and gestational diabetes mellitus. *Pediatrics.* 2005;115(3):e290-6.

11. Boulet SL, Alexander GR, Salihu HM, Pass M. Macrosomic births in the United States: determinants, outcomes, and proposed grades of risk. *Am J Obstet Gynecol.* 2003;188(5):1372-8.

12. Bung P, Artal R, Khodiguian N, Kjos S. Exercise in gestational diabetes: an optional therapeutic approach? *Diabetes.* 1991;40 Suppl 2:182-5.

13. Clapp JF. The morphometric and neurodevelopmental outcome at five years of the offspring of women who continued exercise throughout pregnancy. *J Pediatr.* 1996;129:856-63.

14. Clapp JF. *Exercising through Your Pregnancy.* Omaha (NE): Addicus Books; 2002.

15. Daley A, Jolly K, MacArthur C. The effectiveness of exercise in the management of post-natal depression: systematic review and meta-analysis. *Fam Pract.* 2009;26(2):154-62.

16. Damm P, Breitowicz B, Hegaard H. Exercise, pregnancy, and insulin sensitivity—what is new? *Appl Physiol Nutr Metab.* 2007;32(3):537-40.

17. Duncombe D, Wertheim EH, Skouteris H, Paxton SJ, Kelly L. Factors related to exercise over the course of pregnancy including women's beliefs about the safety of exercise during pregnancy. *Midwifery* 2007;23(4):430-8.

18. Ersek JL, Brunner Huber LR. Physical activity prior to and during pregnancy and risk of postpartum depressive symptoms. *J Obstet Gynecol Neonatal Nurs.* 2009;38(5):556-66.

19. Evenson KR, Siega-Riz AM, Savitz DA, Leiferman JA, Thorp JM, Jr. Vigorous leisure activity and pregnancy outcome. *Epidemiology.* 2002;13(6):653-9.

20. Evenson KR, Savitz DA, Huston SL. Leisure-time physical activity among pregnant women in the US. *Paediatr Perinat Epidemiol.* 2004;18(6):400-7.

21. Evenson KR, Moos MK, Carrier K, Siega-Riz AM. Perceived barriers to physical activity among pregnant women. *Matern Child Health J.* 2009;13(3):364-75.

22. Gavard JA, Artal R. Effect of exercise on pregnancy outcome. *Clin Obstet Gynecol.* 2008;51(2):467-80.

23. Hall DC, Kaufmann DA. Effects of aerobic and strength conditioning on pregnancy outcomes. *Am J Obstet Gynecol.* 1987;157(5):1199-203.

24. Harder T, Rodekamp E, Schellong K, Dudenhausen JW, Plagemann A. Birth weight and subsequent risk of type 2 diabetes: a meta-analysis. *Am J Epidemiol.* 2007;165(8):849-57.

25. Hediger ML, Overpeck MD, McGlynn A, Kuczmarski RJ, Maurer KR, Davis WW. Growth and fatness at three to six years of age of children born small- or large-for-gestational age. *Pediatrics.* 1999;104(3):e33.

26. Hegaard HK, Pedersen BK, Nielsen BB, Damm P. Leisure time physical activity during pregnancy and impact on gestational diabetes mellitus, pre-eclampsia, preterm delivery and birth weight: a review. *Acta Obstet Gynecol Scand.* 2007;86(11):1290-6.

27. Juhl M, Olsen J, Andersen PK, Nohr EA, Andersen AM. Physical exercise during pregnancy and fetal growth measures: a study within the danish national birth cohort. *Am J Obstet Gynecol.* 2010;202(1):63.e1-8.

28. Kaiser L, Allen LH. Position of the American Dietetic Association: nutrition and lifestyle for a healthy pregnancy outcome. *J Am Diet Assoc.* 2008;108(3):553-61.

29. Kramer MS, McDonald SW. Aerobic exercise for women during pregnancy. *Cochrane Database Syst Rev.* 2006;3:CD000180.

30. Mottola MF. Exercise prescription for overweight and obese women: pregnancy and postpartum. *Obstet Gynecol Clin North Am.* 2009;36(2):301-16.

31. Mudd LM, Nechuta S, Pivarnik JM, Paneth N. Factors associated with women's perceptions of physical activity safety during pregnancy. *Prev Med.* 2009;49(2-3):194-9.

32. Narendran S, Nagarathna R, Narendran V, Gunasheela S, Nagendra HR. Efficacy of yoga on pregnancy outcome. *J Altern Complement Med.* 2005;11(2):237-44.

References

33. Ohlin A, Rossner S. Trends in eating patterns, physical activity and socio-demographic factors in relation to postpartum body weight development. *Br J Nutr.* 1994;71(4):457-70.

34. Owe KM, Nystad W, Bo K. Association between regular exercise and excessive newborn birth weight. *Obstet Gynecol.* 2009;114:770-776.

35. Pivarnik JM, Ayres NA, Mauer MB, Cotton DB, Kirshon B, Dildy GA. Effects of maternal aerobic fitness on cardiorespiratory responses to exercise. *Med Sci Sports Exerc.* 1993;25(9):993-8.

36. Pivarnik JM, Mauer MB, Ayres NA, Kirshon B, Dildy GA, Cotton DB. Effects of chronic exercise on blood volume expansion and hematologic indices during pregnancy. *Obstet Gynecol.* 1994;83(2):265-9.

37. Pivarnik JM, Perkins CD, Moyerbrailean T. Athletes and pregnancy. *Clin Obstet Gynecol.* 2003;46(2):403-14.

38. Rasmussen KM, Catalano PM, Yaktine AL. New guidelines for weight gain during pregnancy: what obstetrician/gynecologists should know. *Curr Opin Obstet Gynecol.* 2009;21(6):521-6.

39. Roberts JM, Pearson G, Cutler J, Lindheimer M. Report of the National High Blood Pressure Education Program Working Group on High Blood Pressure in Pregnancy. *Am J Obstet Gynecol.* 2000;183:S1-S21.

40. Sampselle CM, Seng J, Yeo S, Killion C, Oakley D. Physical activity and postpartum well-being. *J Obstet Gynecol Neonatal Nurs.* 1999;28(1):41-9.

41. Serlin DC and Lash RW. Diagnoses and management of gestational diabetes mellitus. *Am Fam Physician.* 2009;80(1):57-62.

42. Stuebe AM, Oken E, Gillman MW. Associations of diet and physical activity during pregnancy with risk for excessive gestational weight gain. *Am J Obstet Gynecol.* 2009;201(1):58 e1-8.

43. Symons Downs D, Hausenblas HA. Women's exercise beliefs and behaviors during their pregnancy and postpartum. *J Midwifery Womens Health.* 2004;49(2):138-44.

44. Symons Downs D, Ulbrecht JS. Understanding exercise beliefs and behaviors in women with gestational diabetes mellitus. *Diabetes Care.* 2006;29(2):236-40.

45. Treuth MS, Butte NF, Puyau M. Pregnancy-related changes in physical activity, fitness, and strength. *Med Sci Sports Exerc.* 2005;37(5):832-7.

46. U.S. Department of Agriculture. MyPyramid Web Site. http://www.mypyramid.gov. Accessed January 29, 2010.

47. U.S. Department of Health and Human Services. *Physical Activity Guidelines for Americans.* http://www.health.gov/paguidelines. ODPHP Publication No. U0036, 2008.

48. Weissgerber TL, Wolfe LA, Davies GA, Mottola MF. Exercise in the prevention and treatment of maternal-fetal disease: a review of the literature. *Appl Physiol Nutr Metab.* 2006;31(6):661-674.

Chapter 19

1. Cummings SR, Karpf DB, Harris F, et al. Improvement in spine bone density and reduction in risk of vertebral fractures during treatment with antiresorptive drugs. *Am J Med.* 2002;112(4): 281-289.

2. Cummings SR, Nevitt MC, Browner WS, et al. Risk factors for hip fracture in white women. Study of Osteoporotic Fractures Research Group. *N Engl J Med.* 1995;332(12): 767-773.

3. Eastell R. Treatment of postmenopausal osteoporosis. *N Engl J Med.* 1998;338:736-746.

4. Grodstein F, Manson JE, Colditz GA, Willett WC, Speizer FE, Stampfer MJ. A prospective, observational study of postmenopausal hormone therapy and primary prevention of cardiovascular disease. *Ann Intern Med.* 2000;133(12): 933-941.

5. Guyatt GH, Cranney A, Griffith L, et al. Summary of meta-analyses of therapies for postmenopausal osteoporosis and the relationship between bone density and fractures. *Endocrinol Metab Clin North Am.* 2002;31(3): 659-679, xii.

6. Hauer K, Specht N, Schuler M, Bartsch P, Oster P. Intensive physical training in geriatric patients after severe falls and hip surgery. *Age Ageing.* 2002;31(1): 49-57.

7. Kannus P, Parkkari J, Sievanen H, Heinonen A, Vuori I, Jarvinen M. Epidemiology of hip fractures. *Bone.* 1996;18(1 Suppl): 57S-63S.

8. Keen R. Osteoporosis: strategies for prevention and management. *Best Pract Res Clin Rheumatol.* 2007;21(1): 109-122.

9. Kohrt WM, Bloomfield SA, Little KD, Nelson ME, Yingling VR. American College of Sports Medicine position stand: physical activity and bone health. *Med Sci Sports Exerc.* 2004;36(11): 1985-1996.

10. Martyn-St James M, Carroll S. A meta-analysis of impact exercise on postmenopausal bone loss: the case for mixed loading exercise programmes. *Br J Sports Med.* 2009;43(12): 898-908.

11. Martyn-St James M, Carroll S. High-intensity resistance training and postmenopausal bone loss: a meta-analysis. *Osteoporosis International.* 2006;17(8): 1225-1240.

12. Martyn-St James M, Carroll S. Progressive high-intensity resistance training and bone mineral density changes among premenopausal women: evidence of discordant site-specific skeletal effects. *Sports Medicine.* 2006;36(8): 683-704.

13. Reginster JY, Seeman E, De Vernejoul MC, et al. Strontium ranelate reduces the risk of nonvertebral fractures in postmenopausal women with osteoporosis: treatment of peripheral osteoporosis (TROPOS) study. *J Clin Endocrinol Metab.* 2005;90(5): 2816-2822.

14. Sambrook P, Cooper C. Osteoporosis. *Lancet.* 2006; 367(9527): 2010-2018.

15. Snow CM, Shaw JM, Winters KM, Witzke KA. Long-term exercise using weighted vests prevents hip bone loss in postmenopausal women. *J Gerontol A Biol Sci Med Sci.* 2000;55(9): M489-491.

16. U.S. Department of Health and Human Services. *Bone Health and Osteoporosis: A Report of the Surgeon General.* Rockville, MD: U.S. Department of Health and Human Services, Office of the Surgeon General; 2004. 436 p. Available from: U.S. GPO, Washington.

17. Weatherall M. A meta-analysis of 25 hydroxyvitamin D in older people with fracture of the proximal femur. *N Z Med J.* 2000;113(1108): 137-140.

18. Winters KM, Snow CM. Detraining reverses positive effects of exercise on the musculoskeletal system in premenopausal women. *J Bone Miner Res.* 2000;15:2495-2503.

Index

Note: Page numbers followed by an italicized *f* or *t* indicate that there is a figure or table on that page, respectively.

About the ACSM

With 35,000 members, the **American College of Sports Medicine** is the largest and most-respected sports medicine and exercise science organization in the world. Founded in 1954, the ACSM works to promote and integrate scientific research, education, and practical applications of sports medicine and exercise science to maintain and enhance physical performance, fitness, health, and quality of life for people worldwide.

About the Editor

Barbara A. Bushman, PhD, FASCM is certified as a program director and exercise specialist through the American College of Sports Medicine (ACSM) and is a professor at Missouri State University. She received her PhD in exercise physiology from the University of Toledo and has teaching experience in identification of health risks, exercise testing and prescription, anatomy, and physiology. Bushman is the senior editor of *ACSM's Resources for the Personal Trainer,* fourth edition, an associate editor for the *ACSM's Health & Fitness Journal,* and a reviewer for ACSM's *Medicine & Science in Sports & Exercise, Women & Health,* and *ACSM's Health & Fitness Journal.* She has been a fellow of the American College of Sports Medicine since 1999, serving on the ACSM Media Referral Network.

Bushman is the lead author of *Action Plan for Menopause* as well as numerous research articles. She resides in Strafford, Missouri, with her husband, Tobin. She participates in numerous activities in her leisure time, including running, cycling, hiking, weightlifting, kayaking, and scuba diving.

About the Contributors

Christopher Berger, PhD, CSCS, is an exercise physiologist formerly with the University of Pittsburgh, but now at The George Washington University where he teaches exercise physiology. He is a certified member of both the American College of Sports Medicine and the National Strength and Conditioning Association. Berger specializes in metabolism and weight management.

Keith Burns, MS, is a graduate student in the department of exercise science at the University of South Carolina. His academic interests are in the area of clinical exercise physiology with a research focus to better understanding how daily physical activity and exercise provide health benefits for people with chronic diseases and disabilities.

Wojtek Chodzko-Zajko, PhD, is with the department of kinesiology and community health at the University of Illinois at Urbana-Champaign. He focuses on the effect of exercise and physical activity on health and quality of life in old age. Chodzko-Zajko is active on several professional advisory boards such as the Scientific Advisory Committee of the World Health Organization, which developed the WHO "Guidelines for Physical Activity Among Older Persons," and the WHO task force charged with developing a strategy for integrating physical activity into a comprehensive program of active aging. Chodzko-Zajko is the principal investigator on projects charged with developing a national strategy for promoting healthy aging in the United States.

Shawn H. Dolan, Ph D, RD, CSSD, is a member of the American College of Sports Medicine and American Dietetic Association (ADA). She is currently the assistant director of Sports Dietetics USA, a subunit of Sports Cardiovascular and Wellness Nutrition, a dietetic practice groups within ADA. Dolan is a sport dietitian and physiologist with the United States Olympic Committee (USOC). She works primarily with the team and technical sports folio. Prior to the USOC, Dolan was an assistant professor of kinesiology at California State University at Long Beach, where she taught sport and wellness nutrition, resistance training program design, exercise physiology, and fundamentals of personal training.

J. Larry Durstine, PhD, is a fellow and past president of the American College of Sports Medicine. He is a distinguished professor at the University of South Carolina and serves as chair of the department of exercise science and director of clinical exercise programs. Durstine has published over 70 refereed research publications, edited 8 books, and written more than 30 book chapters. His research interest includes the effects of physical activity on blood lipid and lipoprotein concentrations. He has examined the relationships between exercise and novel cardiovascular disease risk factors in men, minority women, and people with chronic diseases and disabilities.

Avery Faigenbaum, EdD, is a fellow of the American College of Sports Medicine and of the National Strength and Conditioning Association. He is a professor at the College of New Jersey in the department of health and exercise science. Faigenbaum's research interests include various resistance training techniques as well as the benefits of physical activity for school-age youth. As a researcher and practitioner in the field of exercise science, he has developed successful youth fitness programs and has authored numerous scientific publications, book chapters, and eight books including *Youth Strength Training* (Human Kinetics, 2009).

William B. Farquhar, PhD, is a fellow of the American College of Sports Medicine and is an associate professor in the department of kinesiology and applied physiology at the University of Delaware. Farquhar studies blood pressure regulation in humans and teaches undergraduate and graduate physiology courses. He publishes his research findings in peer-reviewed scientific journals and regularly presents at national meetings.

Amy Fowler, BS, is a member of the American College of Sports Medicine and is an ACSM certified exercise specialist and registered clinical exercise physiologist. She is the manager of preventive cardiology at William Beaumont Hospital in Royal Oak, Michigan. Fowler's professional interests are women's heart health, diabetes management, and patient advocacy.

Barry A. Franklin, PhD, is director of the Cardiac Rehabilitation and Exercise Laboratories at William Beaumont Hospital in Royal Oak, Michigan. He holds adjunct faculty appointments at Oakland University, Wayne State University School of Medicine, and the University of Michigan Medical School. He served as president of the AACVPR in 1988 and president of ACSM in 1999. In 2010, he was appointed to the AHA board of trustees. Franklin is a past editor in chief of the *Journal of Cardiopulmonary Rehabilitation* and currently holds editorial positions with 17 scientific and clinical journals. He has written or edited more than 500 publications, including 27 books.

Anthony Giglio, MS, PA-C, is a physician assistant currently working in endocrinology at St. John's Health System in Springfield, Missouri. He is certified by the National Commission on Certification of Physician Assistants. He is a graduate of the Missouri State University Physician Assistant Program.

Gregory A. Ledger, MD, FACP, FACE, is a fellow of the American College of Physicians and a fellow of the American College of Endocrinology. He is currently section chair for the department of endocrinology, diabetes and metabolism with St. John's Health System in Springfield, Missouri. Ledger is board certified in internal medicine with subspecialty board certification in endocrinology, diabetes, and metabolism. Ledger has a clinical practice with St. John's Clinic and also conducts clinical research in the fields of diabetes, osteoporosis, and hyperlipidemia.

Marcus Kilpatrick, PhD, is an ACSM certified exercise specialist and health fitness specialist. He is an associate professor in exercise science at the University of South Florida and primarily teaches in the areas of exercise psychology and fitness assessment and prescription. Kilpatrick's research interests center on psychological responses to exercise including affect, perceived exertion, and motivation. His research aims to better understand the physical activity experience and facilitate lifelong engagement in sport and exercise.

Laura Kruskall, PhD, RD, CSSD, is a fellow of the American College of Sports Medicine and an ACSM certified health fitness specialist. She is the director of nutrition sciences at the University of Nevada at Las Vegas and teaches in the areas of sports nutrition and medical nutrition therapy. Kruskall's research interests include the effects of exercise and nutritional interventions on body composition and energy metabolism. Kruskall is a member of the editorial board for *ACSM's Health & Fitness Journal* and is a nutrition consultant for Canyon Ranch SpaClub and Cirque du Soleil in Las Vegas.

A. Lynn Millar, PT, PhD, is a fellow of the American College of Sports Medicine. She is a professor in the department of physical therapy at Andrews University, where she supervises all of the graduate research. Millar's areas of interest include arthritis, adolescent sports injuries, and exercise for the patient population. She has published and presented on a wide variety of therapy-related topics and authored the text, *ACSM's Action Plan for Arthritis* in 2003 (Human Kinetics).

Don W. Morgan, PhD, is a professor in the department of health and human performance and director of the Center for Physical Activity and Health in Youth at Middle Tennessee State University. An exercise physiologist, Morgan conducts research focusing on the role physical activity plays in improving the health, fitness, and mobility of youth and adults. Morgan is a fellow of the American College of Sports Medicine and an ACSM certified health fitness instructor. He is also a former president of the North American Society for Pediatric Exercise Medicine.

Lanay Mudd, PhD, holds a dual-major doctoral degree in kinesiology and epidemiology from Michigan State University. She is an assistant professor at Appalachian State University and teaches in the area of health promotion. Mudd's research interests center on the maternal and child health benefits associated with physical activity during pregnancy. Specifically, she investigates the roles of health and physical activity during pregnancy and postpartum on future risk for maternal or child cardiovascular and metabolic disease. She is also an ACSM certified clinical exercise specialist.

Jan Schroeder, PhD, is a professor of kinesiology at California State University at Long Beach. She is the director of the bachelor of science fitness program, which specializes in preparing students for careers in the fitness industry. She is a certified personal trainer and group exercise instructor who teaches weekly in the private sector. Schroeder has authored over 40 research and applied articles in the area of exercise physiology and fitness. Her current line of research focuses on trends within the fitness industry such as programming, equipment, and compensation for fitness professionals.

Andiara Schwingel, PhD, is an assistant professor of kinesiology and community health, working in the area of aging and the effects of lifestyle on health and chronic disease. Her primary research interests focus on how cultural, national, and international factors affect the way people grow older around the world, including the development of chronic diseases and conditions. She is an assistant professor at the University of Illinois at Urbana-Champaign and teaches in the area of aging and international health. She directs the Aging and Diversity Lab, where she is investigating how to promote health in older Latino populations in the United States.

Lucy Sternburgh, MS, is an ACSM registered clinical exercise physiologist. She works in preventive cardiology at Beaumont Hospital in Royal Oak, Michigan, and is also a clinical instructor at Oakland University in Rochester, Michigan, within the Wellness, Health Promotion and Injury Prevention program. She is certified by the NSCA as a certified strength and conditioning specialist, and by the ACSM as a clinical exercise specialist, health fitness specialist, and certified inclusive fitness trainer. She is also a National Wellness Institute certified wellness professional and intrinsic coach.

Stella Lucia Volpe, PhD, RD, LDN is a fellow of the American College of Sports Medicine and is an ACSM certified clinical exercise specialist. She is professor and chair of the department of nutrition sciences at Drexel University. Dr. Volpe conducts intervention studies of exercise and nutrition to prevent obesity and diabetes across the lifespan. Dr. Volpe's work has been published in numerous journals. She speaks internationally and nationally. She is also the lead author of *Fitness Nutrition for Special Dietary Needs* (Human Kinetics, 2007).

Kerri Winters-Stone, PhD, holds appointments as an associate professor in the department of nutrition and exercise science at Oregon State University and the School of Nursing at Oregon Health and Science University and is a fellow of the American College of Sports Medicine. Winters-Stone's research has focused on improving bone health through lifestyle modification across the lifespan, particularly through targeted exercise programs, with a current focus on the effects of cancer treatment on fracture and frailty risk and the ability of exercise to improve health in cancer survivors. Winters-Stone is author of the book *ACSM's Action Plan for Osteoporosis* (Human Kinetics, 2005).

Kara Witzke, PhD, is an associate professor and department chair of kinesiology at California State University at San Marcos. She teaches in the area of exercise physiology for special populations, and her research focuses on exercise to improve bone health across the lifespan. Her current project seeks to determine the dose-response relationship between jumping and bone health in young women, which may translate into a simple recommendation to help women grow and maintain healthy bones. She has published book chapters on the topic for ACSM and the American Council on Exercise, and articles in the journal *Medicine & Science in Sports & Exercise.*